Psychoanalytic Therapy As Health Care

Effectiveness and Economics
In the 21st Century

edited by

HARRIETTE KALEY

MORRIS N. EAGLE

DAVID L. WOLITZKY

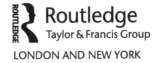

Routledge
Taylor & Francis Group

LONDON AND NEW YORK

First published 1999 by The Analytic Press, Inc.

Published 2014 by Routledge
2 Park Square, Milton Park, Abingdon, Oxfordshire OX14 4RN
711 Third Avenue, New York, NY 10017

Routledge is an imprint of the Taylor & Francis Group, an informa business

First issued in paperback 2014

Typeset in Galliard by EvS Communication Networx, Pt. Pleasant, NJ

Library of Congress Cataloging-in-Publication Data

Psychoanalytic therapy as health care : effectiveness and economics in the
    21st century / edited by Harriette Kaley, Morris N. Eagle, and David L.
Wolitzky.
        p.   cm.
    Includes bibliographic references and index.
    ISBN 978-0-88163-202-6 (hbk)
    ISBN 978-1-13800-527-3 (pbk)
    1. Managed mental health care—Forecasting. 2. Psychotherapy—
Practice—Forecasting.   3. Managed mental health care—Economic
aspects—Forecasting. I. Kaley, Harriette. II. Eagle, Morris N. III.
Wolitzky, David L. (David Leo)
    RC465.5 .P78 1999
    362.2—dc21

                                                           98-47699
                                                              CIP

Contents

Contributors

Drs Julian Abraham, having recently retired from his position as director of an evening and night psychiatric hospital in Amsterdam (De Sluis), is now in full-time private practice.

Neil Altman, Ph.D. is Co-chair, Relational Orientation, Postdoctoral Program in Psychotherapy and Psychoanalysis, New York University. He is an Associate Editor of *Psychoanalytic Dialogues: A Journal of Relational Perspectives.*

Christa Balzert, Ph.D. is a supervisor at New York University, The City University of New York, and the Institute for Child, Adolescent, and Family Studies.

James W. Barron, Ph.D. is Senior Associate in Psychology, Department of Psychiatry, Harvard Medical School, and Faculty, Massachusetts Institute for Psychoanalysis.

Toni Bernay, Ph.D. is Principal, The Leadership Equation Institute in Beverly Hills, California, where she is in private practice.

Sidney J. Blatt, Ph.D. is Professor, Departments of Psychiatry and Psychology, Yale University, and Faculty, Western New England Institute for Psychoanlysis.

Mark Blechner, Ph.D. is Director of the HIV Clinical Service, Supervisor of Psychotherapy, Faculty, and Fellow of the William Alanson White Institute, New York City, and Assistant Clinical Professor of Psychology, New York University.

Dorothy W. Cantor, Psy.D. is in independent practice in Westfield, New Jersey and is a former president of the American Psychoanalytic Association.

Robert R. Cummings, M.D. Ph.D. is Secretary, Board on Professional Standards; Chair, Committee on Peer Review, American Psychoanalytic Association; and Training Analyst, the Southern California Psychoanalytic Institute and the Psychoanalytic Center of California.

Norman Doidge, M.D. is Head, Psychotherapy Centre, Centre for Addictions and Mental Health, Clarke Institute of Psychiatry Division, Toronto; and Assistant Professor of Psychiatry, Faculty of Medicine, University of Toronto.

Morris, N. Eagle, Ph.D. (editor) is Professor, Derner Institute of Advanced Psychology Studies, Adelphi University, Garden City, New York. He is also Faculty, New York University Postdoctoral Program in Psychotherapy and Psychoanalysis.

Ahmed Fayek, Ph.D. is a Training Analyst at the Canadian Psychoanaytic Institute. He is currently in private practice and teaches psychoanalysis in Cairo, Egypt.

Richard Q. Ford, Ph.D. is Coordinator of Psychological Testing, Austen Riggs Center. He is in the private practice of psychotherapy in Williamstown, Masschusetts.

Marvin Hyman, Ph.D. is Associate Professor, Department of Psychiatry and Behavioral Neuroscience, Wayne State University School of Medicine, Detroit, Michigan. He is also a member of the Academy for the Study of the Psychoanalytic Arts, West Bloomfield, Michigan.

Harriette Kaley, Ph.D. (editor) is Professor Emerita and Adjunct Professor, Brooklyn College, The City University of New York Graduate School Psychology Program. She is in private practice in New York City.

Marylou Lionells, Ph.D. is Director, Fellow, Training and Supervising Analyst, Faculty, William Alanson White Institute, New York City.

Stanley Moldawsky, Ph.D. is Training and Supervising Analyst, New York Freudian Society and International Psychoanalytic Association. He is also Faculty, Institute for Psychoanalysis and Psychotherapy of New Jersey.

Russ Newman, J.D., Ph.D. is the Executive Director for Professional Practice of the American Psychological Association. He is also a member of various psychological and bar associations.

Eric M. Plakun, M.D. is Director of Program Development and Research of the Erikson Institute for Education and Research of the Austen Riggs Center. He is also Clinical Instructor in Psychiatry at Harvard Medical School.

Ron Spielman, M.D. is a Training Analyst at the Australian Psychoanalytic Society and a Fellow of the Royal Australian and New Zealand College of Psychiatrists.

David Sundelson, J.D., Ph.D. is an appellate lawyer in private practice in Berkeley, California.

Bryant Welch, J.D., Ph.D. is a member of a law firm in Washington, D.C. specializing in HMO managed care litigation and professional standards and liability. He is also Assistant Professor of Psychology at George Washington University Center for Professional Psychology.

Brent Willock, Ph.D., C.Psych. is President of the Toronto Institute and Society for Contemporary Psychoanalysis. In his private practice, he works with adults, adolescents, and children in psychoanalysis, psychotherapy, and psychological assessment.

David L. Wolitzky, Ph.D. (editor) is Director, New York University Psychology Clinic, and Faculty, Department of Psychology, New York University, and New York University Postdoctoral Program in Psychotherapy and Psychoanalysis.

Editors' Introduction

Health care in general has come under siege in an era of managed care and preoccupation with cutting health costs and maximizing profits. Mental health care has become a special target; and, of the various approaches to mental health care, psychoanalytically oriented treatment has been particularly threatened. The reason is that it is associated with long-term treatment and is not limited to symptom reduction. We as editors join with our contributors, all mental health professionals with a focus on psychoanalysis, in our concern with a variety of questions raised by the current storm raging about our services. Are they health care? Is psychoanalysis a health care profession? Is there a legitimate role for psychoanalytically oriented treatment in the delivery of health care?

It is important to note at the outset that it is not just traditional psychoanalysis that concerns us, but all therapeutic interventions guided by psychoanalytic principles and psychoanalytic understanding. As we understand it, that includes all psychoanalytically informed psychotherapies and most forms of psychodynamic psychotherapy. We conceive of them all as variants of psychoanalytic approaches, and thus all of them are our objects of concern. Questions about their status have great salience in the present climate of flux and uncertainty about how health care in the United States will be provided over the long run.

That psychoanalytic treatment has come in for special scrutiny is not difficult to understand. Psychoanalytic treatment, with the obvious exception of brief psychodynamic psychotherapy, tends to be long-term treatment (but see Bernay, chapter 2) and is therefore anathema to the profit-making and cost-cutting concerns of managed care. In addition, there is a direct clash between psychotherapeutic values, such as the vital importance of privacy and confidentiality and the emphasis on an ongoing, trusting relationship developed over a period of time (see Sundelson, Cummings, and Newman, chapters 8 through 10), versus the demands, intrusions, and interventions of managed health care, which are almost always linked to controlling costs and thereby maximizing profits.[1] In addition, as Barron points out (chapter 3), managed care fails to appreciate the significance of unconscious processes in psychopathology. So serious is this clash of values that at least one of our contributors (Hyman, chapter 5) believes that there is no alternative for psychoanalysis but to remain outside the framework of managed care; however, see Moldawsky (chapter 4) for an opposing point of view. There is little doubt, then, that psychoanalytic treatment, along with other long-term treatment, is seriously threatened. This would be a matter of limited interest—limited, that is, to those practitioners who find it difficult to carry on with their work—were it not for the fact that the threat to psychoanalytic treatments is also a threat to the basic principle that patients should get the treatment they need for as long as they need it. Indeed, as Lionells (chapter 6) points out, managed care represents a challenge to all health care practices, whether generally medical or explicitly psychotherapeutic in nature.

If psychoanalysis and its offshoots are health professions and can contribute to health care, then ways must be found to do what has not hitherto been done: provide effective ways for such forms of health care to be available to those who need it, whether or not they are affluent, as psychoanalytic patients in the past have been reputed to be. But how can we as a nation provide such health care for people without the attendant evils that seem to accompany the currently evolving systems for providing health care: lack of privacy and confidentiality, escalation of administrative bureaucracies and the unintended but inevitable consequent increases in costs, the removal of care-making decisions from the patient–therapist dyad, unending (and unpaid) paperwork, and so on? (See Welch, chapter 1; Barron, chapter 3; Hyman, chapter 5; Sundelson, chapter 8; Cummings, chapter 9; and Newman, chapter 10).

These are the questions that mental health professionals have been struggling with as we as a nation confront and attempt to deal with America's health care needs. Furthermore, as more of us are covered by managed care companies, we come increasingly to experience directly the fact that they are planned as commercial enterprises, as profit-making organizations, whose top officials frequently command staggering compensation packages and whose stockholders demand capital appreciation and

---

[1] It is worth noting that psychoanalytic forms of mental health care are not alone in being questionable treatments in the eyes of managed care. Other forms of extended treatment and potentially life-saving but still experimental treatments, such as bone-marrow transplants, have also been questioned. Some managed care plans still make it difficult for infertility treatments to be covered. The problem, as we see it, is that the concerns of managed care for issues of cost create scotomas that make it hard to see that expensive or extended treatment (or both) is in fact often the treatment best designed to alleviate a patient's problem.

dividends (see Cantor, chapter 7). It has also become clear that political ideologies about the role of government in private life, the value of rugged individualism, and the relative virtues of social welfare and entrepreneurial approaches, color the systems that we develop for delivering—or limiting the delivering of—health care (see Bernay, chapter 2).

When we look at the issues from these points of view, it becomes evident that the fundamental problem may be a basic clash of values. What, really, is important in health care delivery? Is it cost effectiveness in some form or other, or is it optimal patient care? For those engaged in managing health care, the former plays a very large role; for those who care for patients, the latter is the primary concern. Neither group comes to its position without a long and mostly honorable tradition, a philosophy that supports it, and probably, for some, at least, considerable soul-searching. The managed care contingent warns that national resources must be allocated rationally or else the entire system will escalate out of control and ultimately collapse, serving well neither the people in need of services nor the national economy. It presents itself as having to make difficult decisions in an unsentimental manner and claims that its opponents are at best fiscally uninformed and unwise and at worst self-serving and tender-minded (in the least flattering sense of that Jamesian term). For those who treat patients, the managed care position is transparently in basic conflict with the obligation to provide the best possible care, in keeping with a sense of the dignity of the individual and the value of life; to them, the managed care position is a vaguely intellectualized excuse for rationing health care for the ultimate purpose of producing greater corporate profits. They do not accept the notion that this wealthy country, with its expensive advances in medical technology, cannot afford to use its wealth and technology to make life happier, healthier, longer.

Nowhere is this clash of values seen more clearly than when managed care and psychoanalysis meet. The goal of managed care is to return the patient as quickly as possible to a state that we may call serviceability. This is done in the name of a nebulous criterion described as medical necessity. The idea is to get the patient functional in some way, whether or not the underlying problems have been treated and the suffering ameliorated, and to do it with dispatch; if it cannot be done with dispatch, then the patient risks being consigned to some sort of limbo, because his or her problems run more deeply than the concept of medical necessity can contain. Psychoanalytically informed psychotherapy has a different goal; it is to enable the patient to be at his or her best, to be not merely symptom free but internally comfortable and relatively unconflicted, and to live in a fulfilling way. Psychoanalytic treatment seeks not merely symptom relief, but alterations in defense, improved self-esteem, and more gratifying object relations. When corporate values meet the psychoanalytic set of values, there is a clash of cultures wherein politics, power, and money are more likely to be decisive in the outcome than is concern for quality of patient care (Messer and Wachtel, 1997).

At least two considerations have weakened the case that can be made in defense of psychoanalytic treatment. One is the lack of well-designed outcome studies clearly demonstrating the relative effectiveness of long-term psychoanalytic treatment. The other consideration is the equation, in the minds of many, of psychoanalytic and psychodynamic treatment with traditional psychoanalysis (i.e., frequent sessions each week, use of the couch, etc.) and the accompanying, perhaps understandable, assumption that such treatment tends to be limited to relatively well-to-do patients and is not especially relevant to current health care concerns.

The first concern—lack of well-designed outcome studies—is a legitimate and warranted one, and there is no question that the broad psychoanalytic community needs to deal with this concern more fully and effectively than it has up to this point. One should note, however, that attempts have been made within the psychoanalytic community to address this issue (see Doidge, 1997, for an extensive review of studies dealing with the efficacy of psychoanalytic psychotherapies). A brief review is appropriate here of three linked issues associated with studies of psychotherapy outcomes: studies of the efficacy of psychotherapy, of the growing controversy over empirically validated treatments, and of the value of pharmacotherapy.

In the early 1950s, Eysenck's (1955) challenge that the results of therapy were no better than those attributable to spontaneous remission stimulated what has become by now a great number of psychotherapy process and outcome studies. These have been subjected to numerous meta-analyses with frequently similar results. Two main conclusions have emerged from this work: a) psychotherapy is effective, compared with several different kinds of control procedures, and b) no single school of therapy produces consistently superior outcomes (Smith, Glass, and Miller, 1980). These findings are a source of solace to many clinicians, despite the fact that they forced proponents and adherents of rival schools to take a more modest stance. It must be noted, however, that the bulk of the studies used in the various meta-analyses were behavioral or cognitive-behavioral studies. It is therefore not possible at this point to draw conclusions about the relative efficacy of psychoanalytically oriented approaches compared with others. Such uncertainty is especially important when we note that psychotherapy research studies typically use criteria (e.g., elimination of subjects showing comorbidity) and procedures (e.g., random assignment of patients and use of treatment manuals) that are very different from those characterizing routine clinical practice. These considerations limit the generalizability of many psychotherapy outcome studies.

The overall thrust of these findings is, of course, central to the controversy over empirically validated treatments. The conclusions of a Task Force of the American Psychological Association (Task Force on Promotion and Dissemination of Psychological Procedures, 1995), presenting a list of treatments shown on the basis of empirical research to be efficacious for particular clinical syndromes, have been rightly questioned because of the failure to distinguish efficacy in research settings from effectiveness in clinical practice. As Messer and Wachtel (1997) note, different approaches to therapy have different outcome criteria, and in real-life conditions adherence to a treatment manual in dealing with complex, multiproblem patients might retard rather than enhance effective treatment. Even those who are sympathetic to and have been active in efforts to identify empirically validated treatments have expressed concern regarding the possible misuse of the studies and their limited generalizability. For example, Borkovec and Castonguay (1998) write, "Our concern about the empirically supported therapy movement is . . . that we may draw erroneous conclusions from outcome results when applying them to applied questions. . . ." (p. 139). And Goldfried and Wolfe (1998), who explicitly refer to the possible misuse to which insurance companies can put these studies, are gravely concerned that the methodological and other constraints of research designs might translate into clinical constraints for the practicing therapist, to the detriment of practitioners and patients alike.

Additional pertinent data come from pharmacotherapy-and-psychotherapy studies. In the treatment of depression, medication is not more effective than either is alone (Antonuccio, Danton, and DeNelsky, 1995). Nor are the two together more effective than psychotherapy alone is (Greenberg et al., 1994). Medication for depression is only modestly more effective than are placebos, and earlier work (Evans et al., 1992; Hollon, 1990) has shown that antidepressant medication can lead to more rapid improvement than can psychotherapy alone, but the durability of changes is greater if psychotherapy is also part of the treatment plan.

The state of intervention research ought to give committees and managed care companies pause in asserting prescribed forms of treatment for particular psychiatric syndromes. In their search for profits, these companies focus on efficiency and symptom relief, not on the kinds of long-lasting, pervasive, and revitalizing kinds of changes that psychoanalysts emphasize. The practical and economic issue here is whether more liberal mental health benefits would make patients more resilient in the face of future stress and conflict and therefore be more cost effective in the long run (Cummings, 1996; Lazar and Gabbard, 1997). There are, for example, some data to suggest that decreased use of medical services is a consequence of psychotherapy (e.g., Mumford and Schlesinger, 1987), although this is not a uniform finding (Fraser, 1996).

Although there is much room for improvement in the design of such studies and much more to be done (in this volume, see Blatt and Ford, chapter 15, as exemplar), there is enough evidence to suggest that failure to support long-term psychodynamic or psychoanalytic treatment might well deprive many patients of the help they need and from which they can benefit. It seems to us that, given our current state of seriously incomplete knowledge, it is premature to speak about "empirically validated treatments" with any degree of confidence—certainly not with the degree of confidence necessary for the determination of which treatments should or should not be eligible for reimbursement.

We hold that, at this point in our knowledge, it is wiser to provide a broader rather than a narrower range of treatments. If we provide treatments that turn out to be not as economically sound and not as uniformly effective as they could be, we are not cutting costs as well as we might have. If, however, we fail to provide treatments that may be genuinely helpful, at least to some patients, we are putting people's health, well-being, and lives at risk.

The second consideration that may have undermined the case for psychoanalytic or psychodynamic psychotherapy as health care is the view of it as an esoteric treatment suitable only for a limited and highly select group of patients. While this description may conceivably be accurate for traditional or classical psychoanalysis, it is not accurate with regard to psychoanalytically or psychodynamically oriented or informed treatment. It is this second consideration on which the book mainly focuses. The different chapters of this book, taken together, indicate clearly and forcefully the wide range of contexts and populations to which psychoanalytically oriented and psychoanalytically informed treatments are relevant and applicable.

The Division of Psychoanalysis (Division 39)[2] of the American Psychological Association (APA) has been addressing these issues concerning psychoanalytic treatment and health care in an intensive way for several years. In 1994, the Division's meetings at the annual Convention of the APA was devoted to the theme "Psychoanalysis as Health Care." Those meetings, organized by the senior editor of this volume, Harriette Kaley, as part of her responsibilities as president-elect of the Division, helped all

---

[2] In 1994, Division 39 had a membership of about 4200. Because members had to belong to the American Psychological Association (APA), itself a nationwide organization with over 120,000 members, it was, obviously, an organization almost exclusively of psychologists (there were also graduate psychology students and a few people from allied professions whose professional contributions had earned them membership in the APA); the additional requirement was an interest in psychoanalysis. As it turned out, most Division members were clinicians who described themselves as practicing psychoanalysis or psychoanalytic psychotherapy.

of us focus more clearly on the potential opportunities and dangers for psychoanalysis and its related therapies in the emerging health-care delivery systems. Since then, more and more of us in the Division, often in collaboration with our colleagues in psychology and in related mental health professions, have considered the topic in depth. This volume, with the assistance of the two invited coeditors, Morris N. Eagle and David L. Wolitzky, collects some of the most relevant thinking by significant workers in the field. Some of the papers were presented at the 1994 meetings and thus helped define the issues in a focused way; others were invited contributions that the editors believed would help convey a fuller picture of the present state of affairs and the prospects for the future.

The organization of this book reflects our sense of the major topics that must be included in any attempt to view the subject comprehensively. Part I opens the discussion with an overview of the present problems and suggestions for the future. All the chapters in Part 1, except for Cantor's (chapter 7), were presented at the 1994 meetings and were revised for this volume.[3] The chapters in the section pose the question of where psychoanalytic treatments currently stand in relation to health care, offer some ideas about why matters have developed as they have, and consider possible directions for the future.

The second part addresses some of the most critical matters in the attempt to fuse psychotherapy and managed health care: the ethical, legal, and professional issues of confidentiality, privacy, and reporting to third parties. The breach of the "confessional," as Sundelson tellingly terms it, that begins with any kind of reporting to a third party—even so much as whether or not a particular person is in treatment—turns out to have wide-reaching implications that tend to undermine, if not destroy, the basic enterprise. These chapters ask whether it is in principle possible to have managed mental health care, especially when the treatment modality is of the psychoanalytically-informed variety.

Part III takes a larger perspective on the matter. It considers the experiences of psychoanalysts under health care systems in other parts of the world. Willock et al. (chapter 11), in a summary of several presentations at the original meetings, surveys the world scene; in a companion piece written for this volume, Speilman (chapter 12) reviews the history and effects of Australia's very recent adoption of governmental controls over mental health care. These comparative approaches provide much food for thought for America.

The final section, Part IV, brings psychoanalytic approaches to bear

---

[3] Cantor's chapter is taken from a talk originally given to the New Jersey Psychological Association while she was president of the American Psychological Association in 1996 and is published here in virtually its original form to retain its freshness.

on the treatment of a variety of contemporary problems, populations, and questions. The entire section consists of articles written specifically for this volume, and it speaks of the application of psychoanalytic work to such varied and significant populations as AIDS patients (Blechner, chapter 14), seriously disturbed adults (Blatt and Ford, chapter 15), and inner-city populations (Altman, chapter 17). In addition, it considers who the people are today who are analytic patients (Doidge, chapter 13) and describes the encounter between a psychoanalytically run hospital and the constraints of managed care (Plakun, chapter 16). These chapters should, once and for all, dispel the idea that psychoanalytic treatment is only or primarily for the "worried well." The populations to whom psychoanalytically oriented treatment is relevant and applicable are, indeed, worried, but they are in great distress and in that sense are certainly not well. The editors believe that this section, by showing real-life clinical applications of psychoanalytic approaches, puts skin and bones on the skeleton of the arguments rolling around managed care and at the same time demonstrates the continued salience of psychoanalytic thinking to our troubled world.

As editors, we come away from our task of shepherding this volume to completion with a renewed sense of the vigor and applicability of psychoanalytic treatments. We trust that reading this volume will create the same experience in the reader.

REFERENCES

Antonuccio D. O., Danton, W. G. & DeNelsky G. Y. (1995), Psychotherapy versus medication for depression: Challenging the conventional wisdom with data. *Profess. Psychol.*, 26:574–585.

Borkovec, T. D. & Castonguay, L. G. (1998), What is the scientific meaning of empirically supported therapy? *J. Consul. Clin. Psychol.*, 66:136–142.

Cummings, N. A. (1996), Does managed health care offset costs related to medical treatment? In: *Controversies in Managed Health Care*, ed. A. Lazarus. Washington, DC: American Psychiatric Press, pp. 213–227.

Doidge, N. (1997), Empirical evidence for the efficacy of psychoanalytic psychotherapies and psychoanalysis: An overview. *Psychoanal. Inq.*, Suppl:102–150.

Evans, M. D., Hollon, S. D., DeRubeis, R. J., Pasecki, J. M., Grove, W. M., Garvey, M. J. & Tuason, V. B. (1992), Differential relapse following cognitive therapy and pharmacotherapy for depression. *Arch. Gen. Psychiat.*, 49:802–808.

Eysenck, H. (1955), The effects of psychotherapy: A reply. *J. Abn. Psychol.*, 50:147–148.

Fraser, J. S. (1996), All that glitters is not always gold: Medical offset effects and managed behavioral health care. *Profess. Psychol.*, 27:335–344.

Goldfried, M. R. & Wolfe, B. E. (1998), Toward a more clinically valid approach to therapy research. *J. Consult. Clin. Psychol.,* 66:143–150.

Greenberg, R. P., Bornstein, R. F., Zborowski, M. J., Fisher, S. & Greenberg, M. D. (1994), A meta-analysis of fluoxetine outcome in the treatment of depression. *J. Nerv. Ment. Dis.,* 182:547–551.

Hollon, S. D. (1990) Cognitive therapy and pharmacotherapy for depression. *Psychiat. Annals,* 20:249–258.

Lazar, S. G. & Gabbard, G. O. (1997), The cost-effectiveness of psychotherapy. *J. Psychother. Prac. & Res.,* 6:307–314.

Messer, S. B. & Wachtel, P. L. (1997), The contemporary psychotherapeutic landscape: Issues and prospects. In: *Theories of Psychotherapy,* ed. P. L. Wachtel & S. B. Messer. Washington, DC: American Psychological Association, pp. 1–38.

Mumford, E. & Schlesinger, H. J. (1987), Assessing consumer benefit: Cost offset as an incidental effect of psychotherapy. *Gen. Hosp. Psychiat.,* 9:360–363.

Smith, M. L., Glass, G. V. & Miller, T. L. (1980), *The Benefits of Psychotherapy.* Baltimore, MD: Johns Hopkins University Press.

Task force on promotion and dissemination of psychological procedures (1995), Training and dissemination of empirically validated psychological treatments. Report and recommendations. *Clin. Psychol.,* 48:3–23.

PART I

Psychoanalysis and Health Care: Present Problems and Future Prospects

ONE

Psychoanalysis In the Political Arena

The Reality Principle

BRYANT L. WELCH

THE LAWSUIT

In 1985 psychologists took what seemed at the time a very radical approach to the problem psychologists were having obtaining psychoanalytic training. They filed a class action antitrust suit against the American Psychoanalytic Association, the International Psychoanalytic Association, and two of their component institutes.

Psychologists did not take these steps precipitously. In 1983, psychologists felt that at long last the American Psychoanalytic Association was going to change its policy barring psychologists from training in their institutes, from hiring their teachers to set up their own institute, and from admission to the International Psychoanalytic Association.

Unfortunately, in late 1983 the Medical Director of the American Psychiatric Association addressed the American Psychoanalytic Association and strongly cautioned them not to admit psychologists, but, instead, to move closer to their "medical roots." And, in May of 1984, the American Psychoanalytic Association Board of Directors voted to table all proposals to train psychologists.

In the summer of 1984, in the newsletter of the American Psychoanalytic Association, the newly elected president, Ed Joseph, expressed relief that the proposals had been defeated and that during his tenure institutional attention could be directed to other areas. For those psychologists who had been following this issue for 15 years, not only was defeat of the proposals disheartening, but it seemed to them very unlikely that, barring a more radical intervention, psychologists would be able to obtain psychoanalytic training.

While the lawsuit effort was arduous for all, there is little dispute now, even within the American Psychoanalytic Association, that training psychologists has had a wonderful and rejuvenating impact on psychoanalysis in this country. And psychoanalysis is now one of the fastest growing areas of interest within the American Psychological Association, something one would not have imagined just a few decades ago.

The lawsuit's challenge to the long-standing autocratic structure of the American Psychoanalytic Association has at least arguably had a positive impact within the American Psychoanalytic Association. One can now see hope for a reduction in the American's rigidity, as a number of younger analysts realize that one can politically challenge its rules and procedures just as they can with any organization. That one may have a problem with authority does not mean that one has an "authority problem." Indeed, the change has had a salutary effect on freedom of thought within the American Psychoanalytic Association.

It is true that in the early days after the lawsuit many members of the American Psychoanalytic Association responded with a defensive historical revisionism—claiming "We were going to do it anyway." They overlooked the voluminous documents and public statements that were very much to the contrary, not to mention the direct statements made to the lawsuit organizers in presuit meetings between the two groups.

But it is noteworthy that, just a few years later, as psychologists and medical analysts began a perilous reformation period in the nation's health care system, psychology's closest ally was the American Psychoanalytic Association. As both groups confronted the multiple issues that the crisis had raised for them, the analytic community appreciated more fully that, in fighting over psychoanalytic training opportunities, psychologists were testifying to its importance, a value shared by analytically oriented psychologists and psychiatrists but not by many other large segments of society.

It became increasingly important for Division 39 psychologist/psychoanalysts and the American Psychoanalytic Association to articulate their shared values, which often were lost in the health care debate. Psychotherapy is one of the few therapeutic sanctuaries that we provide in our culture. It is founded on a deeply held belief in the importance of the subjective realm of human experience and human emotion. And it inherently depends on a close and intimate relationship that can unfold only over sufficient time and with a degree of intensity sufficient to allow meaningful events to take place.

In 1992, the American Psychoanalytic Association took what were, for it, radical steps—it hired its own lobbying firm and began to participate in the political dialogue in Washington. Psychologist lobbyists were in regular contact with them, and, combined, they added energy geared toward securing a place for intensive psychotherapy and psychoanalysis in the health care reform.

THE HEALTH CARE SYSTEM

While the psychoanalytic community was waging its legal civil war, other major changes were confronting the overall health care system. Costs were escalating exponentially. The percentage of our Gross National Product spent on health care rose from 6% to 15%, and health care became a major political issue in this country. Simply put, we suffered from a system of health care in which patient and provider decided how much of the insurance company's money they wanted to spend. Not surprisingly, their decisions were inflationary. And so we shifted to a system where a fourth private party was given both the money and the power to determine how much of the money to spend on patients and how much to retain for their own corporate profits. (They would like to retain a lot in corporate profits!) This new system became known as managed health care.

By the mid-1990s, the *Wall Street Journal* reported that the CEO of one of the largest managed care companies made a salary of ten million dollars, money that could probably have provided inoculations for most of the nation's children who were not inoculated at the time.

Not surprisingly, long-term psychotherapy was extremely vulnerable in this new system. Therapy's inherent subjectivity, people's fear of and antipathy toward the subjective realm, and the prejudice that exists against mental illness all contributed to the problem and made it very difficult for people to protest when their psychotherapy benefits were removed.

AMERICAN PSYCHOLOGICAL ASSOCIATION PRACTICE DIRECTORATE

Managed care was clearly a political problem that was going to require a massive federal and state lobbying effort. And yet, when psychologists looked to their national trade organization, they found an organization that had been established by research academics, had very little to do with advocacy, and had even less to do with advocacy on behalf of psychoanalytic practitioners. Thus, in 1985, spurred by an insurgent group of young practitioners drawn largely from state psychological associations, the APA established a special tax on its practitioners to raise the three million dollars annually needed to establish an advocacy structure that could begin to tackle the problems that these young psychologists anticipated were going to confront psychology in the not too distant future.

In building the structure, psychologists had to focus on a number of areas. First psychology's scope-of-practice issues, under assault by medical interests, were fought at the state level. Psychologists' state political structures were extraordinarily primitive and ill equipped to meet the major tasks that lay ahead. At the federal level, our health care system appeared to be spiraling out of control and deteriorating so rapidly with managed care that eventually it seemed likely to collapse, forcing the federal government to intervene with some type of quasi-national health insurance system. The United States was one of just two countries that did not have a national health insurance system. (The other was South Africa.)

In response, psychologists did two things. First, they built an infrastructure. Substantial resources were spent building state associations and helping them hire professional staff and equipment. At the federal level, psychologists set up a grass roots network so that psychologists would be able to contact elected officials in their home district. They established a database of information about the value of psychotherapy and psychological services in general. They set up an aggressive political action committee so that psychologists could make contributions to candidates' campaigns and form relationships with elected officials who would support them in legislative chambers. Psychologists set up a public relations arm to advocate their issues in public forums, and they developed a cadre of lobbyists to make their case on Capitol Hill.

The second thing psychologists did while building the infrastructure was to shape emerging legislation to have an impact on inevitable health care reform legislation. When Senator Edward Kennedy (D-MA) and Congressman Henry Waxman (D-CA) proposed the first national health insurance plan, it contained no mention of mental health and no mention of psychology. Psychologists responded aggressively to the proposed legislation and were successful in having both psychology and other mental health care included, albeit with a very limited outpatient benefit.

Psychologists also looked at the Medicare program. Many were predicting that Medicare would be the logical vehicle to extend for national health insurance. Clearly, if psychological treatment were not included in Medicare soon, psychologists would not be eligible for participation in that program in the future, and jockeying for position at a time of expansion to national health insurance would be even more problematic.

HEALTH CARE REFORM

The managed care marketplace continued to deteriorate. We had the worst of all possible worlds: a health care system under which costs of care were escalating dramatically and the number of people not covered by health insurance was also growing rapidly. In his first presidential campaign, President Clinton made health care a major campaign issue, and psychologists knew that with his election would come a major push toward national health insurance. Several questions, of course, then arose. What role would psychoanalysis and psychotherapy play? What could psychologists do to influence the outcome?

One immediate problem that had to be overcome by psychology's leadership was the attitude many of their colleagues had about participation in the political process. Psychologists' traditional passive political postures can be easily fit into personality profiles.

Deniers

Some simply denied that there was any problem. "Health care reform. What's that?" At one Division 39 meeting, a psychologist in the audience raised her hand and said to the speaker, "You seem to be saying that this health care reform issue is something that could affect my practice." The denier!

Narcissists

The narcissist responds to political tension in many ways: "It won't affect me because I'm special," or "Yes, but that's politics and politics is dirty. I'm above that." As Plato said over 2,000 years ago, "The price that wise people pay for not participating in politics is to be governed by the decisions of unwise people."

Infantiles

The third group is the "blatantly infantile." These are the people who look at the health care climate and, in effect, say, "This isn't right," their tone suggesting they have just implemented an action plan.

Escapists

The fourth group—soon to be an extinct species—is the "escapist." "I don't like health care reform. I think I'll fight to get out of it. Then I can survive and prosper." In short, the position suggests that psychologists can simply step "outside" the reimbursement system and do well by their patients and themselves.

That is true for some. But for most psychologists the simple fact is that, if the federal government is going to pour 80 to 100 billion dollars into mental health care, but nothing for intensive psychotherapy or psychoanalysis, psychoanalysis, psychotherapy, patients, and most psychologists will suffer drastically. One can talk about stepping outside the system all they want. Certainly, there are "Gold Coasts" in this country where a few people will maintain practices with the wealthy and the elite. But for most people on a very practical basis it is not a viable option. In reimbursement circles, it was never hard to "get out" of the system. Everybody would let you out. There was no enemy to be met on that battleground. The real battleground was over two issues: benefits structure and managed care.

As for the legislative struggle itself, it was very clear that psychologists wanted to make certain that they had the right to participate in the system. Thanks to the Medicare battle, inclusion of psychologists was not controversial, nor has psychology's scope of practice been threatened in any proposed new systems. The controversy was *all* in the two areas of benefits and managed care.

The health care battle that ensued was remarkable. The psychologists' case was very simple: we can afford good mental health care if we do not waste mental health resources. The areas in which mental health resources were being wasted were inpatient adolescent care and inpatient alcohol and substance abuse. Watch the hospital door carefully, but recognize that it is very cost effective to let people gain access to intensive outpatient treatment. The psychologists also pointed out that the then-current managed care systems' allocation of up to 20 visits for psychotherapy was not sufficient for people who are multiple trauma victims or who have serious personality disorders or severe chronic depression.

Unfortunately, White House staff included one person who espoused a very antipsychotherapy viewpoint and another with an exclusively biological psychiatric perspective. This skew produced a bill with unlimited inpatient care, an unlimited drug benefit at 80% reimbursement, and 30 outpatient visits reimbursed at 50% coverage.

Of course, a major struggle ensued. Thanks to long-time psychologist advocates Senator Inouye (D-HI) and Congressman Ted Strickland (D-OH), psychologists received audiences with Hillary Clinton and with various staff for the Administration's health care reform initiative. Thus, before a more objective tribunal, psychologists were able to present their case for a better outpatient benefit.

One might think that all mental health professionals would be delighted if a better outpatient benefit was obtained. This was not the case. Overlooking the fact that it was private-sector hospitalizations that had deflected money from the states and dominated and misled by the private psychiatric hospitals and later by the duplicitous managed care companies, a vociferous minority of the community argued that outpatient care would block access to treatment for the seriously mentally ill.

As a result of the split in the mental health community, psychologists obtained more limited improvement in the outpatient benefits with the Clinton administration than they would have otherwise. Therefore, they went to the Hill with two objectives: one was to remove from the bill the limits on outpatient care, and the other was to explain the managed care problem to Congress.

By this time psychologists had been through a number of battles. Medicare and other advocacy struggles had seasoned them in the political arena. The psychologists had formed ongoing relationships with key people who would be influential in the health care debate and who psychologists felt would be sympathetic to mental health. The psychologists hired full-time field organizers to go to the states and help organize for political activity. In one week alone, the psychologists sent out 350,000 pieces of mail, including letters to all the members of the American Psychological Association asking them to write and phone their elected officials. The psychologists also sent 35,000 telegrams on critical issues. The psychologists brought in conservative actuaries who said that the benefit model psychologists developed would work and made actuarial sense for health care systems.

Although the overall health reform legislative train stalled, the outcome for psychotherapy was dazzling. Every major bill reported out of committee had an unlimited outpatient psychotherapy benefit. There was no question that psychologists and psychotherapy had made tremendous headway on Capitol Hill. Maybe even more important, there was also a demonstrative attitudinal change in Congress about mental health care. Where once one heard about "the worried well" and the "Woody Allen Syndrome," elected officials now realized that Woody Allen was a far cry from the typical psychotherapy patient.

That was the good news. The second issue, though, managed care reform, was not successful. One can have any size "benefit" one wants, but, if the managed care company will not "authorize" it, patients do not get it.

While psychologists were extremely aggressive with regard to the managed care provisions, there was no question that provisions supporting managed care dominated the legislative proposal brought forth by the Administration. The provisions that the psychologists advocated did not receive serious consideration in the managed care reform effort.

For a period of time, psychologists had succeeded in having a "point of service" option included in the legislation. (A point of service option stipulates that patients who are willing to pay a little higher co-pay are allowed to go outside the system and select providers they want.) Psychologists felt that point-of-service was a good quality check on managed care; if someone was willing to pay more to go outside the system, the implication was that the managed care system may not have been providing quality care. Owing to managed care lobbying, however, that provision was taken out of the Gephardt Bill late in the Congressional session.

A sadly naive mental health lobby fell for the seductive allure of managed health care's argument that, if we just manage care, we can ultimately have "total parity" with insurance coverage for other illnesses. As a result, there was no concerted mental health opposition to managed care other than the combined efforts of the American Psychoanalytic Association, the Private Practice Psychiatrists Association, and the American Psychological Association.

Well, none of the health care bills passed. Was it something more than the interesting history of a failed legislative process? Yes, it was. The change in attitude toward mental health is permanent. The current erosion of health care continues, as does the proliferation of managed care. Gradually, the government will play an increasing role in health care—it will shape the mental health reimbursement of the future.

IT'S PARITY THAT NO ONE UNDERSTANDS

This same naiveté was evident in the euphoria over the mental health "parity" legislation passed in 1996. While the mental health lobby sold it to its members as an "important first step" toward ending discrimination against mental health care, legislative committee language expressly conditioned the legislation on the company's right to comprehensively "manage" the mental health benefit. For psychologists and non-M.D. mental health professionals, it also reopened the whole issue of who provides what service by permitting the Health Care Finance Administration and state governments to define "mental illness" and "treatments."

MANAGED CARE REFORM

The problem confronting the managed care industry is REALITY. As Abraham Lincoln said, "You can fool all the people some of the time and some of the people all of the time. But you can't fool all the people all the time." Reality intrudes and the devastation that managed care has wreaked is now permeating the public consciousness.

And it is with exposure of the deception that the seeds for the destruction of managed care have been sown. Every major media source now appreciates the enormous scandal in our health care system; the stories they encounter pull at the heartstrings of their viewing public.

The simple fact is that the American public has never signed off on inferior health care systems. The American people care about two things: 1) schools for their children and 2) health care. In the early days of managed care, it was easy to promise them more for less. People are gullible and quite willing to believe in such utopian fantasies.

Chickens come home to roost. The growing public relations debacle confronting the managed care industry will not go away. It is inherent to the system, and, as the system grows, more and more abuse will be exposed.

As powerful as the public relations developments are, probably even more significant are changes in the legal system. A Supreme Court Justice once said, "Justice is like a train that is nearly always late." So it is with managed care. From 1985 to 1995, there was very little the courts were able to do about managed care. They were slow to recognize that managed care companies, despite their disavowals, were really practicing medicine when they made determinations of "medical necessity." Further, when they prospectively denied insurance benefits, they effectively denied treatment.

That legal myopia has changed, and attorneys are now able to file suits on the basis of malpractice, bad faith insurance denial, tortuous interference with doctor–patient relationships, breach of contract, and a variety of other traditionally common law causes of action.

Equally important, an arcane federal statute that had been insulating many of the managed care companies from legal liability slowly began to erode. The Employee Retirement Income Security Act (ERISA) of 1974 preempted all state laws that "relate to" employee benefit plans. The phrase "relate to" had been so broadly interpreted by courts that it was virtually impossible to sue ERISA managed care health plans, no matter how egregious their behavior. Since 1995 there have been a number of significant Supreme Court and Federal Circuit Court of Appeals decisions that clarified that the "relate to" clause should not be interpreted so broadly that it wipes out all the aforementioned state causes of action.

These developments in the legal realm, coupled with the public attention the managed care industry received, created a veritable ground swell of interest in managed care litigation in the legal field. It is this combination of public outcry and growing legal pressure that will make it increasingly difficult for employers and political figures to support the once-believed deception of the managed care industry, to wit, that it is saving money by virtue of prevention and careful management.

The truth is out. Having once betrayed the American public, it will be very difficult for the managed care industry to regain that trust. Make no mistake about it, they will try. And be assured that their efforts will be characterized by the very same emphasis on deception that spawned the managed care industry. HMOs advertise their "accreditation" by the National Commission on Quality Assurance (NCQA), a transparent, whitewashing organization established by the managed care industry itself to create the illusion of standard setting.

The NCQA standards pertain largely to demands that the managed care company should make on its providers. Thus, the NCQA, while presented as a quality-control device, is really an insidious means of harassing providers and making it more difficult to provide care. The standards do not address such real quality issues as making appropriate numbers of treatment resources available to patients.

The managed care industry is not going to like its growing legal liability. It is for this reason that they and other large corporate interests in America have been sponsoring efforts to "end frivolous lawsuits." What they are not telling the public is that the specific reform efforts, known as "tort reform," do little to prevent frivolous lawsuits, but, instead, make it very difficult for the average person to obtain any justice from large corporate players not matter how egregious, calculating, or diabolical their behavior.

Managed care will not go quietly into the night. It is, however, terminally ill. The reality principle has to hold sway, and we are already seeing it emerge in the evolution of the managed care industry. How quickly the demise occurs depends on the role that concerned professionals play in forcefully advocating for their patients and exposing the sham of managed care.

If there is one lesson psychologists have learned from the past decade, it is that psychoanalysis will be greatly affected by the political and legal processes. Who can practice? What will the reimbursement and delivery system be like? How much intrusion will there be into the doctor–patient relationship? Will the managed care profiteers be held accountable for the people they hurt, or will their health system continue to reward those who exploit people in need of mental health care?

What can one do? There is only one thing they can do: participate in the political process. What's going to happen with psychology's national organization? How prepared are psychologists to fight a battle about what the American Psychological Association does and does not do to protect patients? How easily beguiled will psychologists be by information that is fed to them?

All those questions have to be answered if psychologists are to be effective participants in the political process. But politics now defines mental health care in this country, and it is going to do so for as long as psychologists are present. Nor will the psychologist's struggle be over even when these current questions have been answered. For their struggle is Sysiphysian in nature—it is never won and is always ongoing. Psychologists can no more avoid and neglect the political realm than they can walk out on their patients in the consulting room. It is the Reality Principle.

TWO

Life After Health Care Reform

A Clinical Solution

TONI BERNAY

When the question of the inclusion of psychological services in proposals for health care reform first loomed large on the political and economic horizons, Division 39 invited me to think about responding to this potential new world of practice. I offer the following program as a "creative, provocative and controversial model" (Bernay, 1994) of psychoanalytically grounded practice. Our concern these days is for a clinical solution that permits psychoanalysis to be embraced within any of the various formats offered for nationwide health care reform. In addition, we require a forward-looking program for the entire field of psychodynamic psychology that enables us to advocate effectively for ourselves.

A PROPOSED CLINICAL SOLUTION

The specific clinical solution I propose follows from an abiding philosophy of the American Psychological Association and of the Division of Psychoanalysis. It was articulated by Dorothy Cantor, the 105th president of the APA, "Psychoanalysis is not just a way of practicing, it's a way of looking at the world. Even with patients I see once a week, psychoanalysis gives me a better handle on how they come to be where they are and how to help them get where they want to be" (personal communication). Similarly, Jonathan Slavin, a former president of the Division, notes: "No other perspective can compete with the way it informs you and your capacity to deal with the whole range of problems" (personal communication). With that sense of the wide applicability of psychoanalysis, let us look to our own historical roots and use our own talents for the answers to our health care reform problems. Let us do what we ask our patients to do—find the familiar in the unfamiliar.

What I am referring to here is the psychoanalytically oriented short-term therapy model born out of the Coconut Grove fire, the disaster that occurred with great loss of life in a Boston nightclub in 1937. In its aftermath, Erich Lindemann (1944), a psychiatrist and psychoanalyst, tended to the victims of the fire. He realized that the ways in which they responded to the crisis and to the trauma they suffered were characteristic for them and were rooted in memories of their past. He called his model for treating crisis victims "crisis intervention." He undergirded crisis intervention with his psychoanalytic understanding that an individual's response to a current crisis springs from his or her historical experiences and unique way of integrating those experiences. Lindemann recognized that the crisis softened the defenses, making psychic processes unusually available and conscious. Using this window of therapeutic opportunity immediately and briefly enabled him to penetrate the traumatic veil, establish a therapeutic bond, and reestablish the patient's equilibrium, perhaps at a higher level than before. Lindemann learned that the more he knew of the idiosyncratic meaning of the crisis, relevant to the victim's earlier experiences, the better the result of the intervention. All this despite the brevity of the intervention and the use of conscious material only.

In Los Angeles a short time later, psychiatrist-psychoanalyst Gerald Jacobson (1966) and psychologist Will Morley followed Lindemann's lead and developed the first walk-in mental health clinic, the Benjamin Rush Center at the Los Angeles Psychiatric Service. The Benjamin Rush Center was anchored in a six-session crisis intervention model that became the paradigm for the country. Speaking in a language created by the recent marriage of business methods and health care that parallels the industrialization of health care, Jacobson and Morley created and then successfully niche-marketed what we would now call a name brand product, a carve-out or a segment. While some providers of mental health care object to such activities, let alone to such labels, considering them crass and unprofessional, it is my contention that at this juncture the best way we can maintain our integrity, offer the best care to our patients, and do our best work, is to use the system to help us maintain our practices as we like them to be, as much as possible. I believe that crisis intervention, or brief short-term therapy, using a psychoanalytic model, demonstrates the efficacy and cost-effectiveness of psychoanalytic thinking. Positioned in the marketplace as a credible, recognizable, name-brand psychoanalytic product, it is going to be one of the best gifts we can give ourself and our patients.

At the Benjamin Rush Center, where I trained, we had six sessions to cure the patient. During the first session, we were required to pinpoint a precipitating event and develop a diagnosis, a psychodynamic formulation, an understanding of the transference, and a treatment plan. In sessions two to five, we treated the patient, and in session six we terminated. By then, of course, we had developed a relationship with the patient and many of us, being the long-term animals we were, wanted to take the patient into long-term therapy and do a great deal more work. This was not allowed. "No, no, no," pronounced Drs. Jacobson and Morley. "Not allowed." On pain of death, a therapist could not take a short-term patient into long-term therapy. If necessary, the patient could be referred to the long-term program at the Center, the Los Angeles Psychiatric Service, since renamed the Didi Hirsch Community Mental Health Center. But the referral had to be to a different therapist.

These were arbitrary boundaries set up to train us in short-term methods. I am eternally grateful for that training. It substantially contributed to my feeling confident that I can provide excellent therapeutic services to a broad range of people, and under a variety of conditions, using techniques that range over crisis intervention or brief short-term therapy, short-term therapy, intermediated-therapy, long-term therapy, and—thanks to my analytic training—psychoanalysis. Psychologists in our division have continued the tradition of developing psychoanalytically based short-term dynamic psychotherapy. Carol Goodheart (1989) and others have contributed to the theory and the technique and have done outcomes research on the topic. Their findings offer us an updated, research-based psychoanalytic short-term therapy model from the perspective of psychologist/psychoanalyst members of the division. It seems a made-to-order opportunity to use this and other members' work as a springboard for our name-brand product and gold-standard positioning efforts.

On the practical side, I know that many psychologist/psychoanalysts share my experience that most analytic cases are conversions from psychotherapy, including from crisis intervention. In today's world, I don't have to stop doing psychoanalysis. Neither do my colleagues. But we are not going to get paid by third-party payers for doing it. That is simply a fact of our professional lives.

In order to maintain our practices in ways that permit us to employ our psychoanalytic skills, we need to use our organizational talents in the service of strategic and creative approaches to mental health care in the current environment. Using our clinical skills and our psychoanalytic understanding of the underpinnings of any effective psychological treatment, we can redesign our analytic practitioner selves and reevaluate and widen the range of conditions under which we can work effectively, both inside and outside of managed care. We can and we need to do this. In addition, we need to define the mental health marketplace using our own models of care and clinicians and our own models of care as credible and recogniz-able, name-brand psychoanalytic "products," such as short-term dynamic psychotherapy, benchmarks, and outcome studies. By doing these things we can:

1. Demonstrate the value, efficacy, and cost-effectiveness of psycho-analytic thinking and products, including the marketing and consumer satisfaction "value added" brought about by psychoanalytic/psychodynamic contributions.[1]
2. Have the tools that speak the federal and state legislatures' own language in order to be effective advocates for our patients and to educate legislators and insurers.
3. Be the premier mental health care consultants to other mental health professional and provider groups.
4. Enter the competitive health care marketplace with a value-added, highly marketable product.

By achieving these four overarching goals, we can not only provide good treatment and consultation, but also build thoughtful, patient-wel-fare-oriented, legitimate feeder systems to keep our practices full. Reach-ing these goals also enables us to be insiders and acknowledged and credible experts in assisting legislators in making changes. While doing so, we can along the way negotiate and advocate for the policies dictated by psycho-analysis. Policy making is a long-term, process-oriented task. Surely we are good at "hanging in" for the long term. It is the very soul of who we are as analysts.

A PROPOSED PROGRAM OF ACTION

The elements of my proposed plan for clinical solution to our national health care problems do not stand alone. They require support from other professional and advocacy activities. We must undertake such activities to provide credibility for our approach, while at the same time expanding our sphere of operations.

Here, in highly skeletonized form, is my recommendation for how psychoanalysis might proceed.

---

[1] In this case, consumers refer to those groups relevant to health and mental health care. Such groups are both inside and outside managed care and its evolving variations, such as capitated arrangements. The groups I refer to include patients, plans and providers, users and purchasers of our direct and consultative services.

Launch a Marketing Campaign Based on the Following Points:

A. Position psychoanalysis as the powerful tool of a boarded (or niche) specialty of the premier mental health profession—psychology. This will become easier to do as we acquire prescriptive privileges, an organized psychology effort now beginning to roll across state and state legislatures. As we obtain prescribing privileges for psychologists, we can offer this service to the public and consult to provider groups on prescribing from the psychoanalytic vantage point. Include prescribing in the marketing campaign as they become a reality.

B. Position psychoanalytic short-term therapy as:

- Credible
- Visible
- Recognizable
- Effective
- Cost Effective
- Name Brand Product

C. Position the outcome data and benchmarks of this signature treatment model as the gold standard of mental health care.

D. Offer consultation and practice management services to other mental health professionals, group practices, and institutions, to help them develop efficacious and cost-effective managed care and niche-marketing psychotherapy programs, again using our name-brand service delivery model as excellent, valuable, and reliable treatment services and our outcome data and benchmarks as gold standards of practice. Practice management services are now a needed and lucrative specialty in and of themselves.

My last point about prescription privileges is obviously the most controversial and deserves some elaboration. I view prescriptive privileges as part of our profession's, our colleagues' and our own—for those who want it—right. Through use of the legislative process, we have the right to expand our professional and clinical boundaries and move into pioneering new areas, as do other professional groups such as podiatrists, who have moved from foot to ankle, and optometrists who have moved into prescribing topical medications. We did just that when, using the courts, we broke the stranglehold of the American Psychoanalytic Association on psychoanalytic training. As a result, psychologist/psychoanalysts have developed a national presence, a nationwide psychoanalytic network, and many training programs for psychologist/psychoanalysts. In the process, we changed the face of American psychoanalysis forever. And psychoanalysis and psychologist/psychoanalysts have flourished. Our nonpsychoanalytic colleagues took a great leap of faith in supporting our efforts to accomplish this. Turnabout is fair play.

It is not just a question of political fair play, however. It is a question of knowing the importance of being able, formally, officially, and competently, to handle medication for our patients. There are some of us who know it now. They include those of us who practice in rural areas, or who serve traditionally underserved populations, or who have more general practices along with our psychoanalytically oriented ones. They include myriads of us who de facto wind up monitoring our patients' medications, perhaps because we see them often, perhaps because we understand mental health issues better than their primary care physicians do. Psychologists who choose not to prescribe need not undertake the specialized and additional training that will be required of prescribing psychologists. But consider the advantages to all psychologist/psychoanalysts of being able to send a patient for medication consultation to a psychologist, with whom we share a more common language! I propose that, as far afield as prescription privileges may seem from the issue of psychoanalytic practice in the current health care climate, it is not. It is a political necessity as well as a practice option. It is something we need to support for the many direct and indirect benefits it brings us.

SUMMARY

That psychoanalytic thinking and treatment are very powerful and effective tools is well-known among us. Our task now is, as the spin doctors put it, to position ourselves properly. We can do this by making psychoanalysis a boarded niche specialty and making the psychoanalytically based clinical model of short-term treatment both a gold standard against which other interventions are measured and a name-brand product on which the public can rely for "the best" treatment. That will give us a basic platform from which we can continue to provide, in managed and other forms, the high quality of care for which our psychoanalytic expertise qualifies us. This is a paradigm shift for us, a sea change that will entail our moving into arenas and activities that are relatively unfamiliar but that are necessary to maintain our lead and prosper in the field of mental health care

The model and program I have outlined will support, not undermine, our identities as psychoanalytic practitioners. We offer our patients the grounding and flexibility to recognize and address the constantly changing patterns and paradigms of the world around them—now a new, faster paced, more competitive 21st-century world. As role models, we can do no less for ourselves. We can serve society at large and continue to give our patients good treatment more easily if we take advantage of the marketplace demands of our time for the benefit of our profession. We will not be less analytic by adopting any of the points I have recommended. We as psychoanalysts are sturdier than that.

REFERENCES

Bernay, T. (1994), Prescribing privileges are good for psychology, including psychoanalysis, *Psychologist-Psychoanalyst,* August, pp. 14–16.

Goodheart, C. D. (1989), Short term dynamic psychotherapy with difficult clients. *Innovations in Clinical Practice, Vol. 8.* Sarasota, FL: Professional Resource Exchange.

Jacobson, G. F. (1996), Crisis theory and treatment strategy: Some sociocultural and psychodynamic considerations, *J. Nerv. & Men. Dis.,* 141:210

Lindemann, E. (1944), Symptomatology and management of acute grief, *Amer. J. Psychiat.,* 101:141–148.

THREE

Managed Mental Health Care and the Denial of Subjectivity

Historical and Philosophical Antecedents

JAMES W. BARRON

ABANDONMENT OF TRADITIONAL VALUES

Despite our tendency to anthropomorphize managed care and project onto it human or at times demonic qualities, it is not a monolithic entity. Instead, managed care is a generally agreed upon shorthand representation of the evolving interlocking health care practices and ideologies of large-scale health care systems, governmental and legislative bodies, regulatory agencies, and insurance organizations. Proponents of managed care simultaneously treat psychoanalysis, along with its derivative theories and therapies, as dangerous aberrations, as enemies of progress, and as quaint, harmless anachronisms destined to wither away. As psychoanalysts, we experience a fundamental antagonism between dynamically based treatment approaches and systems of managed mental health care as currently conceived and organized.

Managed care policies and procedures routinely limit or deny needed mental health care and invade and degrade the psychotherapy treatment relationship. Psychotherapy, as we conceptualize it, requires, above all, a safe interpersonal space in which a trusting, confidential relationship is gradually built and a therapeutic process develops. Managed care practices, as we and our patients experience them, have a corrosive effect on that space.

Vital issues are at stake: preservation of meaningful treatment and

23

maintenance of a high quality of patient care; recognition of the centrality of the therapeutic relationship and protection of the boundaries of that relationship; and survival of our profession in a form that we can recognize and feel proud to identify with. We ask ourselves how it is that so many decision makers and policy planners (in collaboration with many practitioners) are so ready, in some cases so eager, to jettison those values and substitute alternative values compatible with managed care.

STAMPEDE TO MANAGED CARE

We have many persuasive answers near at hand (Barron and Sands, 1996), and we can round up the usual economic and sociopolitical suspects with little difficulty: the sprouting of staff and group model HMOs in the 1960s; the introduction of the federal government as a direct payer with the development of Medicare and Medicaid in 1965; the proposal in 1969 by Paul Ellwood, then executive director of the American Rehabilitation Institute, to establish prepaid systems, which, he argued, would be a competitive, cost-effective alternative to fee-for-service models and would provide incentives for preventive and rehabilitative services; the elaboration and formalization of those incentives by Alain Enthoven, which led to the Nixon administration's endorsement in 1973 of the Health Maintenance Organization Act to counteract the Democrats' advocacy of national health insurance; the recession of the late 1980s combined with concerns about the escalating costs of health care and the gaping holes in the health care safety net; and the forces unleashed by President Clinton's embrace of "managed competition" in his failed attempt to overhaul the nation's health care system.

Other factors affecting mental health services include the comparatively minor role of mental health care in the overall system, that is, its constituting only a small fraction of the trillion dollar health care industry and its being swept along by the managed care tidal wave; the public's limited understanding of psychological disorders and their treatments, as well as the stigma that unfortunately is still attached to them; private practitioners' fear of loss of referrals if they don't jump on the managed care bandwagon; and, perhaps most important, the lure of substantial profits to be reaped by the corporate owners of managed care organizations.

Health care "players" at all levels are frantically positioning themselves so as not to be left out in the cold. Solo practitioners are rushing to form small groups. Small groups are attempting to coalesce into larger networks of providers to salvage some degree of control over their professional destinies, only to discover that they must sacrifice wished-for autonomy so as to be more attractive to the health maintenance organizations that control access to patients. Boards of directors of private hospitals of all sizes are busily buying physicians' practices and scrambling to enter into alliances with other hospitals and outpatient treatment centers to develop large-scale regional health care systems, which they hope will secure their places at negotiating tables and guarantee their survival in the marketplace. The nation's largest insurance companies are developing their own managed care companies or acquiring existing companies. For-profit health care companies with sufficient resources are busily acquiring hospitals and practices throughout the country and beginning to expand internationally.

HISTORICAL ANTECEDENTS

The lure of substantial profits accruing to the corporate owners of large-scale health care systems and the panic of smaller scale players and practitioners drive these frenzied activities and provide a partial answer to our question about the readiness of so many to abandon traditional ways of thinking about and approaching the treatment of patients with psychological problems.

In addition, the rapid growth of biological psychiatry, with its arsenal of psychotropic medications, has captured the public imagination. The proliferation of therapies and specialized support groups has fractured and fragmented the field, leaving the public confused and searching for the quick fix and increasingly disenchanted with dynamic psychotherapies, particularly of the long-term variety, which stress unfolding developmental processes. This fragmentation is also evident in the prevailing diagnostic system, which relies heavily on signs, symptoms, and numerical rating scales of level of stress and degree of adjustment (Barron, 1998). And, of course, in the background, while all these forces exert their influence, various media send out a steady drumbeat of criticism of psychoanalytic theory and its applications.

The more zealous proselytizers of managed care exploit these conditions and caricature psychoanalytic practitioners as dinosaurs unfit to survive and deserving of extinction. We recognize the overall need to control health care costs, but we are aware that mental health care accounts for only a small proportion of those costs and that excessive reliance on inpatient treatment (particularly of adolescents and persons with substance abuse problems) has been the primary cost-driver of mental health care. Outpatient mental health care has been and remains cost effective.

Nevertheless, on the defensive, we are eager to prove our relevance and usefulness. We attempt to gather data to establish that psychodynamically oriented psychotherapy is a good investment, that its cost is more than offset by decreasing illness, absenteeism, accidents and disability claims; that employees and their families receiving adequate care for their psychological problems consume fewer outpatient medical services and require fewer inpatient days of medical or psychiatric treatment.

I am not criticizing those efforts to document our effectiveness. In fact, I think we have done ourselves a disservice by not engaging in that kind of applied research earlier and more systematically.

The assault on mental health care, particularly on psychodynamically based treatments, which frequently extend over longer periods of time than other approaches, does not make rational economic sense. The legislative and judicial branches have taken some small, but important steps in curbing some of the more egregious managed care practices such as "drive-through deliveries" (not paying for reasonable hospital care for mothers and their newborns) and "cherry picking" (excluding those with potentially costly preexisting medical conditions from enrollment in the health care plan). Responding to public pressure and effective lobbying by sectors of the mental health community, Congress determined that discriminatory insurance coverage is counterproductive, and Members passed the mental health parity bill, although managed care organizations have quickly discovered and exploited the loopholes in that bill. The Supreme Court, in *Jaffe vs. Redmond* (1996), reaffirmed the overriding social value of the psychotherapist–patient relationship and strengthened protective confidential boundaries, under certain restrictive conditions, around that relationship. Nevertheless, the value of privacy and confidentiality, essential to psychodynamic treatment, will be seriously challenged by advocates of managed care.

Despite these changes in the health care landscape, vociferous proponents of managed care, supported by critics from both academia and the media, continue their attacks on psychodynamic therapies. Our necessary defense of who we are and what we do makes it difficult, at times impossible, for us to step back from the fray and reflect on the massive changes that are occurring so rapidly and place them in historical context. As psychoanalysts we take seriously the historicity of the individual. We need to apply a similar perspective to the analysis of managed care and its impact on psychodynamic treatment. We need to understand the history of the growth of managed care in general as well as the complex relationship between managed mental health care and the denial of the existence or relevance of unconscious factors in personality development and organization, as well as in the process of therapeutic change.

IRONY OF MANAGED CARE:
RETURN OF THE SUPPRESSED

Experiments in the management of health care go back a long time, and we can trace aspects of contemporary managed care to those origins. Beginning in the 1880s, the Mayo brothers established the first group practice employing an array of specialists. In the early 1900s, the lumbering, mining, transportation, and construction industries experimented with prepaid plans. Farmers, rural, cooperatives, and various town and city governments also tinkered with group practices or prepaid plans, although the two ideas were not combined until 1929. Not surprisingly, mental health benefits of any kind were rarely offered in any of these plans (Bittker, 1992).

Despite some of the similarities between these plans and contemporary systems, there are critical differences. The early experiments were small-scale, fluid parts of the health care landscape. While these experiments were responses to the marketplace, that is, to opportunities in certain urban or rural settings where health care was generally unavailable, they were, in some cases, also infused with social idealism. As Paul Starr (1982) has documented, powerful vested interests, including the American Medical Association, equated these experiments in "contract practice" with socialism and vehemently opposed them.

> [During the early 1900s] . . . physicians became uneasy about various other organizations that potentially threatened their autonomy. Private practitioners wanted to keep their relations with patients unmediated by any corporation. They worried about companies that employed doctors to furnish medical care to their workers. . . . In some areas, employers paid profit-making firms to provide medical services to their workers, and the firms in turn contracted with doctors to give treatment at low rates. These commercial intermediaries were especially distasteful to the medical profession. . . . Reformers, however, viewed these organized health services, particularly the private multi-speciality clinics, as harbingers of a new order in medical care. . . . These expectations were hardly unreasonable, but they proved to be wrong. As occasionally happens, the inevitable did not take place, at least not on schedule: The solo practitioner did not rapidly become extinct. Instead of expanding, organized health services were relegated to the sidelines of the medical system [pp. 198–199].
>
> The dislike of physicians for "socialized medicine" is well known, but their distaste for corporate capitalism in

> medical practice was equally strong. They had no more de-
> sire to be dominated by private corporations than by agen-
> cies of government, and consequently resisted the two forms
> in which business corporations threatened to move into
> medical services—the provision of treatment for their own
> employees through "company doctors" and the marketing
> of services to the public [p. 200].

It is ironic that contemporary (per)versions of these early experiments with "socialized medicine" have become powerful economic engines controlling the lion's share of the health care marketplace and generating huge profits for their corporate owners.

Bennett (1988) has presciently observed:

> There has . . . been a change in the organizational mission
> and its derivative, system values: yesterday's HMO was de-
> signed to organize and deliver health care; today's is likely
> to be a product line, one activity of an organization seeking
> to prosper in the marketplace. Ginzburg (1984) has termed
> this "the monetarization of medical care," i.e., increasing
> domination of health care by those whose primary business
> is the preservation and increase of capital. These changes
> create a crosscurrent that threatens to confuse and inundate
> those who work in such settings [p. 1546].

We have, of course, witnessed the rapid acceleration of these trends in the decade since Bennett made those observations.

PHILOSOPHICAL UNDERPINNINGS

At the turn of the century, psychiatry in this country—in fact, medicine as a whole—was in its infancy, eager to prove its scientific status and to differentiate itself from quackery. Psychology at that time had no involvement at all with health care. Indeed, while experiments in the organization and delivery of health care services were taking place, a handful of psychologists, grounded in the scientific positivism of the turn of the century and trained in the content and methodology of perceptual-physiological research, were laboring to establish psychology as a legitimate domain of inquiry apart from religion and philosophy.

Freud's 1909 Clark lectures exposed American psychologists to psychoanalytic ideas (Jones, 1955, p. 54). The initial response for the first five years ranged from bemusement and mild interest to polite indifference. American psychologists were not at first threatened by psychoanalysis. They felt that it was largely irrelevant and had little if anything to do with science as they conceptualized and practiced it.

> For their part, psychologists initially saw psychoanalysis as just another of the "mind cures" that flashed across the American landscape in the—like Christian Science or the Emmanuel movement—a popular craze that had nothing to do with the scientific study of the mind. Most psychologists who attended Freud's Clark lectures in 1909 saw his speculations about dreams and sex as a pleasant diversion, about as relevant to their work as Mrs. Eddy's epistles [Hornstein, 1992, p. 255].

Within a decade, however, psychoanalytic ideas were penetrating more deeply into American psychology, and the tortuous, frequently tortured relationship between psychoanalysis and psychology had begun in earnest. As Hornstein pointed out in her excellent historical account, what was at stake in this relationship was the fundamental question of subjectivity in science.

> For experimental psychologists, being scientific meant creating distance. It meant opening up a space, a "no man's land," between themselves and the things they studied, a place whose boundary could be patrolled so that needs or desires or feelings could never infiltrate the work itself. Every aspect of the experimental situation was bent toward this goal—the "blind subject," the mechanized recording devices, the quantified measures, and statistically represented results. . . . What united experimental psychologists more than anything else was a distrust of personal experience, a sense that feelings in particular were dangerous and had to be held carefully in check lest they flood in and destroy the very foundations of the work. They were willing to make a number of sacrifices to protect psychology from this threat, including a radical narrowing of the field to include only phenomena that could be studied "objectively" [p. 256].

Ellenberger (1970) characterized early positivism as "the cult of facts . . . [as a search for] the kind of certitude afforded by experimental science and for constant laws such as laws of physics" (p. 225). Ellenberger traced the origins of positivism to Condorcet and the French Encylopedists of the 18th century but pointed out that one of its great systematizers was Auguste Comte, the creator of the term "sociology" and the founder of sociology as a discipline. As I point out later, managed care approaches, dealing conceptually and pragmatically more with aggregates rather than with individuals, are more compatible with sociology than with a subjectivist psychology.

In his novel *Hard Times*, which looks at the human costs of the industrial revolution in England, Dickens (1854) begins his tale with a parody of the positivistic utilitarianism of his day. The title of his first chapter is "The One Thing Needful." The first words are spoken by the character named Thomas Gradgrind, a hard-nosed scientist/industrialist who is addressing a group of children in a classroom.

> Now, what I want is, Facts. Teach these boys and girls nothing but Facts. Facts alone are wanted in life. Plant nothing else, and root out everything else. You can only form the minds of reasoning animals upon Facts: nothing else will ever be of any service to them. This is the principle on which I bring up my own children, and this is the principle on which I bring up these children. Stick to Facts, sir! [p. 47].

DEFINING THE SCIENCE OF HUMAN BEHAVIOR: DRAWING THE BATTLELINES

As a philosophical movement, positivism determined the very definition of science and shaped its content areas and methodologies. Freud himself, the pioneer of radical subjectivity, enshrined the scientific ideals of positivism and materialism exemplified by Helmholtz and Fechner and expressed the fervent wish that human behavior could be understood ultimately as the interplay of physical and chemical forces. Beginning with his "Project for a Scientific Psychology" in 1895, however, Freud discovered that his hypotheses were pushing against the boundaries of that philosophic container. But he was uncomfortable and guilty at the borders as for example, when he apologized that his case histories read less like scientific documents and more like fictive narratives. Students of the history of psychoanalysis have noted these tensions in Freud's writings and have sometimes separated the strands of his thought into two Freuds, mechanistic and humanistic, representative of the philosophical polarities of *Naturwissenschaften* and *Geisteswissenschaften*.

This creative intellectual tension within Freud and therefore within psychoanalysis itself was obscured by the escalating fight between psychoanalysis and psychology in this country over the right to define the science of human behavior. Hornstein (1992) commented:

> The first skirmish actually occurred as early as 1916, when the Princeton philosopher Warner Fite reviewed Jung's *Psychology of the Unconscious* for *The Nation* (Fite, 1916). His

surprisingly nasty tone incited a riot of response from psychologists. In her letter to the editor, Christine Ladd-Franklin, the eminent experimentalist, characterized psychoanalysis as a product of the "undeveloped . . . German mind" (hardly a compliment in 1916), and concluded ominously that "unless means can speedily be found to prevent its spread . . . the prognosis for civilization is unfavorable" (Ladd-Franklin, 1916, p. 374). R. S. Woodworth of Columbia (1916), a bit more circumspect, called psychoanalysis an "uncanny religion" (probably not the psychologist's highest accolade) that led "even apparently sane individuals" to absurd associations and nonsensical conclusions. In a telling illustration, he showed how the words *Freudian principles* led to a train of thought that revealed his own "deep-seated wish . . . for a career of unbridled lust" (p. 396) [pp. 255–256].

Hornstein also noted, "It has been only 70 years since James McKeen Cattell rose from his seat at the annual meeting of the American Psychological Association to castigate a colleague for having mentioned Freud's name at a gathering of scientists" (Dallenbach, 1955, p. 523) [p. 261].

Lest we think that these heated philosophical arguments belong solely to the ancient history of psychology, we can refer to Eysenck's (1993, pp. 3, 68) letter to the editor of the American Psychological Association *Monitor*, in which he exhorted the APA to do all in its power to dissociate itself from psychoanalysis and to "make clear that modern scientific psychology has nothing to do with Freudian psychoanalysis." In a follow-up letter to the editor, Franks (1993) applauded Eysenck for correctly drawing attention "to the glaring deficiencies of psychoanalysis." Franks went on to proclaim, "If science is conceptualized as most behavioral scientists, myself included, view this term, then psychoanalysis is a pseudo-science" (p. 3).

Eysenck and Franks are, of course, not alone in dismissing or questioning the scientific status of psychoanalysis. More sophisticated critics such as Grünbaum (1993) have questioned whether the unique investigatory methods of psychoanalysis can ever be defined with sufficient precision as to be replicable, whether fundamental theories of psychoanalysis can be subject to refutation, and whether its causal propositions and truth claims can be publicly validated. Alan Stone (1997), a psychoanalyst and past president of the American Psychiatric Association, recently declared that psychoanalysis has failed as a science but will survive as an art. John Horgan (1996), senior writer for the *Scientific American*, paid psychoanalysis the backhanded compliment: "Skeptics continue to challenge Sigmund Freud's ideas about the mind. Yet no unquestionably superior

theory or therapy has rendered psychoanalysis completely obsolete"
(p. 107). Some of the most thoughtful researchers within psychoanalysis,
such as Howard Shevrin (1995), grapple forthrightly with the current
limitations of psychoanalysis as a science.

The most shrill critics of psychoanalysis, such as Eysenck and Franks,
arrogate the right to define science along narrow positivistic lines and then
righteously proclaim psychoanalysis to be outside its boundaries, unable
to escape from unscientific subjectivism. Given the rigid positivistic premises with which they begin, such critics are correct when they state that
Freud did not succeed in transforming psychoanalysis into a science. Despite his innovative theory and methodology, Freud was unable then, as
we are unable now, to answer satisfactorily the question: How do we objectively study subjective phenomena in all their depth? Freud's failure,
however, was generative. Succeeding generations of psychoanalysts have
continued to struggle clinically and theoretically with that profoundly
important question.

The situation becomes even more complex when we move away from
Freud's construction of the mind as a more or less self-contained monadic
system to a fuller appreciation of the subtle resonances and determinative
power of the intersubjective field. At its best, psychoanalysis does not pre-
tend to be scientific in the rigid positivistic sense of dealing only with
observable behaviors and precisely defined, clearly replicable interventions.
Nor does psychoanalysis take refuge in the convenient dodge that it is a
purely narrative art form. Instead we remain open to the questions: How
do we continue to improve on our methods of observation and intervention? Where does radical subjectivity fit within a contemporary scientific
framework? And, perhaps most important, in what ways is that framework
itself evolving? In the cognitive sciences, for example, researchers initially
focused on observable, replicable conscious phenomena but are beginning to acknowledge the necessity of developing concepts and techniques
to permit the study of unconscious mental processes. In the spirit of
Winnicott, as psychoanalysts we do not rush to resolve, at least at our
present state of knowledge, unresolvable paradoxes.

MANAGED CARE AND NEO-POSITIVISM

But what is the relevance of this condensed historical/philosophical ex-
cursion to our understanding of contemporary managed mental health
care? I am not suggesting that the corporate purveyors of managed care
and their epigones are agonizing over the philosophical underpinnings of
the health care systems they are constructing. I am proposing, however,
that there is a close link between proponents' dismissal of psychodynamic

treatments and their embrace of other treatment approaches closely allied with a view of science in which intersubjective phenomena have no relevance or scientific standing.

As a case in point, let us consider the experience of one large managed care organization, the Harvard Community Health Plan (HCHP).[1] I am selecting HCHP because it is regarded as one of the premier HMOs in the country and is often cited as a model of managed care, and because its medical directors have articulated a clear philosophy regarding the brief psychological treatments of large numbers of patients.

Since 1984 HCHP has offered a one-year, half-time mental health fellowship for 10–12 psychiatric residents, postdoctoral psychologists, and masters level nurses and social workers. The stated goals of the fellowship are to enhance the trainees' skill in doing efficient and comprehensive mental health evaluations, ability to develop and negotiate focused treatment plans, capacity to perform an array of time-limited therapies, and ability to manage ethically and effectively a large number of patients referred to collectively as a population-based panel (Donovan, Steinberg, and Sabin, 1994, p. 201).

In the training experiences of the HCHP mental health fellows, the influx of new patients invariably creates a crisis.

> By the third month of the year, at a rate of two new patients per week, the fellows will need to discharge one patient for each new intake or they will slowly sink beneath the torrent of new faces. How can they offer high quality care to present patients but retain reasonable access times for new ones? The teachers find themselves in a parallel crisis. If the short-term approaches we teach break down when patient panels fill, we represent false prophets. We take on the challenge of "the crunch" directly in the open sessions we schedule to discuss practice management. First, the students are in no mood for reassurance or to study still another promising brief treatment approach. They feel angry and helpless, scanning the environment for someone to blame—uncaring system, passive patient, or themselves, the inept therapists. Our first and most important step is to acknowledge the pain and despair in the room. Before the students can activate their creativity, they must face their angry pessimism over their apparently unmanageable patient panel.
>
> Next we share some of our own perilous moments in the past, when the system seemed poised to swallow us. We

---

[1] Reflective of the trend to form regional systems, HCHP has recently merged with another large health maintenance organization and is now known as Harvard Pilgrim Health Care.

also gently introduce clinical and fiscal realities of the 1990s. We now know that some patients never improve even with unlimited treatment (Wallerstein, 1986). Managed care often supports more psychotherapy with cheaper premiums than indemnity plans, and no system offers unlimited low-cost psychotherapy. . . .

The "crunch" represents the watershed of the fellowship. In one powerful emotional thrust the students learn perhaps more than they wanted to know about the affective and cognitive demands of working in managed care. This "rite of passage" is harrowing, but high-impact learning about the managed care challenge requires this total immersion [Donovan et al., p. 203].

Those who successfully complete this "rite of passage" presumably can function effectively in a managed care setting such as HCHP.

This means that managed mental health care clinicians, in contrast to traditional practitioners, invest much more of their time in evaluating large numbers of new patients and performing very brief treatment (1–2 sessions) (Manning, Wells & Benjamin, 1987). A full-time equivalent clinician at HCHP, for example, evaluates four new clients a week. Patient requests usually center on acute, specific, present-time conflicts, i.e., should the client leave her chronically unfaithful husband? For the initial therapy, the client may stay only for a few visits, but is likely to return weeks, months, or even years later for follow-up or for more extensive psychotherapy. . . .

Managed mental health care practitioners must arrive at their ethical standards and professional satisfactions by assuming a public health perspective toward a panel of patients rather than developing intimacy with a few (Sabin, 1991). This shift in emotional and professional orientation can be wrenching. When the individual clinician must weigh the valid, competing claims of one person versus another, the internal conflict can be excruciating" [pp. 205–206].

Why should the rite of passage for managed care therapists-in-training be so harrowing, the shift in orientation so wrenching, and the accompanying internal conflict so excruciating? What is a therapist giving up or sacrificing in the course of the journey toward acceptance of the public health perspective? I think the answer is a fuller subjectivity, both the therapist's and the patient's. The managed care/public health perspective attenuates each and sacrifices the intersubjective core of the therapeutic relationship. The experienced loss is profound.

Internal and external realities intertwine to form a complex intrapsychic-interpersonal Gordian knot. Managed mental health care, as currently practiced, wields a positivistic knife to cut through that knot, discard the multilayered subjectivities of therapist and patient, and focus on the remaining target symptoms. In order to perform this economically efficient operation, we need to forget a great deal about who we are and who our patients are. Much of what we mean by subjectivity has to do with memory, fantasy, and desire (conscious and unconscious) and with repetition and re-creation of earlier relational patterns and accompanying affects. When we operate from a public health perspective in a managed care environment, we must forget that past is prologue.

Stone (1997) articulates this perspective:

> If there is no important connection between childhood events and adult psychopathology, then Freudian theories lose much of their explanatory power. If memory cannot be trusted to construct a self-description, what does one do in therapy?
>
> I no longer ask my patients to lie on a couch and free associate, but I certainly have not given up on face-to-face psychotherapy. My focus is almost entirely on the here and now, on problem-solving, and on helping patients find new strategies and new ways of interacting with the important people in their lives . . . [p. 39].

From this perspective, memory and time are foreshortened. We may inquire about the immediate past precipitants of a presenting problem, but we are specifically enjoined from going any further. We must be active and problem solving. We must discourage dependency, while we assume the role of experts who quickly size up the situation and make suggestions and recommendations to our patients, who at the same time are supposed to assume responsibility for their treatments. We must terminate quickly but must expect therapy to be interminable with the understanding that the patient may return "weeks, months, or even years later for follow-up." We are to conceptualize this arrangement as "primary mental health care" akin to that offered by the family physician. When we attempt to escape from subjectivity and deny the existence or relevance of unconscious forces, we find ourselves trapped in multiple contradictions.

Another example of this dilemma can be seen in the crisis intervention treatment guidelines sent by the administration of the Massachusetts-based Pilgrim Health Care prior to its merger with Harvard Community Health Plan.

> Re: Working Definition of Crisis Intervention
> Crisis Intervention is time-limited treatment directed towards the resolution of crises arising as a result of changing life events or biologic processes that have acutely disrupted the patient's pre-morbid adjustment (i.e., adjustment within the preceding 12 months). Therapy is focused on identification of events leading to the crisis, cognitive formulation of the problem, expression of appropriate affect, and the development of coping strategies to deal with the defined problem. Open-ended exploration and/or focus on character pathology or childhood antecedents is inappropriate in this format.
> A. Types of Crises: Developmental (ex.: moving from home, retiring, etc.) or accidental (ex.: fire, etc.)
> B. Goal of Therapy: Re-stabilization and relief of acute crisis symptom. Patient's dynamic understanding or appreciation of contribution of character pathology may not be appropriate.
> C. Techniques of Therapy:
>   1. Establish supportive relationship
>   2. Set reasonable, concrete goals mutually agreed upon at the outset
>   3. Encourage networking to community resources
>   4. Incorporate elements of cognitive therapy (ex.: restructuring of misperceptions)
>   5. Encourage expression of appropriate affect
>   6. Use a problem solving orientation
>   7. Transference and countertransference issues should be avoided where possible
>   8. Make referral for long-term therapy where appropriate
> D. Role of Therapist
>   1. Active and interactive
>   2. Helping ally rather than blank screen
>   3. Real person rather than "as if" relationship
>   4. Must establish rapport quickly

The treatment guidelines specify that these goals should be accomplished within four to six sessions.

To its credit, Pilgrim Health Care did differentiate short-term crisis intervention, which its policy covered, from longer-term psychotherapies, which its policy excluded, while allowing for referral outside the plan. Most health maintenance organizations are not so straightforward.

Although these guidelines are targeted to crisis intervention, they typify the approach taken by most managed care companies, which market their mental health care products in a highly competitive environment to corporations, government agencies, and individual subscribers.

CONCLUSION

A reality-centered approach means that we do not take refuge in the nostalgic idealization of the "good old days" of indemnity insurance before the advent of managed care practices. Returning to those days is neither feasible nor desirable, since they contributed significantly to the inflationary pressures driving up the cost of health care and setting the stage for the managed care revolution. Nevertheless, there were values associated with the older system that remain worth fighting for: the extreme importance of confidentiality which, although not absolute, was not routinely violated; the centrality of the relationship between doctor/therapist and patient, rather than the relationship being viewed as a peripheral attribute in a system of more or less interchangeable parts; and the frequent necessity of an unfolding therapeutic process rather than a quick fix of a patient-fragment or piece of symptomatic behavior.

Extrapolation from present data suggests that the trend toward alliances, mergers, and acquisitions creating large-scale, complex health care systems will continue with linkages among teaching and nonteaching hospitals, community-based hospitals, and urban and rural health care settings. These health care systems will be primarily regional, rather than national, in scope, with allowances made for local differences in patient populations and modes of service delivery. Competition for patients and insurance dollars, already fierce, will intensify, and eventually there will be a relatively small number of large-scale "players" in these regional systems. Physicians will continue to try to leverage their bargaining power by building or joining group practices and networks of physician providers.

As psychoanalysts and psychodynamic practitioners, we tend to work in solo practices or small groups. We fit poorly into the evolving health care systems and will most likely function at the margins of these systems, or outside of them altogether. Nevertheless, we can influence the evolution of these systems by assisting patient advocacy efforts, and providing expert testimony at legislative hearings at national and state levels, leading to the creation of a patient bill of rights to regulate managed care and eliminate its most egregious practices.

Unfortunately, as currently conceived and practiced, managed mental health care frequently fails to meet the needs of distressed, conflicted three-dimensional human beings with rich interior lives. Unwittingly, but not accidentally, the developers and purveyors of managed mental health care have found an ally in a crude version of positivism that allows little or no room for depthful subjectivity and unconscious mental forces.

In addition to our various political and organizational attempts to challenge and shape the health care environment, we can engage in serious ongoing analysis of managed mental health care's historical and philosophical underpinnings, examine its fundamental premises, and strive to provide more realistic, ultimately more practical and cost-effective alternatives that do not sacrifice the subjective core of ourselves and our patients.

As part of our analytic efforts, we can help educate the public and legislators about the necessity of confidentiality in the therapeutic relationship specifically, and about the mounting dangers to the nation's mental health posed by the serious erosions of fundamental rights of privacy at all levels.

REFERENCES

Barron, J. ed. (1998), *Making Diagnosis Meaningful: Enhancing Evaluation and Treatment of Psychological Disorders*. Washington, DC: American Psychological Association.

——— & Sands, H. ed. (1996), *Impact of Managed Care on Psychodynamic Treatment*. Madison, CT: International Universities Press.

Bennett, M. J. (1988), The greening of the HMO: implications for prepaid psychiatry. *Amer. J. Psychiat.*, 145:1544–1549.

Bittker, T. E. (1992), The emergence of prepaid psychiatry. In: *Managed Mental Health Care: Administrative and Clinical Issues*, ed. J. L. Feldman & R. J. Fitzpatrick. Washington, DC: American Psychiatric Press, pp. 3–10.

Dallenbach, K. M. (1955), Phrenology versus psychoanalysis. *Amer. J. Psychol.*, 68:511–525.

Dickens, C. (1854), *Hard Times*. London: Penguin Classics, 1985.

Donovan, J. M., Steinberg, S. M. & Sabin, J. E. (1994), Managed mental health care: An academic seminar. *Psychother.*, 31:201–207.

Ellenberger, H. F. (1970), *The Discovery of the Unconscious*. New York: Basic Books.

Eysenck, H. (1993), Letter to the Editor. *Amer. Psycholog. Assn. Monitor*, 24(8).

Franks, C. (1993), Letter to the Editor. *Amer. Psycholog. Assn. Monitor*, 24(11).

Ginzburg, E. (1984), The monetarization of medical care. *New Eng. J. Med.*, 310:1162–1165.

Grünbaum, A. (1993), *Validation in the Clinical Theory of Psychoanalysis*. Madison, CT: International Universities Press.

Horgan, J. (1996), Why Freud isn't dead. *Scient. Amer.*, 275(6):106–111.

Hornstein, G. (1992), The return of the repressed: Psychology's problematic relations with psychoanalysis, 1909–1960. *Amer. Psychol.*, 47:254–263.

Jones, E. (1955), *The Life and Works of Sigmund Freud*, Vol. 2. New York: Basic Books.

Ladd-Franklin, C. (1916), Letter to the editor. *The Nation,* 103:372–374.

Shevrin, H. (1995), Is psychoanalysis one science, two sciences, or no science at all? A discourse among friendly antagonists. *J. Amer. Psychoanal. Assn.,* 43:963–1049.

Starr, P. (1982), *The Social Transformation of American Medicine.* New York: Basic Books.

Stone, A. A. (1997), Where will psychoanalysis survive: What remains of Freudianism when its scientific center crumbles? *Harvard Mag.,* 99(3):34–39.

FOUR

Is Psychoanalysis Health Care?

The Affirmative Position

STANLEY MOLDAWSKY

PSYCHOANALYSIS AS A FORM OF "ALTERNATIVE HEALTH CARE"

Traditional medicine deals with attempts to cure disease and pathology through the use of medicines, surgeries, manipulations, and technologies in which diagnosis leads to some form of intrusive treatment. It does not deal primarily with *relationship for healing*. Psychoanalysis is a healing modality that depends on a therapeutic relationship (see Grunes, 1984, for a discussion of the "therapeutic object relationship") for the process to unfold and its effects to be felt. It demands that the analysand be an active participant in the therapeutic process. The interactive process (known as the transference–countertransference paradigm) requires cooperation and motivation from the patient that differs from ordinary compliance with medical routines. The focus of the analysis turns to the relationship itself as the process unfolds, and this is never the case—or even necessary—in traditional health care.

Our psychological selves are reflected in our physical selves in important ways. Depression, for example, depletes the immune system. The field of behavioral medicine has burgeoned with the recognition of psychosomatic states in which lifestyles and feelings have an enormous impact on our physiology. When you see the word behavioral, read inner processes, emotions, throughts, unconscious conflict. In other words read Psychology! Traditional medicine and biological psychiatry have ignored the connection between relationship and healing, and therein lies our strength.

Our interpretations in the context of a healing relationship produce changes in the direction of growth and health. Medicine has generally behaved in an arrogant way by making health care and medicine synonymous and then claiming ownership of the health care world. As psychologists we know how hard it has been to claim our piece of the health care world. We have had to fight every step of the way to procure a niche in that world. I can certainly sympathize with the desire to be in a separate world without the turf battles to contend with. But I reject the suggestion that we abandon health care simply because we have to fight politically to make our presence known. Medicine attempts to preempt any treatments by alternative health care groups (such as osteopathy, chiropracty, and the like) and claims them to be part of medicine, as they had controlled psychoanalysis for many years. As each specialty forms its own identity, it breaks free of medical domination and claims legal rights to independence. The famous law suit by four psychologists against the American and International Psychoanalytic Associations claiming discrimination resulted in the opening up of medically dominated training institutions to doctoral level psychologists.

Just because we are now recognized in the world of health care, however, does not make us health care in the usual sense. I still believe we are alternative health care. Because the interaction process is a continuing one, it is clearly different from the authoritative approach of medicine. Most of our patients adapt to this unfamiliar way of working despite the overriding presence of a transference that may keep them in the role of a victim, or passively aggressive, or docilely submissive. In exposing the transference, the analysand has an opportunity to allow reality testing to take place as well as to allow himself or herself to live through the experience of feeling once-repressed affects in a new environment. I believe this living through process is the experience that produces change. Now, it is true that the patient may present with various psychosomatic ailments or depression and may expect the usual medical treatment such as drugs, but as the analytic process unfolds, the necessity for those extra-analytic therapies diminishes.

IS THE ANALYST RESPONSIBLE FOR THE PATIENT?

Hyman (chapter 5) claims that we are responsible only for analyzing and not for taking responsibility for the patient's life. For many patients, the anxiety they come into treatment with or that develops during the treatment may be intolerable or the depression too debilitating. Do we try only to understand what is producing these reactions and work to relieve them with our mutual understanding? Are we responsible for doing more?

I say we must do more. If a patient is suicidal, even if only to bring the analyst to his or her knees, it behooves the analyst to do more than interpret the patient's intent. If in the analyst's best clinical judgment (admittedly a difficult position to be in the light of the usual amount of anxiety in the analyst when confronted with a suicidal patient) hospitalization is indicated, the responsibility is to recommend it, arrange for it if possible. In most hospitals today that usually means having another professional assume responsibility. If our political agenda is successful, psychologists will be able to admit their patients to hospitals and continue caring for them until they return to an outpatient status. Currently to avoid the responsibility of making such a hospitalization decision is unthinkable if not illegal. The courts would certainly find us liable if we stated that we are not responsible for the patient's life but were only analyzing him.

In the same vein, the question of medication comes up when a patient is overly anxious or depressed. Are we responsible for doing more than analyze? I answer in the affirmative and refer my patient to a competent psychopharmacologist. There are many complicated meanings to triangulating medication into the therapy dyad. Those should certainly be explored. But to ignore the patient's distress and to assume that analysis will heal everything sooner or later is to avoid clinical responsibility. When a patient suffers headaches—even if your understanding of the patient's dynamics tells you that the headaches are the solution to the unconscious problem of accepting hostile feelings toward a loved one (the analyst in the transference)—a referral for medication may be indicated if the problem persists. It doesn't mean that you've taken responsibility for the patient's life, but it does mean that you are responsible for some clinical decisions. In alternative health care the patient is always responsible for his or her own life. Referring for medication is not to be taken lightly. Careful preliminary work is necessary before such a referral is made. Is the relationship with the analyst sufficient to reduce the anxiety? It requires time to observe and evaluate the patient's inner resources. How much depression must a patient endure before you call for medication? These are clinical decisions but ones I believe we must responsibly make.

TRAUMA AND RESPONSIBILITY

When dealing with a patient who has suffered early trauma, particularly sexual molestation, it is important that the analyst do more than analyze. There must be an important ingredient in the analyst's behavior that ultimately allows for healing to take place. That is, the analyst must validate the patient's experience. An experienced analyst can recognize flashbacks. This does not mean suggesting that the patient has been abused but, rather, accepting the patient's recall. It is very important to unearth the varying meanings the patient attributes to the abuse suffered. The acknowledgment of the traumas and their existence is important to the health of the analysand, and it is a responsibility of the analyst to use his or her best judgment in validating the patient's experience. Failure to recognize the importance of validating the patient's experience entails the risk of retraumatizing the patient. This is certainly true of people with dissociated states.

One of my supervisees treated a patient for a number of years. In the second year of her once-a-week therapy, she recalled an oral rape that had occurred when she was six years old. A boyfriend of her mother's housekeeper had forced his penis into her mouth. For many years this memory had been repressed. When it emerged, it was resisted, negated, denied, and rejected. The therapist never insisted that the recall was accurate. Soon, however, the patient revealed enough details of the event to complete its recall and force her to confront her feelings about it. It was not until many years later in treatment that she recalled telling her mother about the experience, which her mother dismissed. The greater trauma was, in fact, her mother's attitude toward the matter. And, because of the difficulties with her mother, it took years for that part of the memory to emerge into recall. The mother, long dead, appeared in a dream in which the patient confronted her about her rejecting the little girl's story. The patient yelled at her and accused her of not protecting her. The therapist was also in the dream, as herself, and was simply in the kitchen with the patient while she confronted her mother. With the protection of the therapist, the patient could express her hostility toward the mother in the dream. This dream was overdetermined, and it should be noted that maternal neglect was prominent in the patient's history. In the analyst's acceptance of the patient's recall, rather than assuming it to be a metaphor for the analyst's neglect (which, of course, it was as well), the validation of the patient's experience was necessary to this patient's healing.[1]

HAS PSYCHOANALYSIS CHANGED SINCE FREUD?

Freud taught us that psychoanalysis was 1) a theory of mind, 2) a theory of unconscious processes, and 3) a treatment. It was conceived as a treatment for neuroses. We were advised that, because the vehicle of change is the analysis of transference, only those people capable of forming

---

[1] My comments in this regard are influenced by the writings of Herman (1992), Courtois (1988), Davies and Frawley (1991), and others.

transference relationships are capable of benefiting from the treatment. We know that this concept has been evolving over the years so that other than neurotics can benefit from psychoanalysis. We know much more about nonneurotic transferences, and Freud—who was the least rigid of the Freudians—would have led the way into our new understandings. With the introduction of the concept of parameters, psychoanalytic therapy has been extended to borderline, psychotic, and posttraumatic stress disorder patients. We know that growth takes place in a relationship and that for unconscious conflicts and affects to surface so that the ego can fashion new ways to deal with them, an atmosphere of safety must exist (Schafer, 1983). The analysand dares to experience previously repressed unacceptable feelings and thoughts and begins the process of integration leading to behavior change. Growth in a sense of self, self-esteem, and more genuine relationships and less anxiety occurs slowly. This takes time to develop within the context of a supportive analytic relationship. In Freud's day, analyses were id analyses and lasted a short time, only long enough to discover the id at work. Changes in our theory and developments that have gone beyond Freud (particularly with the advent of ego psychology) have dramatically changed the way we work and the length of time our work requires.

THE WORLD WE LIVE IN

Psychoanalysts know today that the safety of the relationship, which is so crucial to growth, can be attenuated or enhanced by our own anxieties (countertransference). It takes years of intensive training—including a personal analysis, extensive supervision, and didactic course work in personality development, psychopathology, and techniques of psychoanalysis—to prepare us for the delicate yet tough work of psychoanalysis. The environment in which psychoanalysis flourished from the 40s through the 80s was supportive emotionally and financially. Insurance companies recognized and subsidized the treatment. Psychoanalysis in the medical world was flourishing, but psychology, a young profession, had to struggle to establish itself as an autonomous profession. Battles were fought in each state as state psychological associations introduced licensure legislation. We had to fight the medical establishment and in some states even other psychologists, as well as the insurance industry. The associations grew strong as these battles were won. We are now licensed in all 50 states.

Next we moved to enact freedom of choice laws providing that, if a person had a policy covering mental or emotional conditions, then a licensed psychologist could be chosen as the professional to provide those services. Such a law was first enacted in New Jersey, in 1968, and 38 states have followed. For the next 22 years we practiced comfortably. Meanwhile, the rising costs of health care was getting the attention of legislators and the insurance industry. Enter a new adversary, managed care, an intermediate industry created to develop cost-containment mechanisms. The pendulum swung to cost containment and the quality of psychological care deteriorated. Managed care companies coined a buzzword called medical necessity and began a systematic denial of treatment to our analytic patients. The environment had turned hostile, and we were bewildered by the radical changes in the insurance world. We were no longer supported as we had been, and our patients were being forced to accept short shrift instead of intensive therapy. I had a patient, a man who was a trained social worker who became a utilization reviewer for a managed care company. This job paid him almost twice as much as he had earned in a social agency. He was the only reviewer in his office who had had any personal therapy, received any training in therapy, or knew anything about therapy. He and his fellow reviewers would talk among themselves about their successes on the job, literally how many cases they had closed out in a particular week. Although they were not receiving any financial incentive to end treatment, they were doing a good job when they closed out cases. The environment was clearly hostile.

As James Barron (1994) has noted, "Managed care and psychoanalysis are incompatible." I strongly agree. But does this mean that we are not health care providers because the care we offer is being denigrated and marginalized? No—denigration doesn't change what we do or who we are. We are alternative health care providers even though the managed care world is excluding us. They cannot define us! (For an excellent discussion of how managed care impacts on psychodynamic therapy see Barron and Sands, 1996.) Many contributors to the Barron and Sands book describe the negative effects on therapy and in general confirm that managed care and psychoanalysis are incompatible. When the interests of the business community take precedence over the interests of the consumer, we are in deep trouble. Managed care companies' notions of what therapy is does not include the notion of a relationship. It is much more along the lines of the medical model of something you do to the patient. It is cheaper to give the patient a pill than to allow a relationship to develop and uncover unconscious conflicts in an atmosphere of safety.

WHAT ARE OUR OPTIONS

Shall we opt out of the health care system, or shall we try to influence the system to include psychoanalysis? I know the formidable odds of trying to do the latter. I visited my congressman recently with three of my colleagues. We were advocating the inclusion of mental health care in any package of health care that Congress enacted. We were also advocating for psychology. I complained to him about the abuses of managed care and told him that it takes time to build a relationship for a patient to do any growing. I mentioned the well-known case in the news of a brutal murder of a woman by her husband and asked the Congressman how many sessions he thought it would take for the orphaned children to develop trust in a therapist. He replied, "At least two or three sessions." And he thought he understood my point. I told him that it would take years and that those children were badly in need of therapy. I do not believe he was unusual as a legislator. As a matter of fact, he had a good record of caring about his constituency. But his understanding of people's psychological problems was minimal.

Trying to explain to members of Congress how psychoanalysis helps people is a formidable task. At best they can accept the validity of mental health treatment and when they do they support therapies of a short-term variety. The business-driven health economists are willing to support short-term therapies and only reluctantly long-term therapies for the seriously mentally ill. In other words, they are not supportive of psychoanalysis for the treatment of character problems, relationship difficulties, psychosomatic illnesses, and the neuroses. They do not ask the questions we ask. They are satisfied with symptom removal, particularly by way of medication. Managed care reviewers are not supportive of transference analysis. The analogy suggested by a colleague is that a hot appendix would get two sessions of massage therapy rather than surgery because it was "cost effective." With the current *Zeitgeist,* with business now in charge of health care, once again we have to draw the wagons in a circle and prepare our battle strategies. One thing we must be sure to remember is to *point the guns outward.* We must not fight among ourselves. Rather we must support all efforts by practitioners to educate the public about ourselves and what we do, and we must put therapy decisions back in the hands of the professionals rather than the clerks of the managed care companies. They have been sold a bill of goods that short-term therapy solves people's problems, but their short-term model is based on poor science. In this regard see Miller (1996b, c) and Silverman (1995). They argue that science is being inappropriately used to justify limiting treatment.

Efforts of past president of the American Psychological Association Dorothy Cantor to bring together all the mental health association presidents in a "summit" meeting are just beginning to get underway. Presidents of the American Psychiatric Association, National Association of Social Workers, American Association of Marriage and Family Counselors, American Nursing Association, American Psychological Association, and others, as well as their Executive Directors, have issued a Patient's Bill of Rights in order to fight back against managed care companies who are denying patients their rights. These organizations are not stipulating psychoanalysis as such but are casting a wide net to include all professionals who treat people with an array of mental health modalities; they are placing therapy decisions back in the hands of professionals. We must support these efforts. And we need to support the efforts of the Practice Directorate of the American Psychological Association in their lobbying and educating and marketing campaigns. All psychoanalysts do psychotherapy. No longer are prospective patients who come to us seeking psychoanalysis prepared to make the commitment in time and money to undertake the journey. Rather they come with certain problems to be "fixed," and we begin the work, which includes educating our patients to the complexities of their psychic lives and interesting them in undergoing psychoanalysis. A certain percentage of them will accept our suggestions because we offer hope for real changes to take place in their lives. Even before managed care (and limited sessions) analysts educated their patients to realize the advantages of undergoing psychoanalysis Therefore, we must be in the system in order for some of our patients to be available to psychoanalysis.

OUT OF THE SYSTEM

We must also be outside the system and willing to offer psychoanalysis to those who are in a position to elect such an option. Being in and out at the same time may require more battles to be won. We need to advocate on behalf of our patients to allow for psychologists/psychoanalysts to be chosen as "willing providers" and not to be excluded from panels put together by managed care companies. Patients should have the option of selecting us even if we are not on the panel. Managed care companies will ultimately hire those who "do it their way," which means short-term, infrequent visits, and loss of confidentiality. The managed care industry is an unregulated one and is ruthless when it comes to cost containment. There will probably be legal action against them by patients harmed by the denial of adequate treatment. We have had to fight for all our legislative gains in the past, and we cannot stop now if we want our patients to be free to obtain psychoanalytic services. Actively supporting legislation that regulates this unregulated industry and puts clinical decisions back in the hands of the professional is our goal. I realize this is the very issue that has been problematic from the standpoint of the insurance industry. They have felt the providers were taking advantage of the system and that business management has reversed the process. They are now taking advantage of people by denying and limiting treatment.

NEED FOR LEGISLATION

A number of states have been successful in passing legislation that regulates the utilization review process. We should be reviewed only by an independent body in which there is no conflict of interest. Providers should be reviewed by professionals of the same orientation. A bill with those characteristics was written in New Jersey and was supported by the New Jersey Psychiatric Association, New Jersey Association of Clinical Social Workers, Marriage and Family Therapy Association, and New Jersey Psychological Association. Unfortunately, the sponsor lost his election and the bill languished. A new bill was written by the Medical Society but curiously the section about being reviewed by one's peers was changed to being reviewed by two physicians and one of one's peers. Watch out—if you're not minding the store, the medical profession will try to preempt your autonomy. This state of affairs seems to buttress Hyman's (chapter 5) arguments that the whole process of regulation undermines psychoanalysis. I don't like regulation of therapy either. I think psychoanalysis flourishes when the pressure on the patient and therapist is from the process only. That is, pressure from the third-party payor is an unwarranted intrusion into the therapy process and produces mayhem.

I recognize that my statements regarding how to stay in the system and try to influence it legislatively make me appear to be abandoning psychoanalysis. I think I'm being a realist and a pragmatist, but, I'm willing also to be a political infighter. I see no hope for psychoanalysis to be included in the system, but I see how analysts can function in the system as *psychotherapists*. Moses (1992) surveyed Section 1 members of Division 39 as to their practices and discovered that most were doing once- and twice-a-week psychotherapy. These were discouraging results. We are not doing what we were trained to do. But, again, my argument is that if we are doing psychotherapy, and, in the system, some of our patients will choose to intensify their treatment and enter a psychoanalytic relationship. Continuing treatment with such a person takes us out of the system, and the probability is we will adjust our fees in order to accommodate analytic patients because we prefer to practice psychoanalysis.

THE GATEKEEPER ROLE

One of the stumbling blocks in the quest for autonomy has been the role of the Gatekeeper. This has been the traditional domain of the medical community. When physicians are the gatekeepers, psychologists do not fare well. We need to work to introduce legislation that opens this domain up to nonmedical professionals. Psychologists as gatekeepers would naturally recognize the worth of our profession. Thus, the areas we need to be of influence in are:

1) parity of mental health with physical health in all ways (financial limits should not discriminate against mental health);
2) licensed psychologists included wherever mental health is included;
3) substantial outpatient benefits;
4) strong regulation of managed care practices and elimination of abuses;
5) passage of willing provider legislation;
6) passage of point of service options.

These are some of the things we need to work for to make the system respectful of us. How do we opt out of the system? To opt out of the system and operate as lawyers, accountants, and ministers do, without third-party reimbursement, is actually the way psychologists function in Canada. President Clinton has stated he does not want to see any "Harley Street physicians" in our country. Canadian psychologists are able to survive in Canada as private practitioners with a lower fee schedule. They are not in the system as psychiatry is. Some Canadian psychologists think they are better off working outside the system, while others lament the fact they are not in the system. In Ontario activist psychologists have been able to have psychology included in Workman's Compensation benefits at a higher fee than psychiatry. The struggle goes on.

In my practice three of my patients who were undergoing psychoanalysis were terminated by their managed care company. I wrote lengthy reports and appeals after being urged by my patients to do so. "Make me out as sick as possible" said one person in order to keep the reimbursement coming in. I found the process of questionable confidentiality and the collusion with the patient to help them obtain reimbursement distressing. My reviewer (a Chicago psychiatrist, whom I called Al Capone) found no medical necessity for continuing. After all, wasn't four years enough treatment already and the patient wasn't "fixed" yet? He was kind enough to admit he wasn't an analyst and perhaps I should ask for an analyst to review the case. I promptly did that and soon received a letter saying that upon further review, it had been determined that treatment should be terminated. If an analyst reviewed my cases, I was not informed. I must add that the patient is still working with me and growth is slowly taking place. His conflicts are resolving. We kept our sessions at three times per week, and I reduced my fee 25%. The same thing occurred with one of the other patients who was terminated by the "system." Although we were in the system before, we are now operating outside of it. Accepting a lower fee was not hard for me to do.

I believe the golden age is over and younger psychoanalysts will have to get used to lower fees. Moses' study tells us that few of us are doing full-time psychoanalysis. I wish it were not so. I truly believe that resolving the transference is the most thoroughgoing growth experience a person can have in treatment. To "live through" experiencing previously repressed affects in the context of a new relationship with a nonjudgmental, accepting, empathic, and interactive analyst allows for a new integration of those affects to take place within the person, thereby enriching the personality. Change occurs through this living through process. What stops us from just doing psychoanalysis? I believe it is simply the wish to make a living. Can we survive outside the system? Yes. Should we be in the system? Yes, is my answer. We need to protect our patients and ourselves from extinction. This means we need to support political action. Analysts tend not to pursue their agendas in the political arena. Political action is not our usual forte. We are caretakers, nurturers, able to absorb aggression from our patients and tend to be nonaggressive ourselves. Liff (1993) has written that we need to become more politically sophisticated and politically aggressive. I heartily concur. We can't just say that we'll exist (and be passive). We need to organize for political action but be clear about our agenda. And that is: we must work to be in the system as psychotherapists and work to be outside the system as psychoanalysts. I do not think this stretches our identity at all. We are, after all, psychologists/psychoanalysts.

REFERENCES

Barron, J. (1994), Managed care and psychoanalysis are incompatible. *The Psychologist/Psychoanalyst*, 14(2):1–2.
———— & Sands, H. (1996), ed. *The Impact of Managed Care on Psychodynamic Therapy*, Madison, CT: International Universities Press.
Courtois, C. A. (1988), *Healing the Incest Wound*. New York: Norton.
Davies, J. M., & Frawley, G. (1991), Dissociated processes and transference/countertransference paradigms in the psychoanalytically oriented treatment of adult survivors of childhood sexual abuse. *Psychoanal. Dial.*, 2:5–36.
Grunes, M. (1984), The therapeutic object relationship. *Psychoanal. Rev.*, 71:123–145.
Herman, J. L. (1992), *Trauma and Recovery*. New York: Basic Books.
Liff, Z. (1993), Adding a political dimension to our analytic identity. *Round Robin* (Newsletter of Section 1, Division 39, American Psychological Association). 9(3):8–10.

Miller, I. (1996a), Time limited psychotherapy has gone too far. Result: Invisible rationing. *Profess. Psychol.: Res. & Prac.* 27:567–576.

———— (1996b), Some short term values are a formula for invisible rationing. *Profess. Psychol.: Res. & Prac.,* 27:577–582.

———— (1996c), Ethical and liability issues concerning invisible rationing. *Profess. Psychol.: Res. & Prac.,* 27:583–567.

Moses, I, (1992), Survey of psychoanlysts. *Round Robin* (Newsletter of Section 1, Division 39, American Psychological Association).

Schafer, R. (1983), *The Analytic Attitude.* New York: Basic Books.

Silverman, W. (1995), Cookbooks, manuals, and paint by the numbers: Psychotherapy in the 90s. Presented at meeting of American Psychological Association, New York.

FIVE

Why Psychoanalysis Is Not a Health Care Profession

MARVIN HYMAN

The relationship between psychoanalysis and medicine has been a continuing issue in the history of analysis. From the very outset, psychoanalysis was considered as a treatment for a neurological disorder, hysteria, notwithstanding that the treatment was "psychical" in nature rather than physical. Simultaneously, even though many of the earliest psychoanalysts were not medically trained, it was not considered amiss that they undertook the treatment of conditions that were supposedly in the medical domain. Of course, no one took the position that the successful modification of such conditions by psychical means implied that they were phenomena substantially different from those which were appropriately defined as medical. Legal and political circumstances forced a public discussion of this relationship between psychoanalysis and medicine when allegations of quackery were made against Theodore Reik for his practicing medicine without medical training or license by psychoanalyzing. In response, Freud (1926) wrote "The Question of Lay Analysis." In that essay and its postscript, he argued that "psychoanalysis is a part of Psychology; not of medical psychology in the old sense, not of the psychology of morbid processes, but simply of psychology" (p. 262). Nonetheless, he also argued that in the absence of purely psychoanalytic training at that time, medical training was the best available at the moment. At best, as we consider his arguments, we can see that Freud was taking the position that, because of its special nature, "lay" persons should be allowed to practice this medical specialty. Inasmuch as psychoanalysis was considered to be a health care profession, the question of the relationship between psychoanalysis and health care, as it is being considered today, never arose in Freud's essay.

Another discussion of the relationship between medicine and psycho-analysis appeared in Szasz's (1964) book *The Myth of Mental Illness*. Szasz took the position that "mental illness is a myth" and that in actual practice we "deal with personal, social, and ethical problems in living" (p. 308). Further, he argued that the so-called symptom is not a product of a disease process, but, rather, is a form of protolanguage, a system of representational signs or picture language, rebuslike in its form and message. From this view, psychoanalysis is not the treatment of disease, but the semiotical analysis of verbal behavior (associations) and bodily language (e.g., hysterical symptoms).

In 1965, Eissler noted the extraordinary success psychoanalysis had achieved in the United States; it had become the dominant viewpoint in psychiatry and in psychiatric education. He lamented that this success had been achieved, however, at the cost of altering psychoanalysis conceptually and technically in the service of the aims of biological science, that is, reductionistic explanation and the search for cure. As an example of that kind of alteration, Eissler cited Alexander's proposal that psychoanalysis make the "corrective emotional experience" its therapeutic aim. Eissler went on to argue that the phenomena which psychoanalysis investigates cannot, for the most part, be understood through application of the physical sciences—biology, chemistry, and physiology. He contended, therefore, that psychoanalysis should better consider itself an "anthropic" science, dedicated to the study of "man," and that it should designate itself as an "academy for the science of man."

Now, more than 30 years later, it is ironic that we are lamenting the disappearance of psychoanalysis from psychiatric practice and education and its replacement by the biological sciences. And, with equal irony, we observe psychoanalysis struggling to be considered a medical endeavor or, at least, a health care profession. It was not so long ago that Rubinstein (1965) was advocating that psychoanalytic conceptualization become more protoneurophysiological so as to interface better with biological knowledge, which, perhaps reductionistically, was conceptualized as underlying the phenomena studied by psychoanalysis. Now psychoanalysis and its theory and practice have been rejected by the medical and health care establishments. Thus, for those groups, it is irrelevant whether or not psychoanalysis chooses to become more biological.

While it is understandable that, because of political, economic, and organizational pressures, psychoanalysis, until very recently, had not considered fully its relationship to health care, I think that it is important that we begin to do so, systematically and on a continuing basis. Only through an ongoing review of the effects on psychoanalysis of its putative medical affiliation can we gauge the extent to which psychoanalytic thinking has been affected by largely unquestioned and unexamined medical models and practices.

I do not think that many of us in psychoanalysis go to work each day in order to stamp out mental disease. We do not work in the medical model, yet we are often perceived as doing just that. What is the difference? (In what follows, I use the terms health care and medicine as synonymous and the terms physician and health care provider or professional in a like manner, since I believe the models that govern their functioning are identical and defining.)

DIAGNOSIS AND TREATMENT IN THE MEDICAL MODEL

People present themselves for medical care because they have a "problem." The problem is usually a symptom, a manifestation that gives them grounds for believing something is amiss. Pain, fatigue, functional incapacity are examples. Frequently, the symptoms are accompanied by a sign or signs, observed by the physician, such as jaundice or pallor or a particular odor. The symptom reported and the signs observed all are defined as departures from a norm of physical function and, therefore, are deserving of further investigation. Symptoms, in this model, are conceptualized to be the result of some pathological process ongoing in the patient, (e.g., infection), on the basis of which conceptualization further examination is conducted to determine the nature of the pathology.

As pathology is conceived to be causal to symptomatology, so too is etiology causal to pathology. Thus, for example, infection is caused by a particular etiological agent, say, streptococcus B, which is deemed to be the fundamental basis for the manifestations that have appeared in the diagnostic study of the individual and that define that individual as a patient.

This model of a hierarchical relationship of symptomatology, pathology, and etiology has important characteristics. First, it constitutes a theoretical ideal of the diagnostic process. If one can know the three elements of the model, one can understand fully the multiple departures from the norm of the physical processes involved in any disease entity. Further, the model provides an ideal that parallels the ideal model of treatment for disease. One can treat symptoms palliatively, for example, using analgesics for pain. Or one can treat pathology in a general way, for example, using broad-spectrum antibiotics for an infection. Finally, the knowledge of the etiology enables the selection of a specific treatment choice as well as the development of preventative methods for the protection of individuals and, ultimately, the elimination of the etiological agent from nature.

In the treatment model that interfaces the diagnostic model I have just reviewed, the patient is understood to be without responsibility for any of the three aspects of the disease. To be sure, a patient may be responsible for creating conditions of living that make a disease process possible, but once it has begun, the patient's responsibility for it and the power to alter it diminish or disappear. At that point, the health care professional assumes responsibility for prescribing the treatment and implementing its application. The patient, in this model, is limited to complying or not complying with what has been prescribed.

These medical or health care models of diagnosis and treatment work rather well in the case of physical disease processes. A detailed description will enable comparison of these models with alternative ones. Indeed, in those comparisons, the devil is in the details.

A PSYCHOANALYTIC VIEW OF THE MEDICAL MODELS

Consider first the diagnostic model and its utility in approaching "problems" that are presented to the psychoanalytic practitioner. From one psychoanalytic point of view, these problems are not *problems*—they are *solutions* to the intrapsychic, unconscious dilemmas the individual is attempting to solve. But, even if this viewpoint is not adopted, problems or symptoms are not defined by some departure from a societal, statistical, or ideal standard of behavioral functioning; they are defined for the individual by the experience of distress that accompanies them. Problems manifestly presented by analysands are what they state them to be, notwithstanding that the analyst may view them as something more, particularly as indications of some unconscious process, content, or both. Thus, anything can be a "symptom" so long as it is experienced as a discontinuity between the conscious intentions of the individual and the outcome of efforts to implement those intentions. It is part of the analytic process that we demonstrate that those "undesired" effects the individual is experiencing *are* the product of seemingly "unknown" intentions.

Pathology, as I have discussed it as part of the *medical* model, is a concept that has plagued psychoanalysis (and psychiatry) for a long time. Defined as any deviation from a healthy, normal, or efficient condition, it challenges the psychoanalytic view of the human condition in a variety of ways. Freud (1901) called all those manifestations that were unconsciously motivated "psychopathology," as in the "Psychopathology of Everyday Life." Simply put, he took the position that behaviors that are consciously motivated are "normal" and those that are unconsciously motivated are "pathological." In so doing, he left us a legacy that troubles us to this very day. Today I think that there is general agreement that what has been termed psychopathology is better conceived of as psychodynamics. Whatever psychoanalytic orientation we hold, we probably all agree that the dynamic interplay of psychic forces, however conceptualized (e.g., as instincts, defenses, relations to self and object), is an important area of psychoanalytic study in practice, theory, and research. This dynamic interplay of forces is ubiquitous and part of everyday life, including many of its more creative aspects and, therefore, not usefully considered pathological.

The confounding of psychodynamics and psychopathology has led to sometimes odd situations. Take homosexuality, for example. Before 1978, it was considered pathological. One psychoanalyst argued that in his work with homosexuals he had discovered psychodynamic processes that his analysands had in common. He then argued that since psychodynamics equals psychopathology, homosexuality is a disease or, at least, a psychiatric disorder, that is, a manifestation of pathology. Parenthetically, even if his discovery of common dynamics in homosexuals were valid, it would not justify the equating of psychodynamics with psychopathology. It was for this reason, as well as many others, that the American Psychiatric Association disqualified homosexuality as a disorder in 1978.

The skepticism about what is pathological that occasioned that decision in 1978 has, unfortunately, not persisted. At the present time, our society is only too willing to pathologize every behavior with which it is uncomfortable. In a court case, a defendant argued that she was sexually involved with 13-year-old boys because of her "dependent personality," the implication being that she was therefore not guilty of statutory rape by reason of insanity. Appropriately and surprisingly, her argument was rejected in court. I say appropriately because, even if she was psychodynamically a dependent personality, the absence of responsibility that has come to be seen as the product of pathology was defined by the jury. Yet cases such as this, which argue that, because a person is motivated by psychodynamic factors that person is suffering from a pathological condition and is, therefore, without responsibility for the motivated actions, illustrate the weird logic that results in the unjustified disrepute that psychoanalysis has been experiencing.

That which is psychodynamic is not psychopathological. Psychodynamic processes are certainly not "deviations," which are unhealthy, abnormal, or inefficient. People are not sick because they have an Oedipus complex. On the contrary, psychodynamic functions lead to manifestations that are ingenious, creative attempts to adapt to unconscious disturbances in emotional life. To no small degree, psychodynamic processes have been shown to contribute to art, humor, literature, and other such endeavors which our society has, for the most part, valued (e.g., Faber, 1970; Freud, 1905; Sterba and Sterba, 1954).

As pathology underlies symptomatology in the medical model, so psychodynamics underlies the discontinuities experienced by those who come for analysis. While psychodynamics must be inferred from the material provided by the analysand rather than observed directly, it does not follow that psychoanalysis is more an art and less a science. Probably it is both, as art and science come to be seen more and more as interwoven approaches to knowledge. And this is perhaps even more the case when we come to a consideration of etiology as viewed psychoanalytically.

How do people come to have the psychodynamics they are inferred to have and that are discovered in the course of a psychoanalysis? Are there etiological agents that underly the pathology and symptomatology supposedly presented by those we analyze? It used to be that we thought so, and in some cases still do. Just as Stephen Sondheim had the gang members in *West Side Story* proclaiming that they "were depraved because they were deprived," so too did we entertain for a time the concept of the "schizophrenogenic mother," whose characteristic child-rearing practices caused the malignant pathology and bizarre symptomatology of her offspring. Perhaps we still want to think in that etiological fashion as is implied by such current concepts as "the unempathic selfobject" exerting a significant influence during crucial early child development.

Current concepts of "etiology" emphasize "experiences," defined as current reports of "memories," the actuality of which is irrelevant to the analysis since the reports are viewed as thoughts that have come to the analysand's mind in the present moment in order to communicate some ongoing current dynamic. "Experiences" are thus contrasted with "events," defined as actual occurrences that, in the mind of the analyst and the analysand, are remembered exactly as they took place in the "original" situation.

"Experiences" are elements in the analysand's memory and mind, and we seek to learn about such mental events through the experiences of analyst and analysand in the analysis. I do not think that analysis is any longer the search for the "truth" of the "psychic traumas" that analysands are presumed to have undergone in childhood, if for no other reason than that truth is unknowable. Besides, what the analysand thinks and feels and experiences in the analysis constitutes the essential truth of the clinical moment and has embedded in it all the antecedents that come to the analysis with the analysand.

It may well be that in some future "brave new world" we will learn the genetic, chemical, physical, and neurophysiological bases of the infinite varieties of behaviors and mental experiences of which human beings are capable. It may even be that we will learn all the effects of developmental events on the future life of the individual. None of that will, however, provide us with any causal understanding of the specific, concrete, infinitely complex, myriad happenings of the analytic moment as experi-

enced by analyst and analysand. Nor do we need any such causal understanding. The conclusions as to causality at which the participants in the
analysis arrive together suffice: for them, for the moment, for the analysis,
and for however long they wish.

In its essence, psychoanalysis is simultaneously both a "diagnostic"
and a "therapeutic" process. The so-called therapy consists in the participants making together and continuously a so-called diagnosis of each of
the phenomena that make their appearance in the analytic situation. The
therapy consists of making diagnoses. It is for that reason that the legend-
ary analyst who, when asked the diagnosis of his analysand, replied, "I
don't know. We haven't finished the analysis yet."

Psychoanalysis as a therapy is radically different from the health care
model of treatment, and not only because it proceeds from a different
diagnostic framework. As I have noted, the patient seeking health care
consciously defines himself or herself as not responsible for the condition
presented, without sufficient knowledge and training to understand it,
and incapable of doing anything about it. In most instances, the health
care professional shares that point of view. That professional makes the
diagnosis and may or may not share that "truth" with the patient. The
professional may also be sympathetic about the diagnosis, because the patient is perceived to be a "victim" of the disease process that has been
visited upon her. Thus, patient and health care professional collude to
define the patient as incompetent to understand what has been discovered
and to decide what to do about it. It follows, therefore, that the treatment
process proceeds by means of the professional's doing to and for the patient. Prescriptions are made, procedures are performed, and instructions
are given, with each of which the patient is expected to comply.

I believe that most psychoanalytic practitioners do not share this point
of view about the status of the people with whom they are doing analysis.
I am aware that some analysts believe that certain of their patients suffer
from the results of permanently damaging etiological agencies, such as
developmental arrests, infantile traumas, genetically endowed incapacities
of ego function, or anomalies of the central nervous system. These analysts conclude, compassionately, that they have to provide reparative services
to those people, however limited in effect those services must be.

Other analysts, using almost the same model, believe that they are
the knowers of "truth" about their patients, the analytic situation, and the
world in general. This superior knowledge of reality is proven, for them,
by their conviction of their natural endowment, by their possession of
diplomas and certificates, and by their conclusion that transference consists of "distortions of the reality of the analyst" as a result of infantile
trauma. Such analysts see correction of those "distortions" as one of their
major analytic functions. They hold the view that the so-called corrections

are not the responsibility of the analysand and that the analysand cannot use the analytic process to know and effect the needed "corrections," if he or she chooses.

Most of us, however, view the analysand as collaborator, someone with whom the analyst works as a "colleague," each doing her or his task of the analysis. In this view, the analysand is equally responsible for the analysis, something to which we sometimes give insufficient weight as we consider the analytic situation. When we stop to think of it, analysands' responsibilities are many and substantial. They include being responsible for making the contact, for deciding to enter and continue in analysis, and for meeting the minimum requirements of coming to the session, "talking" in it, and paying for it. Other significant responsibilities of analysands are choosing the manifest verbal material and their behaviors, which the participants analyze together; utilizing the interventions of the analyst to effect change, or choosing not to do so; and preserving those important effects of the analytic effort beyond the conclusion of the analysis. The analysand, then, is not perceived as or expected to be the passive, incompetent recipient of those services which are provided by a health care system and its personnel.

In analysis, the status of the analyst is reciprocal to that of the analysand. In contrast to the position held by most physicians and other health care professionals, the analyst is not responsible for the analysand or the analysand's life, however much the latter would like to transfer that responsibility. Trying to assume that responsibility gratuitously risks derogating the analysand by conveying the analyst's belief that the analysand cannot do for himself or herself. People who need another to be responsible for them and for their lives don't need an analyst—they need a guardian. What the analyst is responsible for is analyzing, however that may be individually defined theoretically, technically, or stylistically.

Throughout any analysis, the analyst does more than just analyze. She does not treat the greetings that begin and end the session as thoughts that came to the analysand's mind. She offers appropriate congratulations and condolences, as well as greetings of the season, information of which only she is possessed, and needed assistance when none can be obtained anywhere else. She treats such departures as social conventions that may also be psychodynamically significant but are at the moment not analyzed. Richard Sterba (personal communication) used to compare the analytic method to distilled water in that both could be perceived ideally as being totally pure: the water being without impurities and the analysis being free of anything other than the analysand's associating and the analyst's interpreting, period. Sterba went on, however, to point out that distilled water does not carry an electrical current; it needs impurities in it if it is to do so. The analysis, analogously, needs and has appropriate departures from "just analyzing" if it is to carry an "emotional" current. Thus, even in the most conservative conception of the analytic method, there is a place for human interaction as an integral part of the method. This aspect of analytic work, however, does not support the conclusion of some critics that analysis consists essentially of chatting with the worried well about their sexual hangups. On the other hand, it also does not support the view that analysis is advice-giving by a knowledgeable authority and thus consistent with the medical treatment model.

Psychoanalysis is currently in a state of productive theoretical, conceptual, and technical ferment. Many argue that the effects of psychoanalysis are the result of the analyst's first formulating the psychodynamics that are inferable from the associations in the analytic hour and then presenting them in verbal form to the analysand. Others take the position that the analytic relationship, in its myriad affective and experiential forms, produces the analytic results. Most analysts, in general, believe that it is both. Whatever it is that the analyst provides, interpretation and relationship, the analysand is the only intermediary between that which is provided by the analyst and the results that ensue. And whatever the results may be and however they are described, they occur only with the analysand's active, albeit unconscious, use of that which he encounters in the analysis. This essential aspect of the analysand's active involvement in and responsibility for portions of the processes in the psychoanalysis might appear to the health care professional as improbable as a surgical patient's assisting the surgeon in performing the operation. It is, I believe, one of the aspects of psychoanalysis that is so enigmatic to those who evaluate it using the standards of the currently prevailing health care models.

In much of what I have presented thus far there is an implication that the outcome of the analytic work is essentially the responsibility of the analysand. Further, the only responsibility the analyst can assume in regard to outcome is to analyze it. Most analysands state that they experience significant and early relief from the subjective distress they brought to the analysis. With that objective attained, and as they become better acquainted with the process, their conscious objectives seem to expand in the direction of achieving change in themselves and their lives. Also, they adopt the objective of continuing the satisfaction that is a part of the ongoing analytic work. The outcome of analysis is, therefore, an entirely subjective matter and quite different from that which is expected in a medical model, viz., conformity to a generally accepted state of normality or, at least, a cessation of complaints and symptoms. Indeed, I would argue that one would have to deviate significantly from a psychoanalytic ethos and frame of reference in order to conduct outcome studies of psychoanalysis in a manner that would be acceptable to a health care system and congruent with its model. I urge, therefore, that we be fully content with any belief that we have that our work in a particular analysis has or has not been productive, which belief may or may not be held by the analysand, and that we dismiss any accusations that such conclusions are subjective and, therefore, impossible of validation. If deciding to begin analysis is the prerogative only of the participants, individually and collectively, so too should be any evaluation of outcome. And, finally, it seems to me that any need to consider outcome should better be analyzed, rather than regarded as a truth to be verified.

By way of summary and in support of my arguments that psychoanalysis is not a health care profession, I would like to contrast the health care model and the psychoanalytic one:

Health care is concerned with symptoms; psychoanalysis addresses the whole of an individual's mental life.

Health care pertains to pathology; psychoanalysis, to psychodynamics.

Health care seeks physical, objective, and historical fundamental causes; psychoanalysis studies subjective current experience.

Health care seeks the cure of illness; psychoanalysis only examines the subjective experiences of mental life, including the idea of being ill.

Health care professionals assume responsibility for their patients; psychoanalysts assume responsibility for the analysis.

Health care seeks to reduce the human condition to the biological and chemical; psychoanalysis is content with the psychical.

Health care sees mental illness as an objective fact; psychoanalysis recognizes it as a metaphor.

In health care, the diagnosis determines the treatment; in psychoanalysis the "treatment" is "diagnosing" and vice versa.

Health care emphasizes outcome; psychoanalysis emphasizes process.

In health care, the professional is the responsible authority; in psychoanalysis, the participants are collaborators and share responsibility for the analytic process.

I have understood my assignment in writing this chapter to espouse a particular point of view rather than develop a careful presentation of all sides of the issue. I am cognizant of other positions, but I have left those to the other contributors. In somewhat the same vein, I am mindful of the significance that attaches to being a health care profession in today's world. The organizational, political, legal, and economic benefits that accompany the designation of health care profession are many. I would note, also, that those benefits are costly since they subject the profession to the strangling effects of ever-increasing and enforced rules, regulations, laws, prohibitions, standards, evaluations, intrusions, and the like that compromise and diminish its status and integrity. But discussion of the benefits and costs of being a health care profession should be ongoing for all of us.

REFERENCES

Eissler, K. R. (1965), *Medical Orthodoxy and the Future of Psychoanalysis*. New York: International Universities Press.

Faber, M. D. ed. (1970), *The Design Within: Psychoanalytic Approaches to Shakespeare*. New York: Science House.

Freud, S. (1901), The psychopathology of everyday live. *Standard Edition*, 6:1–290. London: Hogarth Press, 1960.

——— (1905), Jokes and their relation to the unconscious. *Standard Edition*, 8:1–258. London: Hogarth Press, 1960.

——— (1926), The question of lay analysis. *Standard Edition*, 20:179–258. London: Hogarth Press, 1959.

Rubinstein, B. (1965), Psychoanalytic theory and the mind-body problem. In: *Psychoanalysis and Current Biological Thought*, ed. N. S. Greenfield & W. C. Lewis. Madison: University of Wisconsin Press, pp. 35–56.

Sterba, E. & Sterba, R. (1954), *Beethoven and his Nephew*. New York: Pantheon.

Szasz, T. S. (1964), *The Myth of Mental Illness*. New York: Hoeber-Harper.

SIX

Psychoanalytic Education In the Age Of Managed Care

Staying Alive In Shark-Infested Waters

MARYLOU LIONELLS

In its century, long history, psychoanalysis has undergone dramatic growth; it has evolved from a heretical fringe movement into a force that is central to the cultural mindset. Integrated as common sense, the major ideas of psychoanalytic understanding and treatment have become part of our social inheritance. In contemporary America, psychoanalytic ideas define how we know who we are, how to understand what we do, and how to solve many of our problems.

The feat of literally transforming social expectations and understanding in less than 100 years is all the more remarkable when we realize how few centers of psychoanalytic training have been founded and how few individuals have actually been trained as psychoanalysts. The influence of psychoanalytic theory expanded through the writings of academics, journalists, creative artists, and others who either learned its principles from the perspective of the couch or gleaned them from the professional literature. Rather than advertising the virtues of this unique approach to understanding human nature, most psychoanalysts maintained a stance of aloofness bordering on secrecy. Practitioners who are interested in popularizing analytic ideas for a wider audience often meet with disdain from colleagues. They may be considered less serious than is appropriate for promotion to higher rank within the psychoanalytic establishment. Traditional psychoanalysis, following Freud's lead, has remained cloistered and arcane. It is thought to be accessible and understood only by those very few who pursue the arduous path of total immersion in prescribed training.

Until recently, the training practices at all psychoanalytic institutes were remarkably similar. The tripartite pattern of didactic courses, supervision, and personal analysis developed in Europe in the 1920s and 30s became the model used throughout the world. The teaching produced mastery of the theoretical canon; the supervision inculcated how that material should be applied; and the training analysis was intended to uncover personality defects that might interfere with the smooth integration of ideas and techniques into acceptable analytic style. In addition, at most psychoanalytic institutes the course work itself followed fairly similar lines, emphasizing the systematic reading of Freud and including more current literature only after it had become wholly incorporated into accepted dogma.

Psychologists' victory in the ground-breaking lawsuit against the American Psychoanalytic Association in 1988 both coincided with and was responsible for the development of many new psychoanalytic institutes. In the preceding century, new institutes usually emerged out of theoretical dispute, irresolvable personality clashes, or the desire to build a new intellectual empire. But, starting in the 1980s, the founders of many new institutes, in sharp contrast to their historical counterparts, were not motivated by a personal vision of what the content of psychoanalysis should be. They built new organizations to offer professional training to a wider range of students and to expand the psychoanalytic perspective, and they were open to an array of emergent psychoanalytic ideas, including competing and even conflicting theoretical perspectives. While previous training and personal inclination may have oriented them toward one analytic school or another, most of the creators of new institutes in the United States have been unwilling to impose a single conceptual frame, and they have similarly been eager to experiment with new methods, new organizations, and entirely new content for curriculum and training requirements.

The appearance of these various institutes has energized psychoanalytic training with a new vitality. It has posed new questions about what is central to becoming a fully competent practitioner and has raised such complex issues as the impact of eclecticism; the intellectual integrity of mixing divergent conceptual positions; the validity of integrating varied perspectives on countertransference, personal disclosure, and intimate relatedness in the analytic dyad; and the legitimacy of expanding psychoanalytic focus beyond the limited confines of the consulting room.

Among the difficulties posed by current innovations in the content of institute training, the most central is determining and maintaining those practices and beliefs that distinguish such training as psychoanalytic. A new institute must decide what is essential to the core of its training, what must be provided in any program that considers itself psychoanalytic, and what is endangered if changes in the basic paradigm are introduced. While addressing these challenges is critical for the new training centers, established centers are also reconsidering traditional practices. In part, this reassessment is being forced by current competition to meet the interests and needs of students, and in part it is motivated by recognition of the enormous changes in societal expectations and the pressures of the marketplace.

When psychoanalysis was an arcane specialty, restricted to a few practitioners, treating a few, special patients who were diagnosed as suffering from only a few, carefully defined ailments, there was little need or desire to be responsive to wider social concerns. But today psychoanalytic ideas are widely recognized as powerful tools for understanding all levels of human problems, and there is a desire to implement these ideas on the widest societal levels, while, not coincidentally, at the same time facing severe restrictions to the financial demands of traditional psychoanalytic treatment. Training centers, like individual practitioners, are facing powerful pressures to make sweeping changes to meet changing demands.

Managed care, of course, challenges all medical practices, not only those related to mental health. Managed care companies embody the public's resentment and fear of the arrogant possessors of skills that mediate life and death, and business's recognition that in periods of personal peril there is the opportunity for financial gain. They have expanded as a product of societal expectations that there should be answers to every problem and that health care should invariably be successful. The mandates of managed care also represent a noteworthy thrust toward despecialization, assuming that the knowledge of the expert can be knowledge of the general practitioner. Expertise is no longer accepted as the province of those few who achieve special status through extensive training or extraordinary talent.

Interestingly, the emergence of managed care has, in a few short years, affected psychoanalytic training in ways that many decades of diffuse social pressure could not. It has decimated the ranks of applicants to analytic institutes. It has made the image of the full-time, private-practice psychoanalyst a nostalgic relic, like the horse-and-buggy family doctor. And it has forced a timely rethinking of psychoanalysts' avoidance of publicity, our failure to attend to our public image, our ignoring the imperatives of scientific research, and our ostrichlike denial of encroaching political control and financial threat. Institutes must consider the value of continuing to teach skills that may be unusable and practices that are outmoded. Potential candidates question how they will be able to earn a living and whether they will be able to adapt their skills to those forms of treatment that patients will request in the future and that insurers will approve.

Beyond these negative pressures, however, there are potential benefits to the current reevaluation. Many practitioners have long wished to comply with the moral imperative that psychoanalytic training enable students to use their skills to reach a larger population, to deal with a broader range of psychological problems, and to incorporate a wider spectrum of parameters adapted to the specific needs of patients formerly considered unanalyzable. Further, many argue that psychoanalytic tools should be modified to become available to less specially trained professionals. Beyond the multisession, carefully framed, highly charged, rarified psychoanalytic encounter, there are infinite gradations of less intense yet potentially significant psychological interventions. The shrinking availability of analytic control cases has highlighted the necessity for questioning the criteria for a "good analytic patient." Appreciating how effectively new medications can change the patient's quality of life has made the psychopharmacologist a valued partner in many analytic treatments. And the diminished attractiveness of psychoanalytic training among psychiatrists, and even psychologists, has raised provocative questions about what professional background is necessary for competency in analytic training and which aspects of prior education are required to obtain the fullest benefit from an analytic institute.

In the age of managed care, new parameters inevitably enter the psychoanalytic situation. These include involvement with third-party payers, issues of confidentiality, the analyst's willingness to participate in obtaining appropriate insurance payment, questions of fee setting that are contingent on outside resources, and the analyst's advocacy skills and effectiveness in negotiating. In the past, fee setting and payment plans would be considered relatively minor technical issues, categorized as setting the analytic frame and left to individual supervisors to consider as these questions arose in the work with troublesome patients. Now such management issues are involved in virtually every treatment. The analyst's willingness and ability to participate will often determine the feasibility of undertaking the analytic commitment. There are myriad opportunities for acting out and in, for collusion, and even for ethically questionable behavior. But there are likewise many opportunities for productive experiences of collaboration, acceptance of responsibility, and demonstrations of the analyst's availability as a competent caretaker.

Historically, analytic training has remained impervious to what might be considered transient social pressures, political issues, or cultural expectations. Operating from a position that was defined as value neutral and focused solely on the patient's inner life, the analyst could respond to externally generated issues as diversions, resistances, or grist for the cease-less analytic mill. In our contemporary environment, though, it is no longer easy to put aside the issues emerging from managed care. Some analysts have argued from what might be considered a "purist" position. In this view, to adapt to violations of traditional definitions of the analytic frame is to destroy the essence of the analytic setting. From this perspective, analytic process cannot occur unless certain conditions are maintained, including that the analyst remain wholly uninvolved in management of reality issues in the patient's life. Institutes that fail to include discussion of contemporary economic realities are, de facto, subscribing to this position.

On the other side of this question, personal finances press analysts to participate in negotiations with insurers (or with parents, spouses, or other third-party payers). There are, however, serious moral concerns that also argue for such participation. In the 1980s, fees for mental health treat-ment dramatically exploded in the United States in direct proportion to the availability of insurance coverage. We analysts participated in a situa-tion that led to the belief that patients should receive coverage for all medical treatment; and psychoanalysis was defined, by patient and analyst, as a medical subspecialty. We are surely not justified in terminating pa-tients who are so unfortunate as to lose their coverage or run out of ben-efits. Nor is it possible to justify our accepting only those patients who have the good fortune to be able to afford our fees. To do so would result in a population of analysands who are either very wealthy, or are civil ser-vants with unlimited benefits offered by government. It seems a moral imperative that we adapt to the socioeconomic climate and teach our stu-dents how to analytically study their participation in helping patients pay for treatment.

Why should this be so difficult? The answer to that question resides in the prevailing conceptual orientation that grounds most psychoanalytic training. Before I attempt to deal with the specifics of insurance negotia-tions, it is appropriate to move back a step and see this problem in a wider context.

This is a period of flux and turmoil for all psychoanalysts, not only because of the foregoing economic issues, but also because the traditional conceptual foundation has been shaken. From many different quarters, arguments are arising that support the validity of what is being called the "two-person model" of the psychoanalytic situation. Accepting that psy-choanalysis is an interaction between two individuals, rather than a semiscientific examination of just one, has enormous implications for ev-ery facet of traditional theory and practice. Not only are conceptions of the transference and countertransference obviously called into question, but the very nature of the mind, the unconscious, the development of the ego, and the nature of relatedness, is being reconsidered. I believe that the current transition in psychoanalytic thought will have ramifications that surpass the revolution caused by the emergence of ego psychology in the middle of this century. It is too soon to foresee how psychoanalytic education can and should evolve to take into account the shift in the basic model of the psychoanalytic paradigm, but it is clear that major revisions are in order.

First, a working understanding of the two-person model is necessary to deal effectively with matters of the analyst's interventions related to third-party payment and insurance coverage. Decisions concerning what to teach and how to teach it, when to change, expand, and incorporate new ideas, can become points of sharp conflict and even warfare within institutes. Contemporary interest in the uses of countertransference, self-disclosure, working in the relational space, conceptualizations of narcissism, redefinition of the Oedipus complex, and the assault on the theory of reconstruction and the nature of the unconscious, all seem relevant if students are to be prepared for practice in the next century. These topics also, however, raise thorny issues as to how to incorporate them into existing curricula.

A MODEL FOR CONTEMPORARY PSYCHOANALYTIC TRAINING

For more than a half-century, the William Alanson White Institute has struggled with certain of these questions. Two characteristics especially facillitated the institute's ability to respond to change while maintaining its analytic identity. These are its unusual administrative structure and its underlying conceptual orientation. While, as is well known to psychoanalysts, to focus on a single case has certain limitations, it happens that the William Alanson White Institute has several features that recommend it as a model for broader application of practices developed there. These include 1) the length of time it has been in existence; 2) the personal and political characteristics of its founders; 3) its core theoretical/conceptual beliefs; 4) its special organizational structure; and 5) its influence on contemporary psychoanalysis.

Founded over 50 years ago, White has a substantial tradition, a solid economic structure, and a large number of graduates. As is true for most psychoanalytic centers, graduates generally remain deeply involved with the ongoing activities of the institute. Its long history and special political structure has produced several hundred graduates who participate in a very broad range of college and university programs, mental health centers, and other institutes throughout the United States and around the globe. When Clara Thompson remarked that "the Institute is not a home," she meant to encourage graduates to look outside the organization for sources of professional gratification because there is not room for every graduate to participate in the training program. The resulting dispersion of graduates is one source of the profound, yet largely unacknowledged, influence of interpersonal theory in the United States and explains Leston Havens's comment that Sullivan is the most important underground influence in American psychoanalysis. The results of White's training methods, organization, and other practices may be said to have withstood the tests of time and of exposure to diverse conditions and perspectives.

Like many new training centers, the White Institute was founded by a group of radicals and dissidents. Clara Thompson joined Karen Horney in breaking with the New York Psychoanalytic group over its refusal to grant training status to Erich Fromm. When personal difficulties arose between Horney and Fromm, Horney started her own school and Fromm remained at the newly formed William Alanson White Institute. Thompson drew on her relationship with Harry Stack Sullivan to provide an intellectual center for the new institute. Freida Fromm-Reichmann as well as Janet and David Rioch were recruited from the Washington Institute to form the core faculty of the training program.

This group formed an unusual alliance, based more on respect for independence of thought than on unanimity of perspective. What they did agree on was a humanistic concern to alleviate suffering, a political orientation that involved a proactive stance to define social structures to support individualism and personal freedom, and an abiding interest in the manifold interactions between individuals and their interpersonal environment.

Of this group, Erich Fromm was the most committed to political activism and the least comfortable with organizational structure. His influence upon the White Institute and its graduates was a product of his personal magnetism and the force of his ideas, communicated through supervision and seminars and handed down through oral tradition. Fromm soon left the New York area for personal reasons but continued a loose affiliation with the Institute and its students. Students would travel to work with him in Mexico and Europe, and he returned on occasion to offer special workshops.

It is of interest in terms of our discussion of psychoanalytic education that Fromm's theories were not incorporated as part of the formal curriculum of the Institute until very recently, many years after his death. It is usually the case that the stars of the analytic firmament spread their personal gospel through their teaching and lecturing, building a group of adherents and followers within the analytic establishment. Fromm's relationship with White illustrates how a structure that is nondogmatic and pluralistic can accommodate a number of strong, charismatic personalities without fracturing under the pressure of factionalism.

The other founders of the White Institute were particularly interested in extending psychoanalytic ideas to their treatment of schizophrenics
and other deeply disturbed individuals. Their efforts in this area broke
with prevailing theory concerning the nature of pathology and also involved modifications of technique that were labeled deviant. These efforts
offered opportunities for radical experimentation, leading interpersonalists
to discover the implications of working with countertransference as early
as the 1950s. They also expanded analytic technique to include a broad
range of patients who would be considered inappropriate control cases in
traditional institutes.

Perhaps paradoxically, the commitment to innovation and concern
about the vagaries of the human condition in which the individual is understood as entrenched within a given sociocultural milieu gave rise to
both an appreciation of pluralism and heterodoxy and a conviction about
the centrality of environmental impact on the individual personality. The
White Institute prides itself on the breadth of its curriculum, its acceptance of diversity of viewpoints among students and graduates, and its
tolerance of a range of techniques and practices. At the same time, it defines itself as the home of interpersonal psychoanalysis, has established a
journal that is dedicated to the presentation of interpersonal ideas, and has
systematically resisted affiliations with other training centers or organizations that might restrict its freedom to be self-defined. One might argue
that the organization reflects the characteristics of the theory itself (or vice
versa) in that until very recently no one had dared coordinate and integrate
the body of ideas and concepts that represent the interpersonal school.

The personal characteristics of the founders translated into certain
innovative organizational structures. For example, White was among the
first institutes to establish a low-cost clinic for both psychoanalytic treatment and psychoanalytically informed psychotherapy. Students were required to study psychoanalytic psychotherapy as well as psychoanalysis in
order to accommodate the differing needs of varying patient populations.
The appropriate frequency for analytic treatment, including the didactic
analysis and control analyses, was set at three instead of the traditional
minimum of four times per week. These modifications resulted directly
from the founders' experiments in applying psychoanalytic techniques and
testing parameters. In this regard it should be noted that Clara Thompson
had traveled to Budapest to be analyzed by Ferenczi and was deeply impressed by his personal and professional risk taking as well as his openness
to developing new methods.

With few exceptions, psychoanalytic training centers have grown out
of study groups or associations of analysts with common ideas who, once
their numbers reach some critical mass, decide it is time to start educating
others. When educational decisions remain the province of faculty and

graduates, a path is laid toward future factionalism and politization of the training process. The founders of the White Institute were well aware that political intrigue often dominated psychoanalytic societies. Clara Thompson, the first director, considered how to establish an organizational structure that might insulate the Institute from the pressures of personal interests. Thompson decided to establish White as an independent training center governed by a Board of Trustees selected from the lay public. Graduates of the institute, organized into a scientific society, had no direct power over training decisions, including curriculum, personnel, or acceptance of candidates. To maintain a firm connection between graduates and the institute, all faculty are selected from the membership of the graduate society, but administrative control is entirely separated.

This system, unique among analytic groups, protected the internal integrity and coherence of the training process. It was especially tested in the 1960s, when graduates became divided over the question of whether psychologists should be fully equal to psychiatrists in the training process. From the Institute's beginnings MDs and Ph.D.s were trained in the same program, but, under the New York State Board of Education charter they were granted separate certificates. In fact, the official name of the institute was, and remains, the William Alanson White Institute of Psychiatry, Psychoanalysis, and Psychology. Under difficult political and socioeconomic pressures, not unlike those plaguing our field in the 1990s, a group of medical practitioners was opposed to granting full and equal status to psychologists. The debate carried the potential for splitting the institute. Eventually the trustees affirmed the principles on which the institute was founded and, although a small group formally resigned from the Society, the training program remained intact.

This resolution led to important consequences, which, again may offer useful insight into an aspect of traditional psychoanalytic training. Training both academically informed psychologists and medically oriented psychiatrists, the White Institute has necessarily encouraged a dialogue about the medical and psychological viewpoints that inevitably emerge in classes and seminars and that has engaged graduates for over 50 years. This is one of the few forums in the United States where this kind of equality has been practiced and where the consequent issues have been so consistently explored.

For the most part during its long history, the Board of Trustees has been relatively inactive, regarded as more a rubber stamp of decisions made by the professionals than as a sleeping giant. Whenever the possibility of political crisis has appeared, however, the Board has become activated and served to bridge the factions, open channels for dialogue, and maintain the core ideas of the Institute. Other such nodal points, of great concern to any psychoanalytic institute, include a period of potential financial insolvency, the decision to purchase a building, expanding services into nontraditional areas, and increasing involvement of younger graduates in the training process and administration of the Institute.

The creation of a lay Board did protect the early Institute from internecine squabbling. Among the unforseen effects, however, was having established a group of senior administrators that became self-perpetuating. The founders did not anticipate the consequences of unlimited terms of office or the fact that psychoanalysts can practice with undiminished zeal until they are quite elderly, thereby excluding younger colleagues from participating in the decision-making process. Here, again, the Board of Trustees, uninterested in theoretical differences but very concerned about the vitality of the organization, intervened to enable an orderly transition from the "old guard" to the "Young Turks" without need for violent revolution.

Certain of the issues I have described contributed to another feature of the White Institute that is relatively nontraditional. The proactive orientation of its founders, coupled with the practical concerns of the businessmen and community leaders on the Board, fostered an ongoing interest in social issues, humanitarian concerns, and political activism that is rare among psychoanalytic centers. Historically, psychoanalysts have avoided the wider applications of their ideas, focusing interest on the intensive, long-term practice of "pure" technique. Analysts at White, however, applied their skills in mental hospitals and psychiatric facilities and throughout the Institute's history found innovative opportunities to demonstrate the effectiveness of psychoanalytic ideas. In the 1960s, when teenagers were leaving school to "tune in" and "turn on," the Institute sponsored the 'College Drop-Out Project,' an inquiry into the dynamics of adolescence in a changing society. Interest in working with nontraditional populations resulted in the 'Union Therapy Project,' through which a contract was signed with a branch of the United Auto Workers to provide long- and short-term psychoanalytic services to blue-collar workers. An NIMH grant was obtained test the effectiveness of LSD in enhancing analytic treatment. Special clinics have been established for creative and performing artists, for those in midlife crisis and for the elderly, and for Latinos and other minorities.

Recently the institute established the Center for the Study of Psychological Trauma. Under this rubric, graduates and candidates are currently studying patients whose lives have been affected by the AIDS epidemic, victims of sexual abuse, those who have been culturally or socially dislocated through immigration, and those who suffer from infertility. The thrust of the Center is to increase psychoanalytic understanding of the effects of traumatic experience by reconsidering the deep psychological impact of externally induced injury. Such studies might seem a natural extension of the interpersonal position espoused by the Institute, through which life experience is recognized as inevitably interactive with intrapsychic forces in the formation of personality and of psychopathology.

Throughout the history of the psychoanalytic movement there have been splits and divisions among practitioners. Dissidents have left established institutes to start new training centers that would represent their particular vision of psychoanalytic truth, or embodying their own political ideals. Those dissidents who have been able to maintain a dialogue with the mainstream community, such as the Kleinians or the followers of Kohut, have generally survived their break with orthodoxy, and the centers they created eventually flourished. Those who left the establishment completely, or were banished from the ranks of Freud's disciples in the early days of the psychoanalytic movement (including Ferenczi, Jung, Adler, and Horney), tended to become marginalized and represent a very minor force on the analytic scene.

The question may be raised, How has the White Institute managed to retain the singular position of the "loyal opposition" to the psychoanalytic establishment and get financially solid, ideologically secure, widely respected, and wholly independent?

Clearly a multitude of forces contributed to the Institute's success and survival. Two aspects of the training program, however, stand out as pivotal, both involving questions of defining and maintaining standards of quality and excellence. Despite establishing a theoretical position that might be considered to be opposed to traditional psychoanalytic ideas of both theory and technique, training at the White Institute includes a thorough grounding in the teachings of Freud and his followers, as well as an intensive experience of personal analysis and supervision. These standards are virtually identical to those of institutes of the International Psychoanalytic Association (with the noteworthy exception of required frequency of treatment sessions).

The importance of the Institute's adhering to the standard parameters of curriculum and training cannot be overstated. Reformers sometimes believe that in rectifying what are seen as mistakes made in the past, they must reject everything and newly define all aspects of their creation. In the 1970s, universities yielded to pressures for relevance and modernism by offering courses that responded to sociocultural fashion rather than the classical tradition. When informed by a solid intellectual core, such innovations may serve to offer students necessary fundamentals in a topical guise, sugar coating the pill as it were. All too often, however, attempts at relevance result in erosion of key factors in the foundation for future growth.

While in many ways commendable, eclecticism is an extremely difficult and hazardous project. Offering a smorgasbord of courses, a little bit of the modern Kleinians with some Jungian dream analysis and a smattering of self psychology, may result in a curriculum that leaves students confused and ungrounded. The situation is worsened when faculty and administrators do not share a common orientation. Not only are candidates left to integrate disparate teachings and styles into their own work, but they may be penalized if their favorite supervisor does not adhere to the standards represented by the majority on the current training committee.

There is an additional concern that deserves mention in this discussion of contemporary psychoanalytic education. Among the most exciting changes in psychoanalytic theory is the rehabilitation of the concept of countertransference. All analysts now realize that personal reactions offer significant information concerning their patients and the interaction and that the practitioner's inner experience is a key factor in promoting understanding and cure. In traditional analytic training, candidates, through their personal analysis and supervision, have a prolonged opportunity to study and to develop a nuanced appreciation of their own reactions.

Just as the wider culture appropriates analytic concepts in ways that are sometimes meaningful but oftentimes inappropriate, the concept of countertransference is a tool that, in the hands of the untrained, may become a dangerous weapon. Psychoanalysts have always argued that popularizing concepts, without sufficient depth and appreciation of context, can result in applications that are at best erroneous and at worst damaging to those to whom they are applied. The widespread appropriation of countertransference is a situation where those fears may be justified.

The pressures of managed care and cost control in the mental health field, prizing brief treatment and short-term results, have created a frenzied search for powerful methods for affecting on the patient's personality. Even cognitive and behavior therapists, as well as hypnotists and those who work with families and groups, are coming to appreciate the value of the transference–countertransference interface and the utility of working directly with the therapeutic relationship. There is an enticement to psychoanalytic centers to attract students by offering courses and workshops in abbreviated treatment techniques or by exploring applications that are adapted to current economic demands. It is also gratifying to find professionals who previously disdained all that the psychoanalytic tradition might offer are finally acknowledging the power of a psychoanalytically recognized tool. However, this situation may foster potentially treacherous temptations. On one hand, such modifications of analytic technique may be of enormous value if developed out of careful experimentation and prolonged study. But, on the other hand, widespread modifications, attempted in response to social and financial pressures, can fragment a faculty, impoverish the intellectual core of a training center, and deflect resources from the central concern of maintaining analytic standards and integrity.

A related problem is encountered when training centers are pressed to include courses that are adapted to contemporary social conditions or economic pressures. Developing models for rapid change, adapting technical parameters, and condensing intensive treatment require intense and serious study. Such projects, or courses, should not be undertaken lightly lest they result in loose, weak formulations and eclectic, confused methodology. Psychoanalysts are notoriously poor at telescoping their work into short-term treatment, and they can hardly be expected to teach such techniques to students. Conversely, those who are expert in such techniques seldom are deeply committed to psychoanalytic principles. Unless they are very carefully thought through and integrated, introducing alternative therapies into an analytic curriculum opens the way for confusion and controversy. At White, the teaching of psychodynamic psychotherapy is a natural extension of the use of analytic methods. Interpersonal theory provides a conceptual bridge for the continuum between less and more frequent treatment as well between deeper and less serious pathology.

The second factor that contributed to the White Institute's ability to maintain its position of independent prominence in the psychoanalytic world is the circumstance that psychologists were for so long excluded from training at IPA-affiliated institutes in the United States. Selected psychologists were granted waivers to study at American Psychoanalytic Association institutes on the condition that they signed an agreement that their training would be used for research purposes. White offered one of the very few reputable alternatives for psychologists who wished to be fully trained and certified to practice psychoanalysis. Over White's long history, this position has attracted many of the best and brightest psychologists from the New York area and from across the country. White was thereby been able to retain very high standards for entrance, limiting candidacy to a select few chosen from a large applicant pool. This selectivity has had one consequence that also marks the White Institute as different from many other institutes, especially those that are newly formed. Those accepted for training (after the organizational period of the Institute's early years) were medical school graduates having a residency in psychiatry and Ph. D. graduates in clinical psychology with advanced clinical experience. Leaving aside the philosophical question of whether other professional groups should be excluded from the ranks of "lay" analysis, there was virtually no pressure to accept other students since there was always an excess of applicants. Even psychologists trained in the areas of social, experimental, school or counseling were screened for admission only if they presented special situations and extraordinary credentials. This selectivity, perhaps bordering on elitism, fostered a strong sense of community and pride in the training process that contributed to White's position as never seeming marginalized, although wholly excluded from the orthodox club.

Current economic pressures on the profession generated by diminished insurance coverage for psychoanalytic treatment are affecting all training centers. Even as new institutes are forming, bursting with enthusiasm and idealism, the scarcity of candidates and the desire to create innovative programs may lead away from the path of careful screening and stringent credentialing that proved so valuable to White. I maintain that much of its stability and prestige is credited to the White Institute's ability to preserve high standards, being slow to respond to fad and fashion, and depending on a core curriculum that offers a solid grounding in the fundamentals of standard psychoanalytic theory and technique. Surely there is much room for variation from this particular model, but change needs to be carefully considered if we are to protect core values and insure quality training.

In conclusion, in describing the history and development of the White Institute, I have tried to illustrate how certain attributes have permitted it to flourish and how it might serve as a model for other psychoanalytic centers. Its organizational structure, including a lay board of trustees, an independent professional administration, and a strong, loyal, but separate, graduate society, together offer resilience to internal political struggles and external societal pressures. At the same time, it seems imperative that an institute is rooted in a conceptual orientation that offers members a sense of cohesiveness without the requirement of orthodoxy. Committed to certain core ideas that provide a solid yet flexible intellectual center, the White Institute has been able to incorporate advances in psychoanalytic theory and technique without renouncing its fundamental convictions. This position provides students and graduates with a certain grounding that hedges against the confusion of eclecticism and the potential of being swept up in the tidal waves of psychoanalytic fashion. Survival in the treacherous environment of contemporary economic and social constraints requires the ability to remain firmly rooted, while poised for adaptation, accommodation, and change. While this may be a tall order for any educational organization, these qualities essentially define psychoanalytic goals for the healthy personality. It seems fitting to apply them to a psychoanalytic training center.

SEVEN

"There Is a Future For Professional Psychology"

DOROTHY W. CANTOR

Editors' Introductory Note

On November 9, 1996, during Dorothy Cantor's term as President of the American Psychological Association, she addressed the New Jersey Psychological Association at its fall conference. To maintain the color and intensity of its tone, we are publishing her address in as close to its original form as possible. We believe that a contribution like this, complete with its vivid informalities, forcefully conveys the thinking and feeling of a recent president of the association on a topic that is central to the theme of this book.

I bring you good news. There is a healthy, dynamic future for professional psychology. Now this is a prediction that's based on events, not just the fact that, as my family calls me, I'm a Pollyanna. As Marty Seligman[1] would say, I'm an optimist.

Recent events point in the right direction. How many of you are aware that last Tuesday a psychologist was elected to the Congress of the United States? Ted Strickland, from a district in Southeastern Ohio, will be returning to the Congress. He had been elected in 1992, defeated in the Republican sweep in 1994, but is coming back. So, as Congress proceeds with talking about health care, we are going to have our voice there. That's darn good news. He represents the epitome of the private activism that psychology needs to keep that momentum going. What momentum am I talking about? I'm talking about the momentum to end the stranglehold of managed care. Some of you may not have ever heard me say this before, but I hate managed care! I believe that it's passed the peak of its

---

[1] President, American Psychological Association, 1996.

power because the public is catching on to what we've known for years. Let me share with you something that came to me; it's anonymous but it's wonderful. It's called "Managed Care Meets Schubert":

> A managed care company president was given a ticket for a performance of Schubert's *Unfinished Symphony*. Since she was unable to go, she passed the invitation on to one of her managed care reviewers. The next morning the president asked him how he enjoyed it, and instead of a few plausible observations, she was handed a memorandum that read as follows:
>
> 1. For a considerable period, the oboe players have nothing to do. They should reduce their number and spread their work over the whole orchestra, thus avoiding peaks of inactivity
> 2. All 12 violins were playing identical notes. This is unnecessary duplication, and the staff of this section should be drastically cut. If they require the large volume of sound, they could attain this through the use of an amplifier.
> 3. Much effort was involved in playing the 16th notes. This is an excessive refinement, and it is recommended that all notes should be rounded up to the nearest eighth note. If this were done, using paraprofessionals would be possible instead of experienced musicians.
> 4. No useful purpose is served by repeating with horns the passage that has already been handled by the strings. If all such redundant passages were eliminated, they could reduce the concert from two hours to twenty minutes.
> 5. The symphony has two movements. If Schubert didn't achieve his musical goals by the end of the first movement, he should have stopped there. The second movement is unnecessary and should be cut. In light of the above, one could only conclude that had Schubert given attention to these matters, he probably would have had time to finish his symphony.

Humor aside, we know that managed care represents greed and avarice. In 1995, the CEO of U.S. Healthcare earned $3.4 million before his bonus. In its for-profit plan for the year ending June 30, 1996 Aetna had a revenue of $13 billion! In California, two managed care companies, Pacific Care and FHP merged in the spring. The payout for the purchase was $2.1 billion, or $1200 per subscriber. Now, tell me, would a company be willing to pay $1200 for each subscriber if it didn't know it was going to make a heck of a lot of money doing it? And we can't get decent health care! Or deliver services as we would like to! Or get paid reasonably! It's clear that the goal is not good mental health treatment or good treatment, of any kind, but *brief* mental health treatment and low-cost medical treatment.

Did you know that there's a current continuing education course being offered by Merit Behavioral Care (MBC)? I love this title, "Short-Term Therapy for the Long-Term Patient." That's not a joke. It's listed as a course. They are also doing interesting scamming things. I would like to ask any of you who have experienced this particular scam to come up sometime today and let me know because I know I'm not the only one. On behalf of a patient, I did join a manage care network. I avoid managed care companies like the plague, but I joined this for my patient. Up until the time that I applied, I was getting reimbursed at the rate of half my fee and she was paying the other half because I was an out-of-network provider. I applied on May 1. On June 15 they accepted me into the network, and I started getting paid at the rate that they pay in network which was $95.00. When we got back materials from the company, there was a period from May 1 to June 15 that they refused to pay for at all. They said "services hadn't been authorized." So, the patient, not being a passive person, called and said, "Why weren't these services authorized? How could they be? Dr. Cantor wasn't in the Network."

They said, "Oh. We backdated her acceptance into the network." Isn't that cute? They backdate me to May 1, but I don't apply for authorization until June 15 when I'm admitted. So they have a six-week window of opportunity in which they don't pay me at all![2] I know of at least one other practitioner that this has happened to, and, as I said, if this has happened to any of you please let me know, because we don't take any of this sitting down.

As early as September of 1994 economists knew that managed care organizations were not the answer. *The New York Times* headline then said, "To economists, managed care is no cure-all." The point that they made was that the savings that they attributed to managed care would disappear if everyone had it. Cost shifting to people who have fee for service makes up the difference. As there are fewer "fee for service" people, where are you going to shift it to? There's no place to go. So we have to sacrifice quality of care. We certainly know about that. We have to ration care, and we know about that. In fields other than psychology, we have to sacrifice new technology.

The Congressional Budget Office recently reported that, "although HMO's appear to reduce health care costs, there is no credible evidence

---

[2] Months after this talk, under pressure from APA, the company *did* pay.

that they reduce the rate at which costs subsequently increase." I call your attention to the October 1996 issue of *Consumer Reports,* which concluded that cost reductions achieved by a managed care are temporary. *Consumer Reports* notes that 17% of premium dollars are going into marketing. Seventeen percent out of our pockets and out of our patients' treatment is going to market those plans. Sixty-five percent of plans are now for profit, and they spend less on care than the not-for-profit plans. But, again, the public is catching on that managed care is okay as long as you are well.

Managed care sold the public a bill of goods. The HMO's said, "We'll lower your premiums." Well, that sounds good, as long as you don't have to use health care services. As soon as you have to use them, you discover that this is not a very good idea. Public awareness is evident in a number of ways, in consumer behavior, in legislative and regulatory action, and in judicial action. In 1995, US Healthcare recruited six out of ten new policy holders by allowing them to use any provider or hospital. That is, they set up a point of service program. They couldn't sell their old program, where you had to choose your doctor from a panel, to six out of ten purchasers. There's an interesting report that came out of Minneapolis last month; I don't know how many of you are aware of this. Corporations, including General Mills, Honeywell, Pillsbury, and American Express, are cutting out the middle person. Beginning in January they will purchase services for 400,000 people directly from organized groups of doctors, hospitals, and clinics. Minnesota's biggest insurers have control of more than 80% of the marketplace, and they are going to cut out of the managed care market.

So big business is catching on to the idea that they're spending an awful lot of money for a layer of service that does not help anybody. The public doesn't have the control in purchasing health care that it does in purchasing other things. When we buy cars, we are both the buyer and the user. In health care, we very often are not the buyers but we are the users. Consequently, there needs to be regulation in the delivery system. And we do think that the Federal Government is starting to move in, legislatively and regulatorily, to take control of managed care. The story of the "drive-through deliveries" is the most dramatic example, and that started here in New Jersey, where we said new mothers have to be able to stay in the hospital two nights. Then the Federal Government passed legislation that did the same thing. As part of that same "drive though delivery" legislation, Congress passed the first parity bill. Now, it's not the parity bill you were hoping for, but it gets us in the door. It gives us some degree of equity between mental health and medical benefits. In January of 1998 we'll begin a three-year experiment in which the annual cap and lifetime cap for mental health services have to be the equivalent of those for general medical services. The whole country is talking about parity and about having to give mental health benefits to people. The Federal Government also issued rules restricting the ability of HMO's to pay benefits and other financial rewards to doctors as an inducement to limit services to Medicare and Medicaid. Those rules will set the standard for the industry. That's why we want psychologists in government because they'll be there making the rules.

Meanwhile, a lot is happening here in New Jersey. Thanks to Alan Groveman and his work with the Advisory Panel developing revisions to the HMO regulations, we are going to have important provisions such as: only a mental health professional can deny or limit psychological treatment. We are going to be requiring HMO's to give 30 days' notice before terminating a provider or a patient. We are going to have an independent appeals process. Many states are developing legislation to further regulate what has been a runaway industry. According to *American Medical News,* in September of 1996, 35 states took action to control managed care in their last session. There are more than 1000 bills in the legislatures around the country right now that will protect patients, mandate care, and provide access to providers.

Judicially, we have another place where we're able to do things. We can only go to court *some* of the time. As Russ Newman[3] likes to point out, a lot of things that are immoral and hateful are not illegal. So, we can't always say, "Well, let's just sue the bastard." If there's not a law that says the bastard can't do it, we can't sue. Nevertheless, I learned this morning that, following a suit by an individual doctor, the New Hampshire legislature has barred "no-cause terminations." We, of course, with our lawsuit, filed in May of 1996 against MCC, are going after exactly that same point. Because that lawsuit challenges the "no-cause termination," it is going to be a very important case in all of our professional lives. Maybe we haven't told you this, but psychologists are cheap and we have to reach into our pockets and we've got to be supporting actions like the lawsuit and paying our dues and joining the PACs, because that's what's going to keep us strong and keep the momentum moving.

Now everyone needs to be involved. And by being involved, I mean being actively involved, in APA and in your state association. Invest in your future. These organizations are working for you. What's APA doing? Well, in addition to supporting state legislative activity and working very hard to lobby the Congress around health care, you're all aware that we've begun a public relations campaign. A resolution was introduced to the Council of Representatives to put aside $1.5 million for our Public

---

[3] Executive Director, American Psychological Association Practice Directorate.

Education Campaign, and since then the Council has passed additional legislation that will put $1 million a year for the next five years into that campaign.

I'm particularly proud of the work that I've been doing with the presidents of all the other mental health professional associations. I was introduced last winter to Harold Eist, who was then the President-Elect of the American Psychiatric Association. Harold said to me, "Come on, Dorothy, between us, the two APAs can really kill managed care." I said, "You know what, Harold, if you guys get in trouble with managed care, nobody is standing in line behind you. They *have* to use psychiatrists. But if we guys get in trouble with managed care, there are the social workers, psychiatric nurses, counselors, and marriage and family therapists who will be very happy to step in and take over when psychology is in trouble." I said, "So what I want is all of them to be at the table." And that's what we did. We brought together groups now representing ¾ of a million providers of mental health services around the country.

We have developed a document that is still confidential, and the only reason it's confidential is that we're planning to do a big press conference and you don't have news if everybody knows the news. But I will tell you that this document, to which all of the groups have signed on, its called *Principles for the Provision of Mental Health and Substance Abuse Treatment Services—A Bill of Rights.* It covers issues like the patient's right to know about benefits, contractual limitations, and appeals and grievances. It covers confidentiality in terms of our need to protect an individual and not being required to disclose confidential, privileged, or other information. It's very much in keeping with our Peer Review Law. It even speaks to information technology and how those who receive confidential information should treat it.

It talks about choice, the termination of treatment, parity; discrimination (that people who have had mental health treatment should not be discriminated against by other insurance entities); benefits design; accountability; treatment review (we can be reviewed only by professionals trained as we are. My friendly reviewer is named Patrick. Some of you may have spoken with him or someone like him. I asked him the other day what his training was. He said, "Do you mean how did the company train me?" I said, "No. What's your degree?" He said very proudly, "I have a Bachelor's in Psychology." Doesn't it do your heart good to know that we are being reviewed by bachelor-level folks?

Hopefully, this document will be public within the next month or so.[4] We're hoping to have a big press conference on the Hill. At our last

---

[4] That document has since been published in poster and brochure form and is available through APA.

meeting, we brought in all our CEOs and executive directors so that we could get the staffs of the associations working on it. We have an action plan that our attorneys have reviewed for antitrust considerations, but we will be moving forward as a group and we will be far, far stronger. Now, you may wonder, how do you have time to be so involved or how do you manage it? Let me tell you one other secret to my being involved. I work nondirectively, I work psychoanalytically, but in case you haven't noticed, I am an inherently bossy lady. So, this is a very productive place for me to put all this energy, and my patients love it and my family loves it. So, play an active role in policy making by joining committees and having your voice heard. Additionally, start thinking about running for office. I would like in the very near future to see some psychologists in the state legislature as well as in the Federal government. Psychologists in legislatures in other states around the country make a difference.

Finally, let me urge you to be creative. We know you're all smart, or you wouldn't be here today. But, by being creative, I mean finding new ways to use your skills and to deliver services. Start conceptualizing yourself, for example, as a health care provider. Think about working with physicians around surgery and behavioral health, remembering that the seven leading causes of death in this country are behaviorally induced. We need to encourage an understanding of a prevention model. You know that the Federal government thinks that prevention is inoculation, so if we try to get grants for psychological prevention we don't get them because we don't give shots. We need to educate the public and we need to educate the Congress. As a matter of fact, as one of my presidential initiatives, Carol Goodhart, from New Jersey and Sandra Haber from New York have been chairing a series of briefings on the Hill to teach the Congress about the connection between psychological well-being and good health. Thus far we've presented on cancer and heart disease, and we need to bring that same message down to the legislature here in New Jersey and in every state.

We've got hospital privileges now, so use them, get them, start working there, start knowing more people there! We didn't fight this long and hard to get hospital privileges just to say we have them! Use them. Think about working in industry, where the health care system isn't the payor. It's amazing how businesses don't want to pay for health insurance, but they will pay for all kinds of direct services, in stress reduction, for example, because they realize that that reduces accidents and absenteeism. So, reconceptualize how you are going to deliver your services. Think about consulting. My colleague, Toni Bernay, and I, who wrote *Women in Power* have also formed a consulting company. And we are now, in our spare time (she's on the Board of Directors with me too) training executive women to stay in the corporations and move toward breaking the "glass ceiling." We're using our skills. Think about other ways to use them. Think about the forensic system, where the legal system pays, for evaluating capital defendants or doing custody evaluations. We need to create new markets for our services. And marketing isn't a dirty word anymore. We are in a marketplace. You don't have to be tied exclusively to doing psychotherapy. You won't feel as constrained if all of your income isn't coming through the health insurance stream. So the future will be ours— all of ours, if we all take it upon ourselves to be activists. The watchword is: don't be passive.

So, be knowledgeable and don't be passive.

Be involved and don't be passive.

Maintain your professional identity and don't be passive.

Be creative and don't be passive.

Keep in mind, if you want success to fall in your lap, you have to put your lap there. Thank you.

PART II

Legal Issues:
Privacy and Confidentiality

EIGHT

Restoring the Confessional

Reporting Laws and The Destruction Of Confidentiality

DAVID SUNDELSON

Two stories, both true, illustrate the effects of child-abuse reporting laws and their effect on the practice of psychotherapy. At a professional meeting in New York, a candidate at a psychoanalytic institute presented the case of a hysteric patient for discussion by a well-known visiting analyst. The proceedings were videotaped. The candidate reported the patient's statement that she had been "sodomizing" her 15-month-old boy. A few questions from the therapist revealed that the patient did not know what sodomize meant. The patient next declared that she must have been "committing felatio" with the child, but it turned out that she did not know the meaning of that term either.

As the analyst began to discuss the ambiguity of this material, a woman in the audience stood up and interrupted. She began by declaring that New York had a child-abuse reporting law, denounced the candidate angrily for violating it, and finished by asking how she could dare to call herself a psychologist after such a confession. The ensuing uproar subsided only after the analyst suggested turning off the videotape recorder and focused his discussion on the clinical and legal questions the interruption had raised.

The case of *Stecks* v. *Young* in California is an equally disturbing tale. Candace Young was a licensed marriage, family, and child counselor with a doctorate in clinical psychology. She was also a member of the Ritual Abuse Task Force for the San Diego County Commission on Children and Youth.

She began to treat the 29-year-old daughter of the Stecks family, a patient previously diagnosed as schizophrenic and suffering from multiple personality disorder. During her sessions, the patient told Young that her mother and father had sexually molested her when she was a child, practiced satanic worship, abused alcohol and marijuana, and performed human and animal sacrifices and brainwashing. She also told the therapist that she thought her young niece and nephew might be the victims of sexual molestation by her brother-in-law. Two years later, the patient—but not the therapist—informed Child Protective Services of her concerns. More than a year later, the patient told Young that her brother-in-law planned to sacrifice his son at a cult ritual celebration of the fall equinox.

The therapist then spoke directly to an employee of Child Protective Services and also, at his request, sent him a letter. In it, she expressed her concerns about the children, made serious accusations about the Steckses' relationship with their daughter when she was a child and their cult activities, and opined that neither Stecks would be a proper caretaker for their grandchildren. When she sent the letter, Young had had no personal contact with the Steckses, the children, or the children's parents (her patient's sister and brother-in-law). She relied entirely on information her patient provided.

Various employees of Child Protective Services read the letter, as did doctors and individuals within the criminal justice system. As a result, the Steckses sued Young, alleging libel, slander, and intentional infliction of emotional distress. She moved to dismiss the suit, asserting that the California reporting law provides absolute immunity for a report by a health practitioner and mandated reporter, and the trial court agreed.

On appeal, the plaintiffs asserted that immunity did not apply because Young lacked a reasonable suspicion of abuse and had reported irrelevant issues. The Court of Appeal noted that Young had put all her trust in the accusations of a purportedly schizophrenic patient and had not interviewed the alleged victims or abusers or consulted other professionals. It also recognized that "unfounded reports can lead to serious, sometimes devastating consequences" and that the case "presses the outer limits of immunity." Nevertheless, the appellate court affirmed the dismissal, following the rule that "mandated reporters are entitled to absolute immunity even if their reports are negligently prepared or intentionally false."[1]

The angry questioner in my first story and the reckless therapist in the Stecks case represent what Christopher Bollas and I have called "the new informants." Together, these stories say at least two things about the current climate of American psychotherapy and the larger culture that surrounds it. First, psychotherapy and psychoanalysis once took pride in a

---

[1] *Stecks v. Young* (1995) 38 Cal. App. 4th 365.

belief that fantasy was difficult to separate from fact and that the process of clarification, however difficult and prolonged, could bring valuable therapeutic results. Now, as in both illustrations, the line between fantasy and fact is too often unexamined, especially where children and sexuality are concerned. The patient work of clarification and healing gives way to a different sort of action, at once more decisive and more reductive: the telephone call to the police or their agents.

Second, information once thought confidential moves freely from citizens to the state and back again. Here the reporting laws are only part of a larger pattern. California now boasts a "child molester hotline" and an Attorney General who announced proudly that in its first four months, 2,000 citizens had placed telephone calls, at $10 a call, to determine if someone they knew or might hire was a convicted child molester. A federal appeals court in Manhattan recently concluded that many names are placed on state child-abuse registers that do not belong there (N.Y. Times, 1994), but New York will soon offer a similar service, and four other states may soon follow suit.

The erosion of privacy in American life is a large phenomenon whose origins are complex. Our part of the story begins in the 1960s, when reporting laws were passed across the United States with unusual speed and with no opposition worth mentioning. What caused this legislative wave? A complete explanation, I think, would credit persistent and widespread beliefs about children, sexuality, and punishment. I am concerned here with the politics of the reporting laws, with the attitude of the courts, and, most of all, with the response by much of what I will call for lack of a better term the psychological establishment. That response, I submit, begins with inaction and ends with compliance. It reflects at best a disheartening blindness about the ethical implications of the reporting laws and at worst a willing sacrifice of professional identity.

The first opportunity to shape a statute came during the legislative process. In California, the legislative history of the reporting laws reveals that except for one or two formulaic expressions of assent, psychologists and psychiatrists played no advisory role whatsoever, and clinical issues such as confidentiality were never considered.

Instead, the dominant considerations were financial and bureaucratic. In 1974, Congress provided for federal child abuse grants, available only to states that require "reporting of known or suspected instances of child abuse and neglect" by specified persons and that also "require, allow, or encourage all other citizens to report known or suspected abuse."[2] The pursuit of these funds rings like a refrain through the history of California

---

[2] See 45 Code of Federal Regulations section 1340.3(2) (i).

law. With it goes the fear that the reporting law might not be strict enough—for example, with respect to reporting abuse that is only suspected—to satisfy the federal requirements. As Deputy Attorney General Gates put it in 1978 when testifying before a legislative committee: "Only with suspicion. . . . We want them to report things they suspect." The statute was duly amended to guarantee that California would continue to receive the federal funds—in 1993, $1.8 million.

The legislative record also tells of recurrent turf wars between rival professional groups and agencies that compete for the legislative dollar and the prestige that goes with it. The original 1963 reporting law allowed doctors to decide whether or not to report, and a recurrent theme in the 1978 hearings is resentment of such discretion. Various witnesses denounced the "single specialized groups"—there was no need to identify them by name—who "argue that child abuse is not a crime but a non-criminal problem best handled by treatment." (Legislative files, 1978.).

In large part, these witnesses prevailed. The amended statute reflects the firm belief that abuse is a criminal, not a psychological, problem: reports must be made not to an interdisciplinary team that includes doctors, as was once proposed, but to a police or sheriff's department or a county welfare department.[3] Although physicians lost much of their discretion, they were, however, able to defeat one amendment that would have forced them to report any evidence, even a request for birth control pills, that a female patient under the age of 18 had engaged in sexual relations. Similarly, California teachers succeeded in promoting an amendment providing that the term "child abuse" does not apply to efforts to control unruly students.

Psychologists and psychiatrists engaged in no such effort. They did not write letters and did not testify before committees of the legislature. They said nothing about the erosion of confidentiality. The only expression of concern in the legislative record comes from a college student writing a term paper on child abuse. Noting the proposal to add psychologists and marriage counselors to the list of required reporters, she wrote to the assemblyman in charge of the bill: "I am wondering if this would hamper the confidentiality that presently exists between client and therapist."[4] Apparently, this question failed to trouble the California Psychological Association. The Legislative Chairman of that group wrote to the

---

[3] Penal Code sections 11165.9 and 11166.

[4] Letter to Assemblyman Lockyer, of California, regarding proposed AB 1058. There is no copy of a reply in the legislative files.

same assemblyman, but only to make sure that psychologists were included as mandated reporters in the final bill.[5]

Such lobbying has given California a reporting law that turns the principle of confidentiality on its head, as the Stecks case demonstrates. Instead of protection for the patient who discloses his private life to a therapist, there is protection for the therapist (or any other mandated reporter) who tells a tale of abuse, no matter how implausible or unfounded—protection, that is, for the informant.[6] The sadly deficient lobbying is striking, not only in comparison with the greater alertness and effectiveness of other professional groups, but because of the missed opportunity to explain the methods and values of the profession and to enlist the legal system in its defense. That opportunity is readily apparent in a series of judicial opinions on the psychotherapist–patient privilege.

In law, a privilege is an exception to the general rule that requires every person to testify in court. For a variety of reasons, the law recognizes certain relationships as special and therefore exempt from the requirement: those between attorney and client, priest and penitent, doctor and patient, husband and wife.

As the California Supreme Court stated in the leading case, called *In re Lifschutz*,[7] the psychotherapist–patient privilege "won legislative recognition in the face of legal antipathy toward privileges generally." This recognition—one might even call it deference—is explicit in the Legislative Committee comment on Section 1014 of the California Evidence Code.

> A broad privilege should apply to both psychiatrists and certified psychologists. Psychoanalysis and psychotherapy are dependent upon the fullest revelation of the most intimate and embarrassing details of the patient's life. . . . Unless a patient is assured that such information can and will be held in utmost confidence, he will be reluctant to make the full disclosure upon which diagnosis and treatment depends.

In the *Lifschutz* case, Dr. Joseph Lifschutz, a Bay Area psychoanalyst, invoked the privilege at its most absolute. A former patient of his had sued a third party for civil damages resulting from an alleged assault. In addition to physical injuries, the patient claimed that the assault had caused

---

[5] Letter to Assemblyman Lockyer regarding proposed AB 1058.

[6] "The identity of all persons who report . . . shall be confidential and disclosed only between child protective agencies, or to counsel representing a child protective agency. . . ." Penal Code section 11167(d).

[7] (1970) 2 Cal.3d 415, 467 P.2d 557.

"severe mental and emotional distress." The defendant tried to depose Dr. Lifschutz, who appeared for the deposition but refused to answer any questions and would not even state whether or not the plaintiff had been his patient. The Superior Court found him in contempt and sent him to jail, where he spent three days until the California Supreme Court agreed to review his case.

In the Supreme Court, Lifschutz argued that the order to disclose information violated four different rights: first, the privacy rights not just of the particular patient involved in the litigation but of his other patients as well; second, his personal right of privacy; third, his right to practice his profession effectively; and fourth, his right to equal protection of the laws. The ground for this last claim is that unlike a psychotherapist, a clergyman could not be compelled to reveal confidential information in the same circumstances.

The Supreme Court rejected each argument but based its ruling on the narrow factual ground that the patient himself had already revealed that he had been in treatment and had not claimed the privilege when Lifschutz was ordered to testify. Applying what is called the patient-litigant exception to the privilege, the court concluded that the patient had waived his claims to privacy.

More significant than the ruling itself, however, was the court's obvious sympathy for the privilege and also for the claims of psychotherapy. Justice Tobriner, who wrote the opinion, praised psychotherapy as "a profession essential to the preservation of societal health and well-being." He recognized that the patient "confides more utterly than anyone else in the world," and that "[i]t would be too much to expect [patients] to do so if they knew that all they say—and all that the psychiatrist learns from what they say—may be revealed to the whole world from a witness stand." Relying on the landmark United States Supreme Court case of *Griswold* v. *Connecticut*, Tobriner concluded that the United States Constitution protects a patient's interest in retaining the "zone of privacy" that exists in a psychotherapist's office.

Tobriner's vision of the social significance of psychotherapy and the privacy essential for its practice is still cited more that 25 years later in federal as well as California cases. The vision is more than intuitive; it draws on a rich tradition of two professions, the law and the church. At the same time, it is less than theoretical. Tobriner cites an early collection called *Psychiatry and the Law*, but the nature of just what goes on in the patient–therapist "zone of privacy" remains obscure, as does the precise role of confidentiality in the therapeutic process.

This missing understanding, which was apparently not supplied by Lifschutz or his attorneys, may account for the limitations of the opinion. The Supreme Court held that a court may compel disclosure only of matters directly relevant to the specific emotional or mental condition that the patient has voluntarily disclosed in his lawsuit. With its limited understanding of therapy, however, that was as far as the court could go toward protecting confidentiality. Lifschutz tried to defend a duty owed to all his patients collectively, on the basis of the idea that disclosure of one patient's confidence damages a therapist's other patients, but Tobriner did not address it.

The failure to offer a fuller account of how therapy works was also fatal to the argument that a compulsion to disclose made it impossible for Lifshutz to practice his profession. The court's lack of needed expertise appears again and again in the uncertainty of its analysis. "All compelled disclosures may interfere to some extent with an individual's performance of his work"; "we do not know, of course, to what extent patients are deterred from seeking psychotherapeutic treatment"; "we can only surmise that an understanding of the limits of the exception may provide a measure of reassurance to the prospective patient."

The failure to educate the court, to provide a persuasive account of how therapeutic work relies on confidentiality, sank Lifshutz's positions. Nevertheless, the opinion is remarkable as far as it goes. Tobriner's untutored understanding is in some ways more in tune with the purposes and ideals of psychotherapy than is much of what the profession itself has put forth. Psychologists have again and again failed to provide the understanding that might have allowed the Supreme Court to do more to protect a discipline it recognized as crucial to "societal health and well-being." In fact, some of these pronouncements are regressive. They make no effort to defend confidentiality, bowing instead to the rather different interests of law enforcement.

I am thinking, first, of the following statement:

> There was unanimous agreement that the APA should have a clearer policy that strongly supports the basic principle that the social policy of protecting children from the enormous damage to a child's physical and mental well-being and subsequent development inflicted by abuse outweighs the important social policies supporting the protection of confidentiality of the therapy relationship and protection of the projected disruption of the therapy relationship that can result from such mandatory reporting [APA Ad hoc Committee on Child Abuse Policy, 1989].

It is one thing to find such principles in court opinions, where in fact they appear with some frequency. One might wonder, though, how a professional body can take a position so inimical to its most basic tenets, tenets the California Supreme Court was able to recognize and respect.

An answer may be found in Kalichman (1993). The author, a psychologist, pays lip service to the importance of confidentiality. His primary argument is, however, that any "disruption" of therapy can be avoided by telling a patient about reporting obligations at the start of treatment. If the patient's disclosures make reporting necessary, the therapist can remind the patient of that initial notice and take comfort from having given it.

It seems clear that Kalichman is at least as interested in the therapist's psychological and ethical discomfort as in any harm caused to the patient. "Telling parents and children that confidentiality must be breached will be easier," he says, "if they were adequately informed of the limits of confidentiality at the outset of the professional relationship" (p. 126). The word professional is redundant—what else would the relationship be, after all? It suggests a wish to distance the therapist from the patient and from the clinical and ethical obligations of therapy. The euphemism "disruption" (which also appears in the APA) has a similar thrust: it protects the therapist from recognizing just what it means to comply with the law.

Indeed, Kalichman's position is that such compliance has no bad consequences at all. As long as patients have given their informed consent to the therapist's reporting obligations, "breaches in confidentiality are consistent with understood professional roles and responsibilities" (p. 90). For all its bland reassurance, the assertion raises more questions than it answers.

Who is doing the "understanding"—patients or therapists? If patients, one wonders how their "understanding" of the therapist's "professional roles and responsibilities" comes about; one also wonders if such "understanding" is the only kind that treatment requires. Does the author have any notion that, quite apart from conscious, rational "understanding," a patient might have other, unconscious reactions to a request for "informed consent" and the implied threat that goes with it, not to mention actual reporting? If so, his discussion reveals no sign of it.

In fact, his reasoning sweeps such possibilities away: "reporting suspected child abuse may have as much potential benefit as it does potential harm on therapeutic processes; . . . . little evidence exists to support popular perceptions that reporting abuse has detrimental effects on the quality and efficacy of professional services" (p. 54). From here, it is only a small step toward the inevitable conclusions. "A case can be made . . . for the position that mandated reporting is not an ethical dilemma at all" (p. 59).

The theoretical underpinnings of this position can be inferred from Kalichman's vocabulary. He refers to "clients," not "patients," to "services" and "delivery of services," not "treatment" or "psychotherapy" (or, heaven forbid, "psychoanalysis"). Why should we object to these terms? They are, after all, neutral and objective, free of jargon and mystification.

But that is not all, of course. This lexicon turns psychotherapy into something standardized and fungible: a "service" delivered by an active, omniscient therapist to a passive "client." It excludes any notion of transference and countertransference, any idea that patient and therapist are joined in a distinctive collaboration, any idea of unconscious communication—in short, all the theoretical baggage of psychoanalysis. It is therefore ideologically comforting to those who reject this baggage. It is also ethically comforting: it eviscerates the therapist's duty toward the particular patient.

Most disturbing is an unacknowledged shift in professional identity. Kalichman replaces the therapist committed to individual patients with one whose duty is toward society as a whole. The healer is now a cop: his goal is to punish wrongdoers and prevent harm to potential unknown victims. This new role appears in the commentary to his clinical vignettes: Kalichman invariably points out that a decision *not* to report means that some alleged molestor is still in a position to harm other children, even where contact with them is a matter of pure speculation.

I suggest that Kalichman and others like him are responding, whether knowingly or not, to the enormous punitive forces alive in the culture today. These forces produce the insistent cries to get tough on crime, to build more prisons, to make it "three strikes and you're out" or, as a cultivated and prominent San Francisco surgeon suggested to me in a recent conversation, to castrate rapists and molestors.

Lawyers are also subject to these forces, but lawyers have a well-established social role, and the duties that go with it are clearly recognized both inside and outside the profession. It is instructive to compare Kalichman's view with the California statute that defines the lawyer's duty of confidentiality: "To maintain inviolate the confidence, and at every peril to himself or herself, to preserve the secrets of his or her client."[8]

Matters are not so clear for therapists, who have always occupied an uncertain social position. Avidly sought after and often thought of as having enormous, even miraculous powers, they are simultaneously scorned as quacks, pseudo-scientists, and charlatans. At the same time, the profession has suffered from a lack of coherent self-definition. There is an old joke that any three Israelis always have four political opinions. A room full of mental health professionals is likely to offer an equally bewildering range of opinion about what psychotherapy is and how—or even if—it works. At least in theory, Kalichman seems to offer an escape from ideological confusion and social limbo. Therapists can ally themselves with what seem to be

---

[8] Cal. Business and Professions Code sec. 6068(e).

the dominant and respected forces in society, even if those forces are indifferent or even opposed to privacy and healing.

In practice, however, notwithstanding Kalichman's belief that the reporting laws do not undermine "the quality and efficacy" of treatment, the shift of professional identity has given birth to an ugly new hybrid. Too often, today's therapist is torn between a duty to patients and a conflicting duty to third parties or to the state. One result, an unsavory mix of incompetent treatment and Constitutionally unsound law enforcement, is on display in the case of *United States* v. *D.F.* recently decided by the Court of Appeals for the Seventh Circuit.[9]

D.F., identified only by initials because of her age, was a 14-year-old Native American girl who had spent six months in a county mental health facility. She was admitted to the center by her legal guardians in cooperation with a Tribal Court and the state Department of Social Services, but against her own will, because of her history of assaultive behavior and alcohol abuse.

D.F. was first placed in a locked ward for adolescents, where her motion was severely restricted and where she was observed at least every hour. After some time in substance abuse treatment, she was assigned to the so-called Seasons program, intended to treat her behavioral problems. There, she was under the care of a team that included a psychiatrist, a social worker, and various other therapists. Patients in this program received privileges and punishments based on a point system designed to encourage good behavior and active participation. D.F. could earn points by talking regularly to staff members; she lost points for refusing to answer questions or to write in a journal, as required by the program.

Before she was admitted to the Center, D.F. had become a suspect in the deaths of her two young cousins on a Wisconsin reservation. Treatment staff were informed of this suspicion but were divided about how to proceed. Some staff members believed that they were under a legal obligation to report any admissions of child abuse to the authorities. Some, in accord with Kalichman's principles, believed that D.F. would benefit from acknowledging her acts and being held legally responsible for them. Others, fearing that admissions would result in criminal prosecution, tried to protect their patient by arranging for her to speak to a local minister. Their idea was that the disclosures they expected, if made to a clergyman, would be privileged, even if D.F.'s conversations with therapists were not.

The staff told D.F. that any disclosures about hurting or killing a child would have to be reported to the authorities, and she signed a form indicating that she understood. At the same time, they also encouraged

---

[9] *United States* v. *D.F.* (7th Cir. 1995) 63 F.3d 671.

her to write about her problems, to trust the staff, and to speak openly about any harm she had caused to other children. She was questioned directly about whether she had ever murdered anyone and was asked repeatedly to make lists of all the people she had ever harmed.

D.F. did not discuss any of her past assaultive behavior for several months. She told a staff member at one point that she could not talk with staff because they were required to report what she said; she said nothing significant in her interview with the minister. After some time in the Seasons program, however, she admitted that she had abused three of her cousins (not including the two infants whose deaths she was suspected of causing). She signed a release to permit disclosure of her statements, but the county authorities did not prosecute her. Instead, she was told that the Human Services agency had decided tentatively to "shelve" any charges and that no harm would come to her as a result of her admissions as long as she continued to make progress and cooperate with treatment.

Three months later, in a group therapy session directed by her primary social worker, D.F. admitted to having killed her two young cousins. When the social worker reported these statements to the treatment team, another member of the team notified Child Protective Services, which in turn notified the F.B.I. As a result, the United States Attorney brought federal murder charges.

Before trial, D.F.'s counsel moved to suppress the statements she had made at the center on the grounds that they were coerced and therefore violated the Fifth Amendment's protection against self-incrimination and its guarantee of due process. A magistrate recommended suppression of the statements, but on a different ground: that everything D.F. had said was protected by the psychotherapist–patient privilege. The district court agreed with the order but relied on the Fifth Amendment, not the privilege. The Seventh Circuit affirmed both the order and the legal theory, emphasizing that the dual role of the treatment staff violated D.F.'s constitutional rights: "the state, with an eye to prosecution, cannot coerce admissions under the guise of treatment and then prosecute on the basis of those admissions."

Along with the other material I have described, the D.F. case demonstrates what I take to be some of the unfortunate practical consequences, both clinical and legal, of the reporting laws and of a theory like Kalichman's, which justifies them. My objection to these laws comes under several headings. I am first of all a layman and teacher committed to psychoanalysis as an interpretive method and therapeutic process. Thus it seems to me that the reporting laws stifle exploration of the complex relationship between fantasy and reality—an exploration at the heart of psychoanalysis.

These laws also produce a new class of therapists whose divided loyalties make them unworthy of a patient's trust. D.F.'s primary social worker prepared memoranda on her home computer about D.F.'s statements and behavior. Questioned about their purpose, the social worker stated that the idea of helping the police "would be so far removed from my primary therapeutic purpose as to be, yeah, in the back of my mind, but certainly not up front as a major concern at the time I wrote these notes." Not reassured by such testimony, the District Court found extensive evidence of a close relationship among treatment staff at the Center and Child Protective Services, the juvenile court system, and the F.B.I. D.F.'s own description of her treatment as a "mixed message" seems only accurate.

As a lawyer, I also have other objections to the reporting laws. These laws allow the police to sidestep the Fourth Amendment protection against unreasonable searches and seizures. In one recent California incident, a report by private school employees of a suspicious bruise on a child who had come for an admissions interview brought the family a surprise visit by a team of police officers. Disregarding the parents' objections, the officers marched into the family living room to perform a physical examination of the frightened child, and left only when they were shown a doctor's written statement that the bruise was a birthmark.

The reporting laws also reverse the presumption of innocence. Reported molestors like the parents in the *Stecks* case are presumed guilty until proven innocent, even where the reports are unsubstantiated and grotesquely implausible. Most ominous, perhaps, the reporting laws convert psychotherapy into incompetent, unsupervised police work that far too often flouts the Constitution. In the D.F. case, the District Court found that many staff members at the center saw themselves as "an arm of law enforcement." Unfortunately, their warnings to D.F. about the possible consequences of a confession never included any mention of her Fifth Amendment protection against self-incrimination.

As an ordinary citizen, finally, I am appalled by a society that values the informer more than the healer and by the cynicism, the destruction of privacy, and the despair that such a turn represents.

Richard Gardner (1993) has diagnosed the current widespread beliefs about child abuse as a mass hysteria comparable to the Salem witch trials. Gardner proposes to fight this hysteria by changes in federal and state law. He would eliminate mandated reporting, require strict observation of due process protection, and provide funds only to those states which address the issue of false reports instead of those that require reporting of suspected abuse.

I applaud his suggestions and would like to offer my own. I am struck by the missed opportunity in *Lifschutz* and subsequent cases to expand the psychotherapist–patient privilege by defining professional ethics and the clinical rationale that supports them (Bollas and Sundelson, 1995). I am also struck by the equal protection argument raised in *Lifschutz*, based on the greater deference given to lawyer–client and priest–penitent confidentiality in the California evidence code, and by the well-meaning but clumsy attempt to protect D.F. by encouraging her to make her admissions to a clergyman. No statute obliges me, as an attorney if a client tells me that he has molested a child, to pick up the phone and call the district attorney. My duty is toward my client, not toward his victim or other possible victims or "society" as a whole.

These principles are so well established as to be axiomatic. What may be more surprising is that clergymen are similarly protected under the California Evidence Code (§§1030 and 1032). Any "priest, minister, religious denomination or religious organization" has a privilege to refuse to disclose a communication made in confidence where, "under the discipline or tenets of his church, denomination, or organization, [he] has a duty to keep such communications secret." The legislative attitude toward this privilege, as expressed in a written comment by the Law Revision Commission, is a far cry from the intrusive spirit of the reporting laws. "The extent to which a clergyman should keep secret or reveal penitential communications is not an appropriate subject for legislation; the matter is better left to the discretion of the individual clergyman involved and the disciplines of the religious body of which he is a member" (§1034).

In these lines one hears the American deference to religion, a deference even older than that given the legal profession. My view is that psychologists should seize on this perspective and make it their own. Confidentiality is too important to find its only champions in lawyers who represent fathers accused of molestation and in the occasional television special about the consequences of false accusation. Instead of joining the rush to report, psychologists should try to articulate "the discipline of the body" of which they are members. They should justify their right to exercise "the discretion of the individual" psychologist in response to confidential disclosures. These efforts might profitably be directed toward formulating a code of ethics and explaining the clinical reasoning that makes one necessary.

Such a code might have given the *Lifschutz* court a rationale for expanding the psychotherapist–patient privilege. The California Supreme Court is still sympathetic toward the privilege, as it showed in the recent *Menendez* murder case by refusing to expand the reach of the exceptions and by rejecting the lower court's conclusion that the defendants' therapy was "a charade." Moreover, in 1996, in the case of *Jaffee* v. *Redmond*, the United States Supreme Court recognized and applied the privilege for the first time.[10] The factual context is narrow—treatment sought by a police

---

[10] *Jaffee* v. *Redmond* (1996) 116 S.Ct. 1923, 135 L.Ed.2d 337.

officer after she shot and killed a man during an allegedly violent alterca-
tion—and a final footnote undermines the holding: "the privilege must
give way . . . if a serious threat of harm to the patient or to others can be
averted only by means of a disclosure by the therapist." Nevertheless, the
moment seems opportune for a stand by the profession in defense of
confidentiality.

Such a stand would reassert the integrity and dignity of the therapist's
calling. The issues raised by child abuse are not simple. I submit, however,
that, for psychologists, to identify with the police is less meaningful and
ultimately less satisfying than to work toward restoring the confessional: a
space set aside by social and legal agreement for the essential work of psychic
healing.

REFERENCES

Bollas, C. & Sundelson, D. (1995), *The New Informants: The Betrayal of Confi-
dentiality in Psychoanalysis and Psychotherapy.* Northvale, NJ: Aronson.
Gardner, R. (1993), Sexual abuse hysteria: Diagnosis, etiology, pathogenesis, and
treatment. *Acad. Forum*, 37.
Kalichman, S. C. (1993), *Mandated Reporting of Suspected Child Abuse: Ethics,
Law, and Policy.* Washington, DC: American Psychological Association.
Legislative files (1978), California Senate Judiciary Committee. Unpublished.
New York Times (March 6, 1994) ("U.S. Court Faults a New York List on Child
Abusers.") p. 1.

NINE

Psychoanalysis Under Managed Care

The Loss of Analytic Freedom

ROBERT R. CUMMINGS

The various schools of psychoanalytic thought may define specific fundamentals of psychoanalysis somewhat differently, but all recognize a core set of fundamentals of technique (Etchegoyen, 1991) that allow and protect the existence of analytic freedom.

Analytic freedom is essential to the process of successful psychoanalysis. The patient must be allowed analytic freedom to think, to feel, to speak, and to explore his or her inner life. The analyst must be allowed analytic freedom to listen, to reflect, to feel, and to think, unencumbered by preconception, focus, or direction, in order to maintain an even hovering and undivided attention toward the patient in the analytic setting (Stone, 1961; Spruiell, 1983; Etchegoyen, 1991).

Neither the analyst nor the patient is allowed sufficient analytic freedom when a third party is conducting ongoing managed care review within the frame of the analysis. This intrusion forecloses and arrests the unlimited scope of the therapeutic process, which fundamentally distinguishes psychoanalysis from less comprehensive treatments. It disrupts the therapeutic relationship, disrupts the psychoanalytic listening ability of the analyst, and compromises privacy and confidentiality. It destabilizes the analytic situation by placing the analyst and analysand in a constant state of uncertainty whenever the third party has the ability to force an end to the analysis at any point and with little warning (Langs, 1975; Stern, 1993).

Managed care is defined as a method by which a health care insurance entity[1] employs a case-management system that aims to shape medical evaluation and treatment processes according to contractual criteria and policies established to contain costs and continuously monitor the "quality" and "medical necessity" of the treatment. Managed care systems have redefined quality and medical necessity away from their traditional definitions in accepted medical practice,[2] which made the health of the individual patient the central focus of diagnosis and treatment to the fullest extent of the doctor's ability, in keeping with community standards, and aimed to achieve the greatest improvement in the patient's health. (Wilson, 1992a) The managed care redefinition of these terms weakens the central focus on the individual patient, so that the new definitions can also serve cost-containment philosophies that embrace broad, programmed approaches to insure and treat masses of patients. Managed care not only aims to contain costs generally; it also aims to limit financial reward to highly entrepreneurial practitioners who profit financially by overutilizing insurance benefits. (Gray, 1993; Stern, 1993)

In the mental health insurance sphere, managed care defines quality treatment to be minimally time intensive, cost efficient, and focused toward measurable goals and outcomes. Managed care criteria for medical necessity are guided by insurance contract arrangements that usually limit treatment to conditions that demonstrably cause patients to fall below minimal standards of functioning in an occupation or essential social role. For treatment to be authorized and recognized as medically necessary, the patient must be impaired to the extent that he or she cannot perform the basic functions of the occupation or social role. The inability to enjoy work or social roles does not usually constitute medical necessity for treatment; thus ongoing, extended enhancement of a patient's quality of life is not an approved mental health treatment goal under managed care criteria. Managed care often limits mental health treatment to crisis intervention. By redefining quality and medical necessity in a managed-care-friendly context, mental health treatment can be confined more easily to the aim of restoring and maintaining the patient's health; and it can more efficiently halt subsidy when the aim of treatment moves beyond health maintenance to an aim of reconstructing aspects of the patient's personality or

---

[1] It is beyond the scope of this chapter to distinguish, review, and compare the different faces of managed care that are reflected in these various insurance systems, health maintenance organizations, entitlement programs, and the like. Instead, the paper focuses in general on managed care's influence as it is evolving within all of these systems in the United States.

[2] Abraham Flexner's (1910) report marked the beginning of this modern tradition for accepted American medical practice.

promoting higher levels of health and quality of life beyond the patient's prior achievements.

The rapid evolution and public acceptance of these changes of definition in America support Ronald Dworkin's (1994) concept that the "rescue principle" may be permanently replaced by "the prudent insurance ideal" in an active health care reform process driven by various political and economic forces that affect private insurance and government entitlement programs (e.g., Medicare). The rescue principle assumes that health insurance claims be approved to a nearly unlimited degree in the service of maintaining and maximizing health and life expectancy. In contrast, the prudent insurance ideal recognizes that expensive forms of health care, which drive up insurance premiums, include heroic measures to maintain life when the patient is irreversibly demented and elective forms of treatment that extend significantly beyond the restoration of health to enhance quality of life. Rather than pay higher insurance premiums and taxes in order to guarantee that insurance will pay the cost of extreme heroic measures and expensive elective treatments, the prudent insurance ideal assumes that most citizens would rather forego such coverage guarantees in favor of paying lower insurance premiums and taxes, thus being able to apply the resources saved to education, better living conditions, and other measures that they expect will directly increase their quality of life (Hoffman, 1994). Successful marketing of managed care philosophy, particularly when it is being applied to a profit-driven system, is dependent on proponents' ability to avoid use of the term rationing, owing to its negative public- opinion impact. Instead, they emphasize the aim to create more efficient, cost-effective health care delivery systems through a process that discourages subsidy for health care procedures that they assess to be "not medically necessary."

The ongoing, and perhaps endless, process of determining which health care procedures are to be denied significant amounts of insurance money and which are to receive heavy insurance subsidy has become a political and economic process, rather than a medical and scientific one. Through the political process, the premium- and tax-paying public indirectly determines the array of coverage on a continuum. Nearest one pole are those medical procedures which are popular and deemed worthy receiving automatic coverage. Nearest the other pole are those procedures that are deemed suspect and will be thoroughly questioned for accountability before insurance support is provided. Legitimate medical and scientific influence on this political process competes with well-funded, pseudoscientific, political propaganda. The stigma of mental illness in the collective mind of public opinion plays an additional role in causing all mental health treatments to receive managed care's most intensive level of scrutiny (Judd, 1994).

Managed care's application of the term "not medically necessary" is often experienced by health care professionals (among them psychoanalysts) as an insult to their clinical expertise, their patients, their status as professionals, and their livelihood. They understandably respond with aggressive defense of the respectability, efficacy, quality, and medical necessity of the treatment they provide. Many have been eager to do whatever is necessary to maintain and expand insurance coverage for their clinical work. In the spirit of this eagerness, many mental health professionals have been compliant with insurance requests to report in detail that their treatment of the patient meets managed care's criteria medical necessity. As a result, their patients are losing the traditional protection of confidentiality about their treatment as a trade-off for the privilege of being considered for continued insurance subsidy of that care (Lewin, 1996). While considering the various influences that have eroded patients' rights to the protection of confidentiality for their medical records, Bollas and Sundelson (1995) maintain that mental health professionals' collusion with managed care has been the single deadliest blow to confidentiality.

Popular acceptance of managed care by business, government, and the general public, and the willingness of a majority of health care professionals to participate, make managed care the method of cost containment accountability being employed to replace other accountability methods by most private insurance entities. Managed care is likely to undergo reform to curb certain egregious excesses and denials of essential care that are fueled by the profit motive within the private insurance industry. Once evolved and reformed, managed care is expected to endure as the accountability method of choice for most health care insurance systems and government entitlement programs in America (Hiltzink and Olmos, 1995; Smolowe, Perman, and Van Tassell, 1996).

In the evolution of managed care, scrutiny of case manager salaries is leading to their replacement by less expensive methods, such as capitation systems and case-rate arrangements that influence mental health professionals to 'identify with the aggressor' in compliance. By these methods, the role of the case manager is stripped of salary and converted into an introject that conveys the cost containment philosophies of managed care and stands as a shadow in the superego of the professional. This process is driven by market forces that are being focused and intensified by the acquisition and merger of managed care insurance entities (Smolowe et. al., 1996). Market forces carry the managed care message to put pressure on professionals by influencing their educational systems, conditions of their work at university hospitals (which struggle to survive economically), their professional liability insurers, and state and federal legislatures and agencies to encode managed care accountability and cost containment practices into laws and legally enforceable regulations.

Psychoanalytic treatment is well known as a treatment that aims to take patients to improved levels of health that were never previously experienced; it is much less known by the general public as a treatment that also saves lives and offers a cost-effective alternative to serial hospitalizations in some cases. Therefore, if insurance coverage for psychoanalysis is considered within managed care's "prudent insurance ideal," standard treatment through the termination phase would be expected to receive the highest degree of ongoing scrutiny to be thoroughly accountable to managed care criteria that usually limit treatment to health maintenance.

If sufficient motivation were to exist on the part of insurers, reasonable methods to provide accountability and protection of the confidentiality, privacy, and efficacy of psychoanalysis could be developed. For example, insurers could authorize an evaluation prior to the beginning of formal psychoanalytic treatment to determine whether or not psychoanalysis should be prescribed for a given patient. If the evaluation determined that psychoanalysis is the treatment of choice, the insurer could preauthorize subsidy for a significantly lengthy psychoanalytic treatment to proceed as a confidential two-party treatment without imposing ongoing managed care review or requirements for the creation of accountability documentation for future review. While many psychoanalytic cases may not be preapproved under criteria that aim to limit all treatment to health maintenance, some cases might still qualify, particularly if the alternative treatment or treatments for the specific case were noted in the preauthorization evaluation to be more costly than psychoanalysis.[3]

If a managed care approach is applied to psychoanalysis, each of the core set of six fundamentals of technique that establish and protect analytic freedom is violated. These interrelated six fundamentals include the psychoanalytic frame, the therapeutic relationship, confidentiality, analytic listening, neutrality, and abstinence.

---

[3] In comparing these costs, managed care business interests are motivated to consider that their responsibility to pay for the subscriber's health care is limited to the expected time frame in which the average insurance subscriber continues to be insured by one company. They are not motivated to pay the cost of mental health services if the health and cost-savings benefits of those services are expected to be realized in the long term on the next company's watch rather than in the short term on their own watch. They operate in a competitive insurance market wherein a great advantage is realized for companies that charge lower premiums to subscribers. Since subscribers and their employers tend to change insurance carriers when the opportunity to pay lower premiums with another company arises, the time frame that a company considers to be its watch may be as short as two years and seldom more than five years. A single-payer system might be motivated to compare such costs over the entire lifetime of the subscriber.

THE PSYCHOANALYTIC FRAME

The psychoanalytic frame is established to create an environment that facilitates the patient's ability to participate fully in the psychoanalytic treatment process. For psychoanalysis to succeed, the roots of the patient's suffering must be revealed into consciousness within a situation that is sufficiently safe to allow the patient to maintain strong motivation actively to work through and resolve the pathology (Spruiell, 1983).

To insure this safety, the psychoanalytic frame contains certain essential technical features. It is a two-party treatment, held in a setting that is private and free from distraction or intrusion by other people. Practical elements, such as fees, scheduling, frequency, and length of sessions, are arranged by the analyst and the patient. The treatment is established in a manner that best assures continuity and extension until the patient is ready to finish, such that the patient can risk expressing more and more unconscious material while controlling his or her own destiny within the treatment. Everything said within the psychoanalytic frame must be held by the analyst to be strictly confidential (Stone, 1961; Gottschalk and Whitman, 1962; Dewald, 1965; Langs, 1975; Etchegoyen, 1991).

Conducting psychoanalytic treatment under ongoing managed care review changes the standard frame of psychoanalysis from a two-party treatment to a three-party treatment, compromising privacy and confidentiality. This technical violation prevents the development of a sufficiently trusting therapeutic relationship that can properly sustain a successful psychoanalysis (Freud, 1913; Langs, 1975). The case manager[4] becomes a constant absentee participant in the analytic treatment process, erecting nearly impossible barriers to the establishment of a fully analyzable transference, introducing countertransference dilemmas of insoluble proportion, and therefore irrevocably contaminating the treatment (Freud, 1913; Dewald, 1965; Greenson, 1972; Langs 1975, 1976a, b; Gray, 1992). Having thus lost analytic freedom, the patient may not begin to explore the complex of memory-driven thoughts and feelings that unconsciously motivate him or her and create symptoms and character pathology (Stone, 1961; Greenson, 1972). The broad emotional impact of the analytic experience is lost, and the scope of treatment becomes limited to those su-

---

[4] All references to "the case manager" in this chapter are intended to encompass the foreseeable evolutionary process that will transform this influence from being carried in the person of a live case manager into being carried by other vehicles of influence (e.g., case-rate or capitation arrangements) that can produce nearly identical intrusion of managed care treatment philosophies and cost-containment agendas into the psychanalytic treatment situation.

perficially conscious thoughts and feelings which the patient can most easily reveal publicly. If psychoanalysis is subjected to ongoing managed-care review, the resultant violation of the standard psychoanalytic frame produces a form of treatment that is likely to become stalemated rather than satisfactorily concluded through a successful psychoanalytic termination phase (Gray, 1981, 1992, 1993; Arlow and Brenner, 1990).

THE THERAPEUTIC RELATIONSHIP

The nature of the relationship that is formed between analyst and patient contains certain fundamental features (Greenson, 1972; Langs, 1975, 1976a, b). Psychoanalysis is an endeavor in which the patient is involved in a deeply emotional way and in which the greatest degree of trust in the analyst is required. When analytic freedom and trust are sufficiently established, this relationship develops features in common with the early holding environment described by Winnicott (1965, 1970) and allows for exploration of the patient's inner life through a full development and analytic interpretation of transference (Kohut, 1977). Trust in the analyst is also grounded in the realities of the therapeutic alliance, which must be testable and sufficiently strong to produce a stable analytic situation that can sustain and contain the intensity of positive and negative transference (Greenson, 1972; Dewald, 1978; Etchegoyen, 1991). When insufficient analytic freedom stunts the development of the therapeutic alliance, the analytic situation will be destabilized, transference manifestations toward the analyst will not fully develop or be resolved, the unconscious sources of pathology will not emerge, and psychoanalysis will fail (Freud, 1913; Greenson, 1972).

Managed care reporting requirements pressure the analyst to serve as an agent for the third-party payor; thus such requirements act to risk rupture of the therapeutic alliance (Wilson, 1992a; Gray, 1992). The extent to which the analyst functions as an agent for the third-party payor contradicts the role of psychoanalyst within the therapeutic alliance with the patient. This deviation compromises analytic freedom, trust, privacy and confidentiality and distorts the therapeutic relationship to the degree that neither the analyst or the patient can adequately analyze the resulting transference manifestations, which are difficult to distinguish as transference distortions owing to the reality that the analyst is allied with an outside party who actually dictates and limits essential aspects of the analytic treatment (Langs, 1975; Stern, 1993; Gray, 1973, 1990, 1992, 1993). Activities that comply with managed-care charting and reporting requirements force the patient and analyst to bend the analytic work to suit the case manager, who can exercise authority to end the analysis at any time and perhaps without warning (Stern, 1993). This threat of premature ending can consume the therapeutic effort and destabilize the analytic situation. It acts as a constant external hindrance to the analyst's and the patient's efforts to explore troubling conscious and unconscious thoughts and feelings, a hindrance that can be so extreme that it makes psychoanalytic treatment thoroughly impossible (Dewald, 1965).

CONFIDENTIALITY

Properly conducted peer review adequately protects patients' confidentiality (Gray, 1981, 1983, 1990, 1993). Sometimes managed care masquerades as a form of peer review. Gray (1992) maintains, "Neither scientific findings nor metapsychological arguments can neutralize the threat to the therapeutic alliance posed by claims review or quality assurance review conducted in the guise of peer review" (p. 155). Peer review standards require that the reviewer be independent, free from conflict of interest, financially disinterested, and hold professional credentials and experience comparable with those of the treating therapist (Gray, 1983; Mattson and Wilson, 1992; Wilson and Phillips, 1992). Records for peer review are legally protected from public discovery and should be purged of any information that can identify the patient as an individual (Wilson, 1992b.

By contrast, the managed care reviewer is usually a paid agent of the third-party payor and is not usually a professional peer of the psychoanalyst. Managed care documents commonly contain information that can identify patients as individuals and are often screened by office staff—a clear breach of confidentiality. Furthermore, aspects of these records are often converted to computer data bases and are legally available for review by so many outside parties that, for practical purposes, the records are available to anyone who is motivated to do the search (Gray, 1990, 1993; Lewin, 1996). Third-party payors cannot be relied upon to be able to protect these records from unauthorized discovery.

Gray (1992) maintains that, like supervision and case conferences within psychoanalytic educational programs, true peer review may act as an extension of the psychotherapeutic holding environment. However, this assumption does not apply to the development of reports for use by external review programs. When a report will and must circulate outside the traditional circle of confidentiality, basic trust will be impaired even when privacy is maintained (p. 154). Therefore, managed care does not qualify as peer review and breaches patients' confidentiality to such a degree that the strictest legal and ethical standards apply for a psychoanalyst to obtain a patient's informed consent before releasing any clinical information about the patient's treatment externally (Gray, 1992; Mattson and Wilson, 1992; Gray, Beigler, and Goldstein, 1995). If psychoanalysis is conducted under managed care, informed consent standards require that report documents required for managed care review be written in a form that the patient can read, approve, and give fully informed consent before they are released externally (Wolf et al., 1992). Patients should have the opportunity to edit these reports or deny consent to release them because discovery of the information contained in them could effect their career opportunity, advancement, and any of a variety of life issues that are difficult for the analyst alone to predict (Lewin, 1996).

The charting of ongoing progress notes and reports for managed care review, with or without the participation of the patient, introduces a disruptive, deceptive, and confusing procedure into the psychoanalytic treatment situation. The creation of this sort of documentation runs at cross purposes with the broad objectives of psychoanalysis. It pretends that the treatment is linear, focused, and goal-directed toward managed care criteria. It introduces into the therapeutic relationship a foreign element of mistrust that enshrouds the psychoanalytic process and imposes a dubious taint on efforts to interpret and resolve the patient's transference. (Freud, 1912, 1913; Stone, 1961). One professional organization's practice guidelines recommend that psychoanalysts refrain from documenting psychoanalytic treatment session by session (Gray and Cummings, 1995; Cummings and Gray, 1996).

The decision to conduct psychoanalytic treatment under ongoing managed care review and provide adequate opportunity for the patient's informed consent produces an unsolvable confidentiality dilemma. From the perspective of preserving analytic freedom in the therapeutic relationship, the psychoanalytic patient should not have to be responsible to read, edit, and approve documents for release to an outside party. How can the patient give informed consent and at the same time preserve analytic freedom? For the informed-consent process to reliably serve the intended purposes, this consent would need to emerge from thorough analysis of the relevant conscious and unconscious conflicts and concerns of the patient regarding the information to be released and serve the patient and the analyst in the present and future course of the analysis and beyond. This task seems impossible. How can the patient give informed consent that answers unconscious concerns, such that the freely associative psychoanalytic treatment process is not encumbered? The process of review of managed care reports for informed consent would be likely to function as a process of premature analytic interpretation. This process will act as a magnet for unconscious defenses and resistances to analysis, drastically limiting the scope of analysis, especially in the direction of the most salient issues to be analyzed.

ANALYTIC LISTENING

By participating in a psychoanalytic treatment under managed care, the analyst divides attention between the patient and the need to be accountable to the case manager, which is a technical violation of the standard that the analyst maintain an even-hovering and undivided attention to the patient (Stone, 1961). Managed care reviewers press specific criteria for accountability in the direction of symptom focus and goal orientation. This influence forecloses the analyst's capacity for empathic-introspective immersion in the analytic listening process (Kohut, 1977).

Freud (1912) cautioned analysts about this sort of hazard to the psychoanalytic listening process:

> For as soon as anyone deliberately concentrates his attention to a certain degree, he begins to select from the material before him; one point will be fixed in his mind with particular clearness and some other will be correspondingly disregarded, and in making this selection he will be following his expectations or inclinations. This, however, is precisely what must not be done. In making this selection, if he follows his expectations he is in danger of never finding anything but what he already knows; and if he follows his inclinations he will certainly falsify what he may perceive. It must not be forgotten that the things one hears are for the most part things whose meaning is only recognized later on [p. 112].

The aim of the analyst is to listen to the patient in an openly receptive fashion that is empathic and unencumbered by preconception, focus or direction (Spruiell, 1983). The neutral, empathic recognition that the patient experiences through the process of analytic listening is a powerful therapeutic source from which can emerge a new integration, continuity and hope (Schwaber, 1990). The listening process is part of the art of psychoanalysis that encourages and allows the patient to explore transference manifestations and elucidate wishes, fears, fantasies, defenses, moral imperatives, and realistic concerns (Loewald, 1975).

This quality standard for analytic listening is violated by the intrusion of the case manager, who imposes different, nonpsychoanalytic criteria for treating and listening to the patient.

NEUTRALITY

Unlike most forms of psychotherapy, psychoanalysis does not restrict or focus the scope of the therapeutic endeavor. To do so would defeat the objective of a free and deep unconscious reach to shed light and reveal the unconscious roots of pathology. Objectives of psychoanalytic treatment must be regarded in very broad terms. A narrow definition of "objectives" is a technical violation of the psychoanalyst's essential technical neutrality and serves an antitherapeutic function by strengthening the patient's unconscious resistances that oppose analytic progress in treatment (Freud, 1913).

Analytic freedom is enhanced and sustained by the analyst's neutral, empathic-introspective approach to the patient (Kohut, 1977). This quality of analytic listening enhances the patient's freedom to say anything that comes to mind and to choose whether or not he or she will resolve symptoms or change patterns of behavior or choices in life (Stone, 1961; Greenson, 1972; Spruiell, 1983)

The philosophy of managed care aims to focus the analyst and the therapeutic task on those symptoms or behaviors which the third party agrees are important and away from those which the third party trivializes. The contamination of neutrality standards by managed care involvement in psychoanalysis is analogous to the danger visited upon a surgical procedure if a case manager were to intrude, stand beside the surgeon, break aseptic technique, frenetically bump the surgeon's arm to direct changes in surgical approach at moments when delicate surgical skill is required, and insist that the surgeon divert the use of one hand to write notes on the progress of the surgery and simultaneously perform single-handed surgery with the other.

ABSTINENCE

It is common that transference manifestations develop within the analytic setting at an early stage and replace troubling symptoms and behaviors that simultaneously improve or disappear in the extraanalytic arena. It is essential for the success of the analysis that this early symptomatic improvement be understood as temporary and dependent for ultimate resolution on the effective resolution of the transference phenomena within the analytic setting (Freud, 1909, 1913).

Managed care views treatment as complete and ready to end when troubling symptoms and behaviors resolve; managed care will urge a premature ending to psychoanalytic treatment at this early symptom-relief stage, when the patient is most emotionally vulnerable to betrayal, to relapse, and to suggestion that further analysis need not proceed (Stern, 1993). The delays and uncertainty that accompany appeals to higher managed care authorities will further erode the patient's trust and ability to participate actively in the psychoanalytic treatment process.

Subjecting patients to the foregoing intrusions and violations of core fundamentals of psychoanalytic technique that result from managed care involvement in psychoanalysis disrupts the analyst's ability to abstain from responding or behaving toward the patient in a manner that confirms and justifies the patient's neurotic childhood fears, wishes, and past pathological object relationships (Greenson, 1972; Gray, 1973, 1981; Langs, 1975; Arlow and Brenner, 1990; Etchegoyen, 1991)

When applied to psychoanalysis, managed care destroys the treatment it intends to review. According to Lawrence Friedman (1988), an effort to combine and integrate managed care philosophy and its reporting requirements with psychoanalysis is not an honest challenge for psychoanalysts to accept. He feels that all psychotherapy, including psychoanalysis, "runs counter to the needs of [cost containment] quality control," and he explains further:

> Architects can cater to society's demands while independent principles of engineering ensure that buildings do not collapse. Psychotherapy has no independent tool to safeguard treatment while styles of thinking go in search of money. Thinking is the only tool a psychotherapist has. . . . Inspectors have a different competence.
> Bureaucratic reality concerns what we must write in a record. It has nothing to do with what we think about what we write. Considerations of bookkeeping and social policy are properly involved in choosing patient and illness priorities, allocations of public monies, even modalities of treatment. But they have absolutely no jurisdiction over the principles of psychotherapy. . . . [However], because the profession does not agree on those principles, it is ill equipped to respond to nonprofessional demands in a principled manner. Psychotherapy is endangered by its unformed state, which leaves it open to inadvertent decisions based on irrelevant considerations. It has to be more on guard than any comparable practice. (Psychoanalysis enjoys a much greater consensus, but it is doubtful that even analysis would have survived without its private institutes [pp. 537–539].

Friedman's warning suggests that psychoanalysts must concern themselves with the preservation of the private base of practice and education if psychoanalysis as a profession is to survive efforts to contain and regulate it under insurance and entitlement programs that employ managed care. The legal and ethical responsibility for the decision to conduct psychoanalytic treatment under managed care conditions rests with the psychoanalyst (*respondeat superior*). Eagerness for the perceived security of insurance compensation for psychoanalysis and intensive psychotherapy is an example of what Eric Fromm (1941) termed an "escape from freedom". This eagerness threatens the loss, perhaps the extinction, of analytic freedom, and with it the profession of psychoanalysis, unless a substantial and sustainable private base for practice and education can be maintained outside the jurisdiction of the bureaucratic controllers.

Analytic freedom is vital but fragile. It must be assiduously protected. The history of psychoanalytic progress in the 20th century reveals bleak and often horrific episodes of analytic freedom's being lost through military occupation and war. In Vienna, in Budapest, in Prague, psychoanalysts were imprisoned and killed, or fled for their lives. A few remained. Some were reeducated to serve the interests of the state. Others practiced psychoanalysis in clandestine conditions where analytic freedom, abstinence, and neutrality in the treatment relationship were superseded by the role of analyst as de facto underground resistance fighter. Absent the horrors of occupation or war, the threat to analytic freedom in America comes by more subtle reaches for a greater market share.

Will American psychoanalysts retain analytic freedom and continue to make this country a safe harbor and a fountainhead for psychoanalytic thought, education, influence, and practice; or will American psychoanalysts become the next refugees from land where analytic freedom has been lost?

REERENCES

Arlow, J. & Brenner, C. (1990), The psychoanalytic process. *Psychoanal. Quart.*, 59:678–691.

Bollas, C. & Sundelson D. (1995), *The New Informants*. Northvale, NJ: Aronson.

Cummings, R. & Gray, S. H. (1996), Charting psychoanalysis, A clarification. Approved by Executive Council, American Psychoanalytic Association.

Dewald, P. (1965), Reactions to the forced termination of therapy. *Psychiat. Quart.*, 39: 102–126.

——— (1978), The psychoanalytic process in adult patients. *The Psychoanalytic Study of the Child*, 33:323-332. New Haven, CT: Yale University Press.

Dworkin, R. (1994), Will Clinton's plan be fair?—Health Security Act. *The New York Review of Books*, January 13, pp. 20–25.

Etchegoyen, R. H. (1991), *The Fundamentals of Psychoanalytic Technique*. London: Karnac Books.

Flexner, A. (1910), *The Flexner Report on Medical Education in the United States and Canada*. North Stratford, NH: Ayer, 1972.

Freud, S. (1909), Five lectures on psychoanalysis. *Standard Edition*, 11:50–52. London: Hogarth Press, 1957.

———— (1912), Recommendations to the physician practicing psycho-analysis. *Standard Edition*, 12:109–120. London: Hogarth Press, 1958.

———— (1913) On beginning the treatment. *Standard Edition*, 12:130-144. London: Hogarth Press, 1958.

Friedman, L. (1988) *The Anatomy of Psychotherapy.* Hillsdale, NJ: The Analytic Press.

Fromm, E. (1941) *Escape from Freedom.* New York: Holt, Rinehart & Winston, pp. 123–126, 157–230.

Gottschalk, L. and Whitman, R. (1962), Some typical complications mobilized by the psycho-analytic procedure. *Internat. J. Psycho-Anal.*, 43: 142–150.

Gray, S. H. (1973), Does insurance affect psychoanalytic practice? *Bull. Phil. Assn. Psychoanal.* 23:101-110.

———— (1981), Oral presentation to Psychoanalytic Association of New York. New York City, April.

———— (1983), Peer review in psychiatry. Presented to Delaware Psychiatric Society, Wilmington, March.

———— (1990), Utilization and managed care review: The psychoanalyst's perspective. Presented to American Psychoanalytic Association., Miami Beach, FL, December.

———— (1992), Quality assurance and utilization review of individual medical psychotherapies. *The Manual of Psychiatric Quality Assurance*, ed. M. R. Mattson. Washington DC: American Psychiatric Association, pp. 153–159.

———— (1993), Preauthorization of long-term medical psychotherapy. Presented to American Psychiatric Association. Philadelphia, PA, May.

Gray, S. H. & Beigler, J. & Goldstein, J. (1995), Informed consent to review. *Amer. Psychoanalyst*, 29(1):3a–4a.

———— & Cummings, R. (1995), Charting psychoanalysis. *Amer. Psychoanalyst*, 29(2): 3a–6a›.

Greenson, R. (1972), *The Technique and Practice of Psychoanalysis, Vol. 1.* New York: International Universities Press.

Hiltzink, M. & Olmos, D. (1995), The health care revolution: remaking medicine in California. *Los Angeles Times*, August 27, pp. 1, 20–22.

Hoffman, L. (1994), Open letter to the executive committee, American Psychoanalytic Association. January 9.

Judd, L. (1994), Understanding the politics of mental illness. *Psychiatric Times*, March, pp. 46–47.

Kohut, H. (1977), *The Restoration of the Self.* New York: International Universities Press.

Langs, R. (1975), The therapeutic relationship and deviations in technique. *Internat. J. Psychoanal. Psychother.* 4:106–141.

———— (1976a), *The Bipersonal Field.* New York: Aronson.

———— (1976b), *The Therapeutic Interaction.* New York: Aronson.

Lewin, T. (1996), Questions of privacy roil arena of psychotherapy. *New York Times*, May 22, pp. 1, 10.

Loewald, H. W. (1975), Psychoanalysis as an art and the fantasy character of the psychoanalytic situation. *J. Amer. Psychoanal. Assn.*, 23:277–299.

Mattson, M. R. & Wilson, G. F. (1992), Ethics of peer review. In: *The Manual of Psychiatric Quality Assurance*, ed. M. R. Mattson. Washington, DC: American Psychiatric Assn., pp. 37–39.

Schwaber, E. A. (1990), Interpretation and the therapeutic action of psychoanalysis. *Internat. J. Psycho–Anal.*, 71: 229–240.

Smolowe, J. & Perman, S. & Van Tassel, J. (1996), A healthy merger? *Time*, April 15, pp. 77–78.

Spruiell, V. (1983), The rules and frames of the psychoanalytic situation. *Psychoanal. Quart.*, 52:1–33.

Stern, S. (1993), Managed care, brief therapy, and therapeutic integrity. *Psychother.*, 30:162–175

Stone, L. (1961), *The Psychoanalytic Situation*. New York: International Universities Press.

Wilson, G. F. (1992a), Defining and measuring quality. In: *The Manual of Psychiatric Quality Assurance*, ed. M. R. Mattson. Washington, DC: American Psychiatric Assn., pp. 19–21.

———— (1992b), Legal aspects of quality assurance. In: *The Manual of Psychiatric Quality Assurance*, ed. M. R. Mattson. Washington, DC: American Psychiatric Assn., pp. 31–36.

Wilson, G. F. & Phillips, K. L. (1992), Concepts and definitions used in quality assurance and utilization review. In: *The Manual of Psychiatric Quality Assurance*, ed. M. R. Mattson. Washington, DC: American Psychiatric Assn., pp. 23–30.

Winnicott, D. W. (1965), *The Maturational Processes and the Facilitating Environment*. London: Hogarth Press.

———— (1970), The mother-infant experience of mutuality. In: *Parenthood*, ed. E. J. Anthony & T. Benedek. Boston: Little, Brown, pp. 245–56.

Wolf, A., Bridburg, R., Ciccone, J. R., Kirby, E., Deutschman, D., Reading, A., Caesar, G., Rose, C. Beigler, J. & Deutschman, D. (1987), Confidentiality. In: *The Manual Psychiatric Quality Assurance*, ed. M. R. Mattson. Washington, DC: American Psychiatric Assn., 1992, pp. 44–46.

TEN

Privacy and Confidentiality

Issues in Psychoanalysis
In the 90s

RUSS NEWMAN

In their chapters, Sundelson and Cummings have presented two instances of outside intrusion into the confidential and private realm of psychotherapy, one dealing with child abuse-reporting laws and the other with managed care cost-containment strategies. In an attempt to determine what lessons may be learned from the two overlapping but different situations, an analysis of significant similarities may be of benefit.

To begin with, both mandated reporting laws and managed care cost-containment techniques appear to be overreactions to real problems in need of remedies. Additionally, each appears to be an overly simplified reaction to actual problems. The real problems inherent in potential child abuse are, without question, the danger of abuses occurring and injury inflicted on the victim. Responding to these problems, however, by mandating a law that treats every actual and potential instance of child abuse as though they all were identical, leaves much to be desired of this so-called solution. In fact, responding to all instances in the same manner, when involved individuals are already receiving psychotherapy or other forms of treatment, poses a high risk of interfering with the very interventions intended to help deal with the problem of child abuse. In other words, reflexively requiring a psychotherapist to report any suspected child abuse to outside authorities runs the risk of interfering with a treatment perhaps already attempting to prevent any further instances of abuse.

Similarly, managed care cost-containment is an attempt to respond to the real problem of rising health care costs in this country. Yet, it is an overly simplified attempt to solve this problem by focusing only on cost while ignoring the quality of treatment being provided. To the extent that quality treatment is interfered with or lost, the so-called remedy to the cost problem may actually contribute to the problem rather than help solve it. In fact, the continued application of managed care strategies that attempt to contain costs in the short term but do not, in the long run, contain costs at all is a common occurrence consequent to what may be referred to as this country's "cost-containment neurosis." Neurosis—in the conventional sense of defensive coping mechanisms and styles—is defined as a self-defeating attempt to solve an immediate problem and alleviate current anxiety while actually perpetuating the very problem the neurotic behavior is intended to address. Overaggressive attempts to contain costs through managed care strategies that sacrifice quality follow the same pattern. There is perhaps no more expensive treatment than inadequate treatment or no treatment when treatment is necessary, as it results in the need for more intensive and more costly treatment in the long run. Yet the anxiety created by the increasing cost of health care in this country appears to perpetuate the use of this self-defeating strategy, providing positive short-term bottom line results, but a long-term increase in treatment cost.

Managed care cost-containment strategies and mandated reporting laws alike clearly share a consequent interference with the psychotherapeutic and psychoanalytic processes. The interference in each case is the result of society's having balanced the various priorities and interests involved and determining that the treatment process is a lesser priority. The legal system provides various mechanisms for balancing these competing priorities. In the area of child abuse reporting, the constitutional test of a mandatory reporting statute is whether or not the government can demonstrate a "compelling state interest" to warrant the intrusion into otherwise protected individual privacy. In other words, the interests of the state are balanced against the individual citizen's right to privacy. At first blush and assuming a constitutionally valid reporting law, it appears that the state's interest is compelling and outweighs the individual's right to privacy. On closer inspection, however, it may actually be that even the state's interest is not adequately served by mandatory child abuse reporting laws, which further compound the problems created by sacrificing individual privacy as the following analysis demonstrates.

Most legislatures that have advanced child abuse reporting laws identify two state interests to be served: protection of the child and providing an abuser or potential abuser with the necessary services or treatment to prevent future instances of abuse. The oversimplification of mandatory child abuse reporting laws to address a complex problem is exemplified by the fact that the reporting law applies similarly to persons already in treatment and to persons not in treatment, despite the different "policy implications" inherent in each. In other words, no determination is made as to which interest is the priority in each case despite actual differences in the weight of the interests to be balanced. If one of the interests to be served by mandatory reporting is securing treatment and the relevant individual is already in treatment, questions should at least be raised as to the appropriateness of applying the law in that instance. It may be that the relevant interests are not really balanced at all; that is, sacrificing the individual's right to privacy may not be justified if the state's interest is not served. Even more problematic, the mandatory reporting solution to the child abuse problem may actually interfere with the very treatment the law intends to secure and, therefore, works against the state's public protection interest.

The intrusion and interference of treatment by managed care cost-containment strategies is more difficult to understand in the context of a direct legal analysis, but perhaps an analogous legal analysis will be instructive. While such cost-containment strategies do not, for the most part, present constitutional issues of privacy, they do present some similarities to the issues involved in the duty to protect doctrine created by the California courts in the case of *Tarasoff v. Regents of the University of California* (1976).[1] The civil liabilities and legal duties of the therapist in *Tarasoff*-type situations are the result of the court's attempts to balance the interests involved. According to the court in *Tarasoff*, "the protective privilege ends where public peril begins." In effect, the court balanced a public protection interest against the patient's right to privileged communication in treatment. The court also acknowledged an individual's right to receive treatment as a necessary part of the balancing process in determining the legal obligation imposed on the therapist.

The significance of striking the correct balance between an individual's right to treatment and privacy, on one hand, and the public's right to be protected, on the other, is paradoxically best exemplified by what may happen if the balance is incorrectly struck and the therapist is inappropriately obliged to breach the patient's confidentiality. The result is likely to be that people who have problems with aggression and who are in need of treatment will not seek it for fear of having to communicate problems that their therapists will be forced to disclose to the authorities. Alternatively, a person who does seek treatment may be unwilling to talk about the very problem for which treatment is needed for fear of triggering the therapist's disclosure to the authorities. Or people who do seek treatment and discuss their difficulties with aggressive thoughts and feelings may find the therapy intruded on by outside authorities in such a way that effective treatment becomes impossible.

---

[1] Tarasoff v. Regents of the University of California, 17 Cal. 3d 425, 551 P.2d 334, 131. Rptr. 14 (1976).

To extend this type of legal analysis to managed care cost-containment strategies, a person's right to quality treatment must be balanced with the need to contain costs in a health care system under which costs are spiraling out of control. The courts have, in fact, begun to do just such a balancing of interests; where the interest in cost-containment has so outweighed an interest in quality care that patients are injured, managed care entities can be held liable for those injuries. Beginning with the California cases of *Wickline v. State of California* (1987)[2] and *Wilson v. Blue Cross of Southern California* (1990),[3] courts have held that a third-party payer or managed care entity can be held responsible for negligently designed or implemented cost-containment strategies that result in patient injury. It can be argued, then, that if managed care cost-containment has foreclosed the ability to provide treatment and resulting injury to patients can be demonstrated, liability to managed care entitles will occur. Further, in a government-sponsored managed care plan, like a federal or state health reform plan relying on managed care strategies, a violation of an individual's constitutional right to be free of government intrusion may be found.

What is apparent from both child abuse reporting laws and the development of managed care cost-containment strategies is an increasing intrusion of outside influences on the heretofore protected and private treatment process. More problematic, however, is the apparently forced transformation of the therapist's role from agent of change on behalf of the individual to agent on behalf of other societal interests. Nowhere is this clearer than with child abuse reporting mandates under which the therapist in effect becomes an agent of the state who is privy to information about an individual that the state is otherwise unable to obtain. Where managed care cost-containment strategies are concerned, the therapist is being forced to act on behalf of society's economic interests, or perhaps even as an agent of industrialization, rather than solely on behalf of the individual patient's best interests.

Consistent with this forced role-transformation of the therapist, there occurs an alteration of function by the therapist under the press of either child abuse reporting mandates or managed care cost-containment. This alteration is perhaps best described as the negation of the therapist's ability to behave truly objectively or to function as an "observing ego" during the therapeutic process. In fact, it can be argued that reporting laws not only negate the therapist's observing ego function but also force the thera-

---

[2] Wickline v. State of California, 239 Cal. Rptr. 805, 741 P.2d 613 (1987).

[3] Wilson v. Blue Cross of Southern California, 271 Cal. Rptr. 876 (Cal. App. 2 Dist.).

pist to function more in a superego role. In any event, the requisite neutrality of the therapist and the therapeutic process is contaminated.

From a slightly different perspective, what results from mandatory reporting laws and managed care cost-containment strategies is a breach of the therapeutic boundary and containment by forces external to the patient–therapist relationship. Reports of suspected child abuse disclose otherwise confidential communications from patient to therapist and invite further denigration of the containment from outside investigatory authorities. What results from cost-containment strategies is perhaps best illustrated by the effects on confidentiality when the third-party payer is able to intrude into the psychotherapy process. The adverse effects on the containment of the therapy and the neutrality of the therapist are likely to go well beyond the need to provide information about the psychotherapy and the patient to a party outside the therapeutic dyad.

In the end, the key to preserving the therapeutic process in these instances will, of course, be the adequacy with which relevant interests are balanced—an individual's interest in privacy and effective treatment, on one hand, with society's interests in public protection and economic stability on the other. While each of us in our role as therapist must do what we can to maintain this balance, we are also obliged as a profession to press to ensure that Congress, state legislatures, and the courts provide the necessary foundation for maintaining an adequate balance (Newman, 1987).

REFERENCES

Newman, R. (1987, August), The psychotherapist's duty to report child abuse and the legislature's duty to strike a better balance. Presented at annual meeting of American Psychological Association, New York City.

PART III

International Perspectives

ELEVEN

National Health Insurance Coverage of Psychoanalysis and Psychotherapy

An International Review Highlighting Some Current Problems

BRENT WILLOCK

CHRISTA BALZERT

AHMED FAYEK

JULIAN ABRAHAM

GLOBAL PERSPECTIVE

As citizens and psychoanalysts, we live increasingly in the global village anticipated by Marshall McLuhan. Most analysts now belong to one or more of the growing number of transnational associations, such as the International Psychoanalytic Association, the International Federation of Psychoanalytic Societies, or the International Federation for Psychoanalytic Education. An increasing number of analysts simultaneously hold teaching appointments in more than one country. Trade restrictions and other boundaries between nations are being relaxed, even dissolved. Goods and services move between countries more expeditiously than ever before. Information is transmitted almost instantaneously on the electronic "information superhighway." Ideas, such as those in this book, can be conveyed with unprecedented speed to interested parties anywhere on the planet. Such knowledge may be used by health care researchers, administrators, professional organizations, and consumer groups to inform policy development and support crucial policy changes.

Despite the accelerated rate of global interconnectedness and information exchange, in some areas, including health care, it sometimes feels as if true progress is elusive, or agonizingly slow. At times, the balance between progressive and regressive forces seems seriously askew. Bad news, such as the rapid growth of managed care in the United States (Barron and Sands, 1996), sometimes appears to travel faster than good news. In a global village, current practice in one area may soon be implemented in other jurisdictions. In challenging economic times, such changes may be highly undesirable from the point of view of increasing accessibility to high quality mental health care. It is, therefore, very much in the interests of both the public and professionals to become more aware of how psychoanalysts and psychotherapists manage and are managed around the world.

Some national health insurance plans can be regarded as generally positive models. Citizens, analysts, and therapists will want to incorporate the best features of these schemes into the systems evolving in their own countries. Other plans can serve as negative models; they have features whose incorporation into their countries' plans citizens, analysts, and therapists would, no doubt, strenuously want to oppose. Whether a health system is predominantly good or bad, there is much to be learned from it.

Each health insurance plan has many idiosyncratic characteristics. It is important to understand these features not just as isolated peculiarities, but as often representing the outcome of dynamic struggles between competing forces. National health insurance schemes can be regarded as compromise formations, some of which are more far more creative, integrative, flexible, and adaptive than others are.

It is our hope that both the good news and the bad news in this chapter will move far, fast, and wide, contributing to the expansion of consciousness of what is transpiring, and what could happen, in relation to public funding of two very important aspects of national health care, namely psychoanalysis and psychotherapy.

ONE PSYCHOANALYSIS OR MANY?

During the past decade, there have been animated discussions in the analytic literature on the topic "One psychoanalysis or many?" (Wallerstein, 1988). This debate typically refers to the question of whether or not distinctive psychoanalytic perspectives (such as ego psychology, Kleinian analysis, self psychology) can be integrated into a single body of psychoanalytic theory and practice. The query is sometimes raised as to whether certain of these orientations are actually psychoanalytic.

Similar to the global village situation described previously, an integrationist viewpoint is currently gaining momentum in our discipline. Some of the bitter feuds that have long divided some psychoanalytic groups appear to be lessening. This reduced fragmentation seems to reflect a healthy maturational process as psychoanalysis enters its second century. This promising trend toward greater cohesion may also be facilitated by a feeling among analysts in the current political, economic, and sociocultural climate of managed care and "Freud bashing" that united we stand, divided we fall.

There is another version of the "one psychoanalysis or many" debate which is rarely discussed in the analytic literature. Nonetheless, it constitutes a major topic that is sometimes passionately discussed in small groups, in informal settings, and in professional newsletters. This shadow version of the more customary query could be stated as follows: Is there simply one psychoanalysis, or is there medical psychoanalysis, psychological psychoanalysis, and perhaps a variety of other psychoanalyses, like social work psychoanalysis, theological or pastoral psychoanalysis, sociological psychoanalysis, philosophical psychoanalysis, and so forth?

Such questions generated controversy even in Freud's day. Freud (1926) viewed psychoanalysis as "part of psychology; not of medical psychology in the old sense, not of the psychology of morbid processes, but simply of psychology" (p. 252). He feared the potentially adverse effects of excessive medical influence on the development of the discipline that he had founded and about which he cared so deeply. In his musings on the ideal psychoanalytic curriculum, Freud envisioned analysis as being tremendously enriched by contributions from many related fields: "We do not consider it at all desirable for psychoanalysis to be swallowed up by medicine and to find its last resting-place in a text-book of psychiatry under the heading "Methods of Treatment' . . . It deserves a better fate and, it may be hoped, will meet with one" (p. 248).

The manner in which psychoanalysis is treated under national health insurance plans is a major factor influencing the destiny of the discipline. If psychoanalysis is understood as a multifaceted intellectual discipline bridging the sciences and the humanities and constituting a powerful, sophisticated means of psychological health care, then the fate of analysis may be a positive one, as Freud so ardently hoped. If, however, national health insurance plans construe psychoanalysis as nothing but a, perhaps questionable, medical method of treatment, then the fate of analysis may move increasingly in the dismal direction Freud feared.

Government and private insurers are not very interested in the debate about which psychoanalysts organize symposia and publish papers, that is, the controversy concerning theoretical monism versus pluralism. If insurance plans do cover analysis, they typically do not care whether those conducting the treatments have a classical, object relational, or Kohutian perspective. Insurers can, however, take considerable interest in the question, one psychoanalysis or many, when it refers to the thorny problem that analysts do not write much about. Insuring bodies adopt positions on this matter and create policies that have major repercussions in the real world. Thus some countries fund analytic treatment, but only when it is provided by physicians; these health plan authorities evidently believe there is but one true psychoanalysis, namely, medical psychoanalysis. Other countries fund analysis when it is conducted by either psychologists or medical doctors; these countries believe there are two psychoanalyses, not many. In rare instances, a nation acts according to the belief that there is one psychoanalysis composed of many professionals having diverse academic backgrounds prior to pursuing formal analytic training; these exceptional states provide coverage for psychoanalytic treatment regardless of the earlier academic background of the qualified analyst.

In reviewing the national health insurance plans of a number of countries, we must not lose sight of this important variant of the question concerning one psychoanalysis or many. Bearing in mind the need to provide some redress to this hitherto relatively neglected issue, we can, from this perspective, divide national health insurance plans that cover analysis and psychotherapy into two basic types: the reasonably progressive, rational, equitable plans and the more irrational, antiquated, inequitable schemes. It is our hope that, by our contrasting these systems, in future deliberations and revisions of outdated insurance arrangements, the progressive plans may have a greater chance of positively influencing the more archaic schemes.

REASONABLY RATIONAL, PROGRESSIVE, EQUITABLE PLANS

Finland

Sjodin (1994) described psychoanalysis in Finland. There, analysis is covered by the national health insurance plan, regardless of the academic specialization the analyst had before undertaking psychoanalytic training. Educational facilities, like the Therapeia Institute, accept persons from such disciplines as psychiatry, psychology, and theology into their psychoanalytic training programs. There is no law restricting the right to practice therapy or analysis to those who have had formal training in these areas. Only analysts (and therapists) who have graduated and received a certificate from an authorized training institute, however, are eligible to be on the register of competent analysts that is administered by the national authorities. Only patients treated by these therapists and analysts can receive public funding for their treatment.

Analysands must be referred for treatment by a psychiatrist. (This gatekeeping role assigned to one profession or specialty would not be acceptable to all analysts in all countries.) The referring psychiatrist must attest to the patient's "failing working capacity." The system makes treatment available for the entire working population. Citizens who are unable to work at all are not covered under this plan. They may obtain treatment at public clinics. Seventy percent of analytic treatments are financed by the National Medical Insurance or some other insurance system; 30% of patients pay personally for their treatment.

Check up reports by the analyst and a psychiatrist have to be provided annually. This feature would not be palatable to all analysts as it has potential to be a disruptive influence on the treatment, may constitute unnecessary expense, and privileges one mental health discipline over others.

The Finnish plan pays for up to three years of treatment at a frequency of up to three sessions per week. Patients may pay for additional sessions and may thus be able to create a more "classical," long-term, intensive (four or five times per week) analysis. This freedom for patients to obtain additional sessions is extremely important. As we shall see, there are countries, or jurisdictions within countries, that will not permit citizens to use their discretionary income to purchase more intensive treatment. Some jurisdictions discourage, or actually forbid, analysts from providing additional sessions, even for free.

In summary, the Finnish system has many highly desirable features. While no plan is absolutely perfect, the Finns have created a model for the delivery of psychoanalytic treatment that should be carefully studied by those concerned with health care policy in every country.

The Czech Republic

Sociocultural, historical, and political factors are always important for understanding the position of psychology and psychoanalysis in any nation. In countries behind the Iron Curtain, these disciplines were officially devalued as bourgeois science. Czech history shows particularly clearly how the well-being of psychology in general, and psychoanalysis in particular, depends on the relationship these fields of inquiry and intervention have with the wider sociopolitical system in which they are embedded.

Sebek (1993) described how psychoanalysis was developing nicely in Czechoslovakia until the Nazis seized control. Some analysts continued to work illegally during the fascist occupation. During the brief interval of freedom from 1945 to 1948, some positive developments took place. This promising period was terminated when the Communists declared psycho-analysis illegal, and for the next 41 years analysis continued to be practiced only in secret, to a limited degree, in defiance of the law. Within months after the revolution of November 1989, the Czechoslovakian Psychoana-lytical Society was established, officially ending the dark age in which analysis could be studied and conducted only underground.

During the recent revolution, Czech psychologists treated citizens who had been beaten and traumatized. Their efforts became widely known, and people came to see psychology in a new light, markedly different from the devaluing perspective promulgated by the totalitarian government. Many psychologists and other therapists worked in the political under-ground prior to the revolution and developed close relationships with political figures who later came to hold influential positions in the new government. A prime example among such personages is President Vaclav Havel, a leader who holds psychology in high esteem. After liberation, psychologists had the opportunity to work vigorously with the new gov-ernment to reform the entire health care system. They struggled to create a system that would optimally respond to patients' needs. They developed a reputation for being reliable professionals with a broad commitment to human welfare rather than merely being practitioners dedicated to their own interests.

The outcome of all these efforts by Czech therapists and analysts has been very encouraging. Health care is now financed through insurance companies. Everyone is insured. There are no differences in psychotherapy coverage among the various companies. Analysis and therapy are fully cov-ered when performed by qualified practitioners, who include social work-ers if they have the appropriate training and have passed mental health specialist examinations set by the Ministry of Health.

Three levels of psychotherapy are recognized: 1) psychotherapy sup-port—any psychologist or medical doctor is considered to have adequate training to provide up to 10 hours of psychotherapy to a patient in a year; 2) nonspecific psychotherapy—any clinical psychologist or psychiatrist is considered to have sufficient training to treat a patient for up to 100 ses-sions per year; and 3) psychoanalysis—qualified analysts can see patients up to five days a week for as many years as is necessary.

This recognition of levels of qualification is far superior to the com-paratively backward, outdated systems prevalent in such countries as Canada and Australia, which, as we shall see, fail to recognize even the grossest differences in professional training and skill between highly trained clini-cal psychologists and psychiatrists, with or without psychoanalytic qualifi-cations, on one hand, and relatively untrained, general practitioners practicing psychotherapy on the other hand. The Czech plan, in marked contrast, appears to be both rational and equitable.

Czech psychologists and their patients won the right to initiate treatment without medical referral, but later lost that privilege, except for patients in crisis or after trauma. Czech psychologists are fighting to restore this important right. There is a lesson here for citizens, therapists, and analysts in all countries. The struggle between progressive and regressive forces never ends. Citizens and mental health professionals have to be constantly on guard to preserve improvements achieved in health care systems. We will see how the experience of analysts in other countries strongly supports this conclusion.

Czech therapists almost succeeded in establishing psychotherapy as one of the seven basic specializations, like internal medicine, gynecology, and surgery. It is now considered a secondary specialization. One has to be a specialist first, then achieve certification in psychotherapy. Jiri Ruzicka (1994, personal communication), a leading Czech psychoanalyst, was extremely helpful in providing me (Willock) with greater understanding of these developments in his country. He believed the situation in neighbouring Slovakia was similar, although the medical influence there appeared slightly stronger. Ruzicka thought the situation in Poland was similar. According to Pawlak and Sokolik (1992), there are about 30 people in Poland with close affiliations to psychoanalysis. These individuals all belong to the Psychoanalytic Section of the Polish Psychological Society.

Norway

The Norwegian system, as described by Sjodin (1994), appears reasonably equitable. Citizens have the right to have their treatment paid by the national social insurance system, fully or partly, depending on the contract their therapist has with the local authorities. Some psychologists and psychiatrists in private practice are paid partly by the National Medical Insurance and partly by the local community. Other practitioners do not have a contract with the local community. They are paid by the National Insurance and the patient. There is no private insurance.

Unfortunately, patients treated by practitioners who set up their practice after October 1992 have to pay for their treatments completely by themselves. It is expected that this limitation may have a choking effect on the private practice of psychotherapy. Again, there is a message here for all citizens, therapists, and analysts. Good systems will be weakened or even destroyed unless we continuously struggle to improve them. Many situations in other countries underscore how economic concerns can lead to significant cutbacks in the availability of psychotherapy and psychoanalysis.

Germany[1]

Germany's health and social welfare system has changed only slightly since it was introduced over one hundred years ago. Ninety percent of the citizens are covered by the unified public health insurance system, every student, worker, and retiree has health insurance. Employers withhold a sum from each paycheck and contribute a matching amount to the national health agency. Each citizen may request on a quarterly basis a referral from the regional health agency for a consultation with a primary care physician. The physician may, in turn, refer the patient to a specialist or a hospital. Health care providers are reimbursed directly. No additional copayment is required from the patient. Providers follow a fee structure agreed on by the German Medical Association and the Affiliation of Providers of the Health Administration. Citizens may purchase additional insurance from private companies to cover special needs.

The public health insurance system consumes 8.6% of the gross national product. In comparison, the United States spends 14.2% of its GNP on health care. Germany is in the middle range of health care spending, after the United States, Canada, France, Austria, Switzerland, and Italy (according to figures from the Organization for Economic Cooperation and Development, cited in the German newspaper, *Ruhr Nachrichten,* Jan. 29, 1997).

From the beginning, the place of psychotherapy was poorly defined within the health insurance system. There have, however, been some very interesting developments in this area over the past three decades. Legislative guidelines for psychotherapy were established in 1967. Originally, therapy was covered only if the symptoms of an acute neurotic disorder were targeted. The guidelines required the therapist to demonstrate, in a detailed report, that such an illness was present and that psychotherapy was a treatment method necessary, appropriate, and sufficiently promising as to outcome.

In the late 1970s, political liberalization and increased efforts by psychologists and other therapists and analysts led to greater recognition of the importance of psychotherapy for the health of society. From 1976 onward, structural changes (e.g., the analysis of character neuroses without acute symptoms) came to be regarded as constituting acceptable treatment goals within the scope of the guidelines for psychotherapy. This development represented a major breakthrough.

According to the psychotherapy guidelines, only therapists with a

---

[1] This discussion is drawn largely from Balzert (1994 and subsequent personal communications) and, to a much lesser extent, Sjodin (1994).

degree in medicine or psychology were eligible for reimbursement, even though professionals with other degrees were trained and accredited by the German Psychoanalytic Association. In comparison to a country like Finland, there continues to be in Germany, to a much greater extent, a category of analysts whose patients do not have access to state insurance reimbursement. Germany is, nonetheless, far more advanced in this regard than Canada and Australia.

Until recently, a psychologist could only treat patients who had been referred by a physician. Under this referral procedure, a physician had to request the treatment and, at least in principle, remain responsible for the therapy; the physician charged the insurance agency for the services rendered by the psychologist and justified the ongoing treatment via extensive reports at regular intervals.

The German psychoanalytic community, the largest in the world after the United States, is composed of approximately equal numbers of psychologists and psychiatrists. (It is notable how much this composition differs from that of the American Psychoanalytic Association, although the imbalance in the United States is changing as a result of the successful lawsuit brought against the American and International Psychoanalytic Associations by American psychologists.) Collegial relationships among German analysts from different disciplinary backgrounds have historically been good. Consequently, the referral procedure did not create too much difficulty. Recently, however, that aspect of the guidelines did become a greater source of conflict and controversy between medical and nonmedical psychotherapists.

Under the psychotherapy guidelines, a panel of consultants appointed by the National Insurance Agency renders a decision concerning the treatment modality proposed by the therapist. Their judgment is based on a catalogue of guidelines. No connection is made between diagnosis and permissible number of sessions. Treatment can be approved for 80 sessions at a time, with a limit of 300 sessions. (Under a recent health care reform movement, however, there appeared to be a trend toward reducing the total number of sessions, as well as the number certified at each request.)

The limitation of 300 sessions posed a problem when psychoanalysis was the treatment of choice. The German health care system embraces the principle that, as long a treatment has the potential to ameliorate a disorder, it should be funded. There was, for years, a silent understanding between the health authorities and psychoanalysts that created an illusion that each party was fulfilling its mandate. The panel of consultants affirmed the possibility of improvement up to the 300th session, but not beyond. Analysts made private arrangements with their patients after the 300-session limit had been reached. (This system thus had some com-

monalities with the Finnish system, although the latter plan, which funds
three sessions per week for three years, is significantly more supportive of
patients needing analytic treatment.) Eighty-five percent of psychoanalytic treatments are funded by the National Insurance Agency; 15% are
funded by private insurance. Only 15% of patients pay for continuing
treatment once their insurance limit has been reached.

Various problems in the psychotherapy guidelines created increasing
strain that eventually led to bitter struggles between consumers and providers on one side and the health administration on the other. There was
also polarization among provider groups, which were accorded different
status under the guidelines. It became obvious that new mental health
regulations were needed. After several years of discussion between consumers, providers, and the Department of Health, a new bill, commonly
referred to as the Psychotherapists' Law, was introduced in 1993. This bill
included, for the first time, two nonmedical professions—the psycholo-
gist/psychotherapist and the child and adolescent psychotherapist—as
independent providers.

Reimbursement was to be restricted to procedures believed to have
been empirically validated. This criterion was said to have been met by
depth psychological/psychoanalytic therapy and behavior therapy, but not
by Rogerian, Gestalt, or art therapy. (Given the well-known research done
by Carl Rogers and his colleagues, one wonders how much political clout
had to do with decisions regarding what has been empirically validated.)
High frequency psychoanalysis was originally included as one of the empirically validated methods. Later it was rejected and, later still, reincluded,
as we shall see.

German analysts welcomed some of the changes proposed in the Psychotherapists' Law. They were, however, also becoming increasingly concerned about state control over the choice of therapeutic method and
frequency of sessions. The independent psychoanalytic institutes feared
that training and accreditation would be increasingly determined by the
government, with the possibility of state boards of examiners being instituted that were ignorant of, or hostile to, the analytic approach. The proposed inclusion of two new independent provider groups constituted
significant progress, although the exclusion of other provider groups was
a continuing problem.

This bill failed to pass in the 1993 legislative period because of two
main obstacles. First, the federal government proposed a 40% copayment
for psychotherapy. This amount was eventually reduced to 25%, with an
exemption for children and adolescents. Aiming to bring psychotherapy
coverage more in line with the coverage provided for other medical conditions, the political opposition, the states, and consumer and other interest
groups insisted on either no copayment or a maximum of 10%. They ar-

gued that high copayments discriminated against citizens with mental health problems and that the poor would likely be treated with cheaper (psychopharmacological) methods. The second obstacle confronting the bill was that the amount allotted for nonmedical providers of psychotherapy, 1.25% of the total health care budget, was considered too low, given the number of practitioners and the need for mental health services.

The arrangement based on the illusion that psychoanalysis could characteristically be conducted within a 300-session limit, and the associated denial of the existence of treatable illness beyond that point, created a strained compromise that eventually broke down. The arrangement was challenged by a group of patients and analysts who must have felt it was not in the spirit of truth for which psychoanalysis stands, nor in their interests, to support the fiction that gains in all cases accrue only before the 300th session. In response, in December 1992, the National Insurance Agency decided that only "psychoanalytic therapy" with a limit of three sessions per week would be covered under the guidelines. The agency claimed that it could no longer support higher frequency psychoanalysis, as the need for more frequent sessions had not, they claimed, been demonstrated empirically. At this reduced frequency, the length of analytic treatment could be extended somewhat, with no additional cost to the system. The agency was supported in this policy change by one faction of the divided psychoanalytic community. Another faction opposed this alteration vehemently.

By this time, it had become painfully clear to the German Psychoanalytic Association that the psychotherapy guidelines were interfering with clinical decisions made by analysts and that the State Board was making judgments on the scientific merits of psychoanalysis as a theory and as a method of treatment. The president of the GPA reported (Gattig, 1996) that requests were being made by the State Board for German institutes to change their training guidelines so that three sessions per week would become standard for students' control cases. The GPA refused to comply. Since 1992, candidates have often provided the required fourth weekly session without receiving remuneration for it.

German analysts decided to challenge in court the exclusion of high frequency psychoanalysis from insurance coverage. They gathered evidence for its medical necessity, appropriateness, and economic soundness. Two volumes of case histories were published documenting the efficacy of long-term psychoanalytic treatment (Henseler and Wegner, 1993). In an effort to make psychoanalysis more transparent and accessible, a manual was published describing the analytic method, including the high frequency version, in a language corresponding to the criteria of the insurance system (Danckward and Gattig, 1995). This threatened class action suit ended in a settlement. Fourth sessions that had not been funded were reimbursed retroactively. The health plan administration revoked their judgment that long-term treatment with four or more sessions per week was unscientific. Henceforth, more than three sessions per week would be covered for a certain period of time when substantiated in special applications. The norm in analytic psychotherapy continues, however, to be two or three weekly sessions, with a 300-session limit.

The most recent crisis in the efforts to arrive at a Psychotherapists' Law related to the refusal by the powerful association of medical health insurance providers (*Kassenaerztliche Vereinigung*) to include qualified psychologists on an equal level with medical psychotherapists in the national insurance system. Over the last few years, the different professional groups, in discussions with the government, seemed to have arrived at an "Integration Model." At a meeting in September 1997, however, representatives of the medical establishment voted 50 against 42 to exclude psychologists from equal status in the national health care system.

Fortunately, the antiprogressive stance of the association of medical health insurance providers was ultimately defeated. A new "Law about the professions of the psychological psychotherapist and the child- and adolescent therapist" was publicized in the federal *Law Journal* on June 16, 1998. This "Psychotherapists Law" is effective January, 1, 1999.

The new law recognizes two new, independent professions. These therapists must have postgraduate training in scientifically recognized psychotherapeutic technique from a federally approved institution. Psychologists will no longer require "delegation" by medical doctors. They will be able, instead, to determine independently the indication for treatment. Decisions concerning eligibility for insurance will be made by regional representatives regulating the federal health insurance. These representatives may restrict the number of psychotherapists practicing in overserviced areas, just as they do with medical specialists. There continues to be some controversy concerning the required co-payment of 10 DM (approximately U.S. $4).

It has been exciting to follow the struggle between the progressive and the regressive forces in the German health care system as they have fought to try to win the day for their vision of how psychological treatment should be offered, and denied, to the public. It has been particularly exhilerating to see some real, concrete advances achieved by those who have advocated for the public's need to have increased access to a greater number and variety of highly trained psychological health care professionals. It is especially noteworthy that the German health care system has been able to secure these improvements during challenging economic times.

Since the beginning of this decade, German analysts have made themselves increasingly heard in the public health care debate. Most analysts wish to practice within the system, and for good reasons. Participation gives analysts a strong voice with respect to mental health issues. It allows for a clear differentiation of the specific contributions of psychoanalysis in comparison with other methods, and such involvement may be essential for the economic security of the practising analyst. The challenge is how to participate in a national health care system, with its unavoidable regulations, without losing one's identity and independence. In this negotiation process to date, a good deal of external and internal conflict and acrimony has arisen. Some of these problems might have been avoided if German analysts as a group had entered the political debate at an earlier point. For a long time, only a handful participated actively in the public discussion. Many analysts felt they were poorly represented in these debates.

On the positive side, the recent developments in the German health care system have created not only greater access to a wider variety of highly trained professionals, but also increased awareness and activism by psychoanalysts. They now understand that their participation in the national health care system offers the opportunity to show that analysis is the most effective treatment for certain pathologies and that, as a body of knowledge and way of thinking, it contributes invaluably to the understanding of conditions outside its immediate scope. On the negative side, being part of the system may bring with it unpalatable regulations concerning how analysts may practice, think, and educate future analysts, thereby threatening their autonomy and integrity.

The developments of recent years have shown that whether German analysts will retain a strong influence in the mental health field or whether they will lose the freedom to work as they would like depends to a large extent on their own initiative. In the future, it will be very important, particularly for the newly recognized psychotherapeutic professionals to take an active role in professional politics which, with the new developments have become much more clearly linked to state and federal politics. The necessity for this activism is underscored by the fact that concern about escalating healthcare is already a significant political issue.

DISCRIMINATORY PLANS

Australia

Australia provides a striking illustration of an inequitable system that, nonetheless, has some good features, despite its glaring limitations. Psychoanalysis and psychotherapy are insured under the national health insurance plan, but only when provided by medical doctors. These procedures are not funded when conducted by psychologist/psychoanalysts. Australian psychologists have tried to overcome their government's systematic discrimination against their patients and their profession. They have, however, tended to use a rather soft approach (like the somewhat inconsistent efforts of Canadian psychologists and their patients). They have not been able to change the system (Waterhouse, 1994, personal communication).

Physician/analysts typically charge somewhat more than the national insurance plan provides. Patients pay for missed sessions on their own. Some private insurance companies provide limited coverage for services provided by clinical psychologists. (See the chapter by Spielman, this volume, for a detailed description of the Australian system.)

Canada[2]

The Canadian arrangement is an outdated, discriminatory one, similar to the Australian. As with the Australian plan, there are, nonetheless, some very good aspects to the Canadian health care system despite its glaringly backward features, which are particularly obvious in the realm of psychological health care.

The federal government guarantees universality of health insurance throughout the nation. Each province or territory has considerable influence over the shape of the plan in its particular jurisdiction. Some provinces (like Finland) limit the number of sessions per week. No region puts any limits on the total duration of treatment in a patient's lifetime (unlike Finland and Germany). Only Ontario places no limitations on the number of sessions per week. Alberta requires the physician/psychotherapists to provide information and explanation for psychotherapies that exceed three sessions at any particular time. When that is done, permission is automatically granted for unlimited psychotherapy. Quebec restricts coverage to three sessions per week (like Finland); greater frequency is permitted only in a few designated teaching hospitals in Quebec.

All provinces fund the private practice of psychotherapy when it is conducted by medical practitioners. No province supports such treatment when it is provided by practitioners from any other background, such as psychology. It does not matter how many years or even decades of pre- and postdoctoral training and experience a psychologist may have had, or how many books or articles he or she may have published. The treatments conducted by those professionals, no matter how necessary they are, no matter how unavailable alternative treatment is, simply will not be funded. In contrast, medical practitioners need show no particular evidence of any training or competence in psychodiagnosis and psychotherapy. They will

---

[2] This discussion of Canada's national health insurance plan is based on Fayek (1994, 1996) and Willock's (1994, 1995) knowledge of the Canadian system.

be fully funded if they wish to diagnose and treat psychological disorders, even if they have had no more than a few weeks' exposure to such concepts, years ago, in medical school.

Inadequate, discriminatory systems, like the Canadian model, are rarely exposed. When they are, those individuals and groups who are in a position to address the fundamental inequities invariably opt instead, to obfuscate matters, maintaining the status quo. It is instructive to look at a couple of examples of this process. A particularly impressive illustration of the completely irrational nature of the government's approach to the issue of qualifications, of who is authorized and who is excluded from providing psychological health care under the national health insurance plan, came to light in a recent, routine review of physician billings by the Ontario Ministry of Health. It was discovered that a Toronto cardiologist had a record of submitting one of the highest billings for psychotherapy ($1,250,000 between January 1993 and August 1997). In the most recent fiscal year, his billings for psychotherapy were the seventh largest in the province. While this physician spent most of his day conducting tests in cardiology (11 a.m. to 6 p.m.), he frequently billed the insurance plan for an additional eight hours of psychotherapy. In three instances, he charged for more than 24 hours of psychotherapy per day. When Ministry officials interviewed some of his patients, the patients said they had only had heart tests from this physician and had never received any psychotherapy from him. These shenanigans were reported in Canada's national newspaper (*The Globe and Mail*, 1997).

What is crucial about the preceding illustration is not just that the physician so easily got away with this colossal fraud for more than four and a half years before anyone noticed that anything odd was going on, but that he would probably not have come to anyone's attention if he had been less extravagantly outrageous in his billings. In all likelihood, no one would have questioned whether he was providing psychotherapy or whether he was qualified to do so, if he had not allowed himself to be quite so carried away by greed. No doubt he felt fully protected by the government-sponsored illusion that all physicians are qualified to provide any kind of psychological health care under the health insurance plan and the corresponding illusion that other highly trained practitioners, such as psychologists, are not qualified to do so. This sense of privileged immunity to rational thought served this physician's purposes well for several years, but eventually the extremity of his behavior, if not the paucity of his qualifications, aroused suspicions.

That little newspaper article exposing this intriguing instance of fraud noted that it was unusual for a cardiologist to bill for large amounts of psychotherapy. The newspaper noted that "the list of those billing for psychotherapy would normally include psychiatrists, psychotherapists, and psychologists." This statement is, of course, blatantly false. No psychologist can bill any of the provincial health insurance plans for anything, no matter how badly a patient may need the treatment. Nor can most psychotherapists. Such untrue statements are all too common in Canada, which harbors such a deceptively inequitable insurance scheme. These kinds of false assertions convey an erroneous impression that the system is rational and equitable, except for occasional individual cases of excess. (In a less corrupt world, one might like to interpret the journalist's statement that the list of those billing for psychotherapy would "normally" include psychologists as meaning that this *surely* would be the case if the system were not so grossly *abnormal*.)

The extreme irrationality of the Canadian system has given momentum to a phenomenon known as "GP psychotherapy." Particularly in jurisdictions where there appears to be an oversupply of general practitioners, an increasing number of physicians have begun to devote some or all of their practice to psychotherapy. Some of these physicians seek training and supervision. Others do not.

Many Canadians who favor the public's right to select the qualified practitioners of their choice are deeply distressed by their government's inflexible, outdated policies in the field of psychological health care. Successive governments have consistently elected to deprive citizens (except for the relatively affluent) of freedom of choice in this realm. In communities that might have a psychologist, but no psychiatrist, the government's policy virtually amounts to depriving the populace of all mental health care. The consequences of the government's rigid, unchanging policy has been extremely deleterious for both the public and many, if not all, professions.

The government seems unmoved by the public's plight. The government appears unperturbed by repeated findings, such as those of the Ontario Health Study described on the front page of *The Globe and Mail* (Coutts, 1994) indicating that approximately 20% of the population has a mental disorder. Government inertia seems unaffected by the fact that only a small minority of this large group receives any form of treatment whatsoever for their psychological disorders.

Psychoanalysis is not insured as a specific act under any provincial health plan. Only in Ontario is it mentioned as an acceptable modality of treatment. It is, however, not billed separately. Rather, charges are submitted under the category of psychotherapy. Ontario patients can receive as many sessions per week as they wish, for as many years as they need, as long as the practitioner of this psychological health care is a physician, not a psychologist or any other sort of psychoanalyst.

Needless to say, such conditions make it extremely difficult, if not impossible, for psychologist/psychoanalysts to practice the profession for which they have spent years of their lives studying. It is even difficult for such people to practice psychotherapy, particularly with patients who need long-term, intensive treatment. The spectrum of sophisticated diagnostic and therapeutic services in which they have been trained and for which they are regulated by statutes and professional colleges to provide to the public is, consequently, not available to the general population. (Some psychological services are available to the public in hospitals, particularly in major urban centers, although even these resources have been cut back drastically over the past several years.) Psychologists in independent practice can generally see only those few patients who are blessed with uncommonly good private insurance plans (and such plans are becoming increasingly rare) or whose personal resources permit them the freedom to consult the practitioner of their choice. Other professionals, such as clinical social workers or child and adolescent psychotherapists, are often in even more difficult circumstances, as it is even rarer for their services to be covered by private insurance plans

As can be imagined, psychologists and other nonmedical mental health professionals are deeply discouraged from seeking lengthy, costly training in complex modes of diagnosis and treatment which they are unlikely to be able to practice on completion of training. This deleterious impact on motivation for advanced training has, until recently, been compounded by a long-standing perception that such persons are not welcome for training at some of the major, medically controlled psychoanalytic institutes. Discriminatory government funding, coupled with such factors as the likelihood that many medically trained analysts may have felt more comfortable evaluating and training candidates from their own discipline, has led to a situation that has been profoundly biased against psychologists and the public whom they serve. The end result is that the situation for nonmedical analysts in Canada has been as unfavorable as in the United States (before the historic American event known as "The Lawsuit"). In Ontario, for example, Fayek (1994) reported there were only seven nonmedical analysts practicing, or rather trying to practice, compared with 178 medical analysts. In the vast domain of Western Canada (British Columbia, Alberta, Saskatchewan, Manitoba) there are no nonmedical analysts at all. In marked contrast, in Germany, which has a government health insurance plan that is not designed to discriminate totally against psychologists and their patients, there are approximately equal numbers of psychologists and psychiatrists practicing psychoanalysis.

Just as interest in analysis has survived in other adverse circumstances, such as under hostile, totalitarian regimes, so, too, in jurisdictions like Ontario have a few nonmedical practitioners persevered in spite of serious obstacles to psychoanalytic interest and training. In the last few years, there have been some very important developments in Ontario, particularly in the Toronto region. For example, with the establishment of the Toronto Institute for Contemporary Psychoanalysis, there are now far more opportunities for psychologists and others coming from academic backgrounds different from medicine to pursue psychoanalytic training. There are also educational opportunities for nonmedical practitioners at the Institute for the Advancement of Self Psychology, and now even at the older Toronto Psychoanalytic Institute. Funding, however, has not improved at all for the patients of psychologists and other nonmedical analysts. The situation thus lags behind the far more equitable conditions found in more enlightened jurisdictions, such as in certain European countries.

Only one Canadian province, Manitoba, specifically excludes psychoanalysis from its health plan. This exclusion was instituted just a few years ago, as part of an effort to contain costs in the recessionary economic climate. Similar action was subsequently considered in Ontario, but vigorous lobbying by analysts and analysands succeeded in preventing the Ontario cutback. These analysts and patients, are, however, worried that, with current governmental commitments to cost cutting and deficit reduction, such lobbying may fail in the future.

In provinces that do not allow physicians to bill for unlimited frequency of sessions per week, it is illegal for a physician/analyst to bill the government for the number of covered sessions (say three), then charge the analysand for extra sessions (say one or two more) to reach the frequency of a more "classical" analysis. Because of this provision, there used to be some possibility for nonmedical analysts (in Quebec), particularly if they were training analysts, to practice their profession, usually with candidates. This is becoming less possible, however, as it appears that more physicians/analysts are starting to defy the law, providing and charging analysands for the extra sessions required for a more intensive analysis.

In Ontario, in contrast to Quebec, it has never been very feasible even for those who have achieved training analyst status, if they are not physicians, to practice the method of treatment that they have spent such a long time learning. Candidates training to become analysts in Ontario almost always pursue their personal analyses with medical analysts because this required didactic analysis can be billed to the taxpayers under the "psychotherapy" code. The law does not actually allow training analyses to be paid for by the state, but this difficulty is easily circumvented by commencing analysis prior to beginning formal analytic training. Virtually all training analyses are paid for by the state. This practice, illegal in other jurisdictions (such as Australia), has been scrutinized by cost-conscious bureaucrats. They have decided not to make a fuss about it at this time.

It is illegal to charge patients any fee beyond that which is provided by the plan (approximately $100 per session in Ontario and about 30% less in Quebec). This law is circumvented by many analysts who feel the fee is less than it should be. Years of training, experience, and accomplishments are not recognized by the system. A recently graduated psychiatrist receives the same fee as a senior training analyst. Some analysts also justify "extra billing" with the argument that out-of-pocket payment creates better patient motivation.

One hopes that psychoanalytic societies would vigorously lobby the government, not only to maintain the situation that they and their patients currently enjoy, but also to extend these benefits in a nondiscriminatory manner to all analysts in their group. This latter aspect does not happen to any significant degree, if at all. Knowing that the government has traditionally been unwilling to facilitate the public's receiving high quality psychological health care, (at least not from the professional group that is arguably the most suitable to provide it, namely psychologists) and also knowing that government institutions are drastically reducing what little accessibility the public ever had to psychologists, medical analysts have probably been unwilling to risk rocking the boat they are in, which, for them at least, is as good as or better than any situation in which analysts function anywhere in the world.

Not long ago, the Canadian government introduced a Goods and Services Tax (GST), which was to be added on top of existing provincial sales taxes (PST) and extended, for the first time, to all services (rather than just "goods"). Nonmedical analysts and therapists would be in the position of having to charge their patients an additional 7% to 10% for the services they provided. Psychologists campaigned vigorously and ultimately succeeded in defeating this proposal, which could have made their services even less accessible to the public. That campaign, led by psychologists, eventuated in the exemption of all other regulated health care providers from the hated tax.

Nonmedical, nonpsychologist analysts lobbied the Progressive Conservative government and achieved a similar exemption, albeit with the troubling proviso that they would enjoy this exemption only as long as the Canadian Psychoanalytic Society continued to be at least two-thirds medical. Recently, however, after several years of this exemption, the Liberal government decided to repeal it. Analysts in Ontario who are neither physicians nor psychologists must now charge their patients an additional 7% GST or else pay that amount themselves. The situation is even worse in Quebec, where the GST has been "harmonized" with the 6.5% Provincial Sales Tax. This cheery term means that these analysts in Quebec must charge the 7% GST, then levy the 6.5% PST on top of that. The total surcharge is therefore nearly 15%. On gross private practice earnings of $50,000, for example, one would have to remit about $7,500 in "sales tax" to the government. One then pays income tax on the remaining amount. (If one operates a very small business or, in this case, a small private practice generating less than $30,000 per annum, one does not have to pay GST. If one earns more than this amount, say $31,000, then one must pay tax on the entire $31,000.)

Canadian practitioners are becoming used to being taxed to, and perhaps beyond, the limit. Canadian therapists, for example, were used to paying a business tax on their offices. This would usually be about one thousand dollars per annum. Now with the GST, the must pay a 7% tax on this tax!

SPLITTING PROCESSES IN NATIONAL HEALTH INSURANCE PLANS

The glaring differences between the reasonably rational, admirable health care plans in countries like Finland and the Czech Republic as opposed to the outdated, discriminatory plans in countries like Australia and Canada warrant a pause to reflect on such gross disparities before we proceed to discuss some intermediate cases. Exemplars of the discriminatory tradition—nations like Canada and Australia—deny their people the freedom to choose from among the full array of qualified health care providers. Astoundingly, citizens are allowed to consult whomever they wish ("GP psychotherapist," psychiatrist, or any other physician) for psychological health care, as long as they do not select a professional from the group with the lengthiest training in the understanding of both normal and abnormal psychological processes—psychologists. In some instances, this is tantamount to denying the public access to any competent mental health care at all.

Aspects of the funding of psychological health care in countries like Canada and Australia are organized according to a logic suitable to Alice in Wonderland. The situation is comparable to an insurance plan generously funding the work of Neurosurgeon B, but refusing to fund the work of similarly, or even better, qualified Neurosurgeon A. The government apparently feels it is acceptable to say you must have your operation done by Neurosurgeon B, or perhaps by a general practitioner with an interest in neurosurgery, but you cannot have it done by Neurosurgeon A, even though he or she has comparable or superior training, may practice much nearer to where you live, or be the only qualified practitioner in your area, etc.

Countries like Canada and Australia do facilitate access to some mental health care workers, many of whom are well trained, even if some are not. Generally speaking, however, only the relatively well-to-do, and those few citizens with good private insurance, have the freedom to choose from among the available psychological health care providers for the expert diagnosis and treatment they may require. In such countries, the well-being of citizens, and issues like professional competence, comprehensive diagnosis, and quality of treatment are, evidently, considered relatively unimportant

Cost containment has, of course, become an increasingly dominant consideration in government policy deliberations. Concern with the short-term bottom line does not, however, seem to be the only factor in government decision making. For example, several years ago, when billings for GP Psychotherapy in Ontario were approximately $75 million per annum, the Ontario Psychological Association (1991) presented the results of an independent, actuarial study to the government indicating that the public could have full access to the approximately 2000 psychologists in the province for about $75 million per year. Furthermore, American studies (e.g., Jones and Vischi, 1979; Cummings and VandenBos, 1981; Mumford et al., 1984) have indicated that most of such expenditures would actually be offset by savings in the medical sector, where patients would no longer seek help for essentially psychological ailments. The government ignored this proposal to increase public accessibility to psychological health care in Ontario. Meanwhile, billings for GP Psychotherapy have been allowed to soar beyond $150 million per annum.

Several years ago, Australian psychologists informed me (Willock, 1988, personal communications) that they, too, had presented a study to their government indicating that providing citizens access to psychologists would increase government expenditures only temporarily. After two years, cost-offset factors would nullify these initial outlays. The Australian proposal, like the Canadian one, was ignored by the government.

Antiquated systems, where patients of one group of highly qualified practitioners are denied coverage while patients of a similarly, or less, qualified group have excellent coverage, might fruitfully be regarded as *minor* apartheid systems. This evocative phrase captures the mean spirited nature of splitting operations manifest on the level of social group process. The term is a composite of "apart," meaning separate, and "heid," related to the English suffix "hood," found in concepts like nationhood and falsehood, derived from older variants meaning person, rank, order, condition, manner. Needless to say, the condition of persons who have been ranked, separated, and deprived in a systematic manner is not pleasant, regardless of the basis or extent of the segregation.

When discrimination is culturally syntonic, thinking tends to be black and white. There is not much room for more complex thought processes. In cultures that like to feel they have evolved beyond segregated modes of thinking, splitting processes can continue comfortably only in circumscribed areas where "no one knows" anything is amiss. Highly developed, selective inattention is a must.

Writing about a completely different topic—attitudes toward sexual abuse—Bennett Simon (1992) argued that we have always known and not known, avowed and disavowed, the traumatic reality of incest. Similar processes of concurrently knowing and not knowing appear to manifest themselves in the way that certain psychoanalytic groups and larger governmental bodies that conceive and perpetuate problematic health insurance plans may simultaneously recognize and not recognize the importance of discriminatory practices towards certain disciplines (such as psychology) and their patients. There seems to be a certain amount of collusion, turning blind eyes toward certain practices and policies.

In these delimited domains of state discrimination, when one makes inquiries to find out why things seem to be so irrationally arranged, one encounters the most startling forms of confused, obfuscatory thought. For example, I (Willock) made a presentation a few years ago to the annual convention of the Ontario Psychological Association on the impact of the public's being denied freedom of choice in the area of psychological health care. A journalist in the audience from Canada's national newspaper, *The Globe and Mail* (Mickleburgh, 1991), considered the issues raised to be of sufficient importance to bring them to the public's attention in a prominent article. This journalist had an ear for the absurd and oppressive. At about the same time, he (1990) wrote an important piece exposing the fact that the discipline committee of the Ontario College of Physicians and Surgeons had cleared one of its members on charges of sexual impropriety. In the guise of practicing psychotherapy, this physician had evidently been encouraging female patients to perform what sounded like oral sex on him. The College felt compelled by a patient's complaint to hold a hearing. They were however, satisfied when the doctor explained that he had just been practicing a form of therapy that he called "pelvic bonding."

The patient was being treated for insomnia and emotional difficulties. According to the patient's testimony, after 10 months of weekly sessions, the doctor ushered her into a small room with a mattress on the floor. He administered acupuncture and then, while she lay on the mattress, removed his pants. He always worked without shoes and socks. Now she learned that he did not wear underwear. The Doctor lay on his back, with his hands behind his head. Uttering peculiar sounds and making rippling movements with this body, he pressed his pelvis into her face, telling her to do whatever she wanted. After awhile, the physician left, annoyed, because the experience had not been successful for the patient. On a second occasion, when the pelvic bonding ended, the doctor was "very upset" with her.

The physician dismissed the first encounter as a "bonding incident." He described how the patient's hand had gradually ascended from his leg to his pelvic region. He denied that the second episode had ever taken place. The doctor explained that his therapeutic practices had evolved over the years into a combination of acupuncture, bioenergetics, and martial arts. He felt "it was not improper for a female patient to bury her head in his pelvic region" during treatment. A former patient and a colleague testified in support of the practice.

Since the College of Physicians and Surgeons evidently had, in common with the government, massive ignorance of what constitutes psychotherapy, of who is trained to provide it, and of who should be funded to practice psychological diagnosis and treatment, the College concluded that the psychological health care provided by this physician did not warrant penalty. In a system where patients (and professions) are, in the vernacular, "screwed" daily by the health insurance system, it is perhaps not surprising that the body which the government approves to monitor and evaluate allegations of abuse could see nothing profoundly amiss with a physician's indulging in a little pelvic bonding with his patients.

In defense of the College, it might be stated that, although they did dismiss the woman's complaint, cleared the physician of all charges of sexual impropriety, and imposed no penalty, they did, nonetheless, criticize the doctor's pelvic bonding technique. The College went so far as to refer to his particular technique as "dangerous and inappropriate *in that it is liable to be misconstrued*." Presumably the College felt that the female complainant had misconstrued the doctor's intent.

The journalist must have been perplexed, perhaps perturbed, by these peculiar proceedings. He apparently contacted the College of Physicians and Surgeons for enlightenment. The director of communications for the College assured him that the College treats sexual complaints "very seriously." She assured him that they have a high rate of convictions on sexual cases and generally impose "heavy penalties." Apparently they did not regard the complaints against this doctor as being all that serious, hence not requiring even a light penalty, let alone a heavy one.

This journalist was also perturbed and puzzled by the discriminatory exclusion of the patients of psychologist from the health insurance plan. Consequently, he contacted the government in search of illumination. A senior spokesperson for the Ministry of Health explained to him why psychologists, despite having achieved the highest educational degree bestowed by society (the doctorate) and being registered to practice by the state as a regulated health care profession, were still not deemed suitable to be funded. The reasons were so blatantly untrue (alleging that Ontario psychologists did not have a professional college, standard examinations, or uniform standards) that the following day the *Globe and Mail* (1991) had to publish a prominent article in which the Ministry of Health apologized for having transmitted such gross misinformation. Interestingly, in retracting its misinformation, the Ministry of Health did not attempt to create any new rationalizations for denying coverage to the patients of psychologists. They merely acknowledged that the rationalizations they had given had absolutely no basis in fact. The Ministry seemed content to deal in false-hoods and to rescind them when necessary, that is, when found out and put under sufficient pressure. Skillful at obfuscation, the government did not seem to feel the slightest need to deal with the actual, gross inequities. The situation was "handled" as usual. No modifications were made to the status quo.

The journalist's article on pelvic bonding resulted in a public outcry (fuelled significantly by feminist consciousness). This uproar by the citi-zenry resulted in official reconsideration of how allegations of sexual abuse of patients are processed. Ultimately this led to a policy of zero tolerance. While the journalist's article on physician malpractice had been highly ef-fective, his piece on patients seeking assistance from psychologists did not result in sufficient public response to move the government. Whereas gov-ernments can sometimes be influenced by large exertions of power, it is evidently very difficult to sway ruling bodies by straightforward appeals to logic, equity, truth, and other such supposedly time-honored values.

MODIFIED INEQUITABLE PLANS

Sweden

Sweden affords an example of a system that has attempted to soften the impact of its fundamental inequities. Analysands working with Swedish psychiatrists can have as many sessions as they want for as many years as they wish. No regular reports are required, although occasionally they may be (Sjodin, 1994). There is a nominal user fee of about $5.00 per session (Birchard, 1994).

Patients of Swedish psychologists can sometimes get a seat at the back of the health care bus if a psychiatrist sponsors them. The way this is ar-ranged is that in some parts of the country there are special provisions whereby the government gives, say $125,000, to the local health author-ity to provide for patients of psychologists. Certain hospitals administer these funds and decide who gets them. There are long waiting lists and restrictions on how often and for how long such patients can see their psychologists. Treatment can sometimes be intensive (e.g., three times per week). One has to apply each year for continued treatment. Funding may cover only a portion of each visit, say 30% (Carlsson, 1993, personal communication). On the very day in November 1993 when I (Willock) spoke with a Swedish psychologist/psychoanalyst, Dr. Jan Stensson, government funding for that year had just run out for these patients at the back of the bus.

It used to be that certain Swedish state employees (for example, at universities) received some assistance if they wished to obtain psychotherapy from a psychologist. The government might pay 1/2 to 2/3 of the psychologist's fee (Carlsson, 1993, personal communication). With the economic downturn, the state no longer provides this support. Access to psychologists is now much more difficult. Meanwhile, there are waiting lists of three to five years to see medical psychoanalysts.

The Swedish experience with health care cutbacks triggered by an economic downturn is not unique. Earlier we saw similar factors disturbing the practice of psychotherapy in Norway. Sweden, like other Nordic nations, had a prosperous economy in the early 1990s. By 1994, this had changed; Sweden by then had the highest per capita budget deficit of any industrialized country (Birchard, 1994). Unemployment, almost nonexistent in 1989, was close to 14% by 1994. From 1991 to 1994, Sweden went from being one of Europe's biggest spenders on health care to being one of the smallest. Health service expenditures were reduced by more than a billion dollars. The government has given doctors more incentive to operate privately, yet still receive some public funding. Ninety-five percent of Swedish physicians work for the state, mostly in neighborhood clinics. The remaining 5% are in private practice.

Switzerland

Switzerland provides another example of a modified discriminatory system. Organized along federalist lines, health care is run largely at the canton (provincial) level. As in the Canadian system, this means there can be differences in plans in different regions.

In 1991, 269 health insurance companies provided psychotherapy coverage in 26 cantons. Historically, coverage for depth analytic therapy had been, according to federal law and the wish of most Freudian analysts, an optional benefit, usually modest. Moser (1992) reported that the restriction that payment be only for certain forms of psychotherapy has been dropped. (Such a limitation continues in some other countries, such as Germany.) That qualitative restriction has been replaced by a quantitative arrangement. The Federal government recommended that two weekly sessions be covered for three years, then one session per week for an additional three years (Condrau, 1994). A common plan, however, seems to be to cover two sessions per week for two years, with extension possible under certain circumstances (Moser, 1992). Psychoanalysts see opportunities in these new developments, as well as unsolved problems.

Historically, insurance payment was only for medical practitioners.

During the past several years, some insurance companies have begun to consider the radical possibility that psychological health care could be provided by psychologists. These companies now pay (lower fees) for "delegated psychotherapy" conducted by psychologists, in medical doctors' consulting rooms, under physician control (like the schemes under which Dutch and German psychologists practiced until recently) With these modifications, the Swiss people have gained access to a much greater variety of well-trained and regulated practitioners.

The Netherlands[3]

The Dutch Society for Psychoanalysis, founded in 1917, initially kept its doors firmly closed to nonmedical analysts. This policy was applied to the extent of denying membership to the four German-Jewish analysts (Reik, Landauer, Levi-Suhl, and Waterman) who escaped to Holland in 1933 and 1934. Ironically, three of these immigrants were medically qualified in Germany but did not possess Dutch medical diplomas. A new psychoanalytic society was eventually established, and these refugees became members of it.

In 1938, the concept of "lay" analysis was finally accepted by the Dutch Psychoanalytic Society. Since analysis had been legally defined as a medical procedure, psychologist/psychoanalysts had to have their diagnostic assessments checked by physicians. The president of the Psychoanalytic Society had to be medically qualified. Late legislative changes have resulted in a less oppressive climate. In 1990, the Dutch Psychoanalytic Society changed its charter to allow a nonphysician to become president. Other legislative and administrative changes have, however, been less facilitative. Possibilities for private practice have been restricted and salaries of nonpsychiatric analysts in mental health centres have been reduced (since 1980).

With respect to the financing of analysis and therapy, the situation had been that a psychiatrist had to reinterview a psychologist's patient to approve the diagnostic assessment and treatment recommendations. The psychologist then had to continue working in association with the psychiatrist. The psychiatrist received 20% to 25% of the psychologist's fee throughout the course of the treatment. This arrangement was referred to colloquially as the long-arm system. Recent changes have brought some progress, and the long-arm system has almost been abolished; it continues only for patients whose treatment began prior to March 1994.

---

[3] This section is based primarily on the detailed contributions of Abraham (1994) and, to a lesser extent, on Groen-Prakken and de Nobel (1992).

As in several jurisdictions around the world, the Dutch National Health Care system planned to stop reimbursement for psychoanalytic treatment owing to questions of cost and efficiency. Similar concerns were raised with respect to psychotherapy. Political lobbying by analysts was successful in maintaining coverage for psychoanalysis (as it was in the province of Ontario, Canada, but not in the Canadian province of Manitoba, which delisted analysis from the schedule of insured services).

Separate budgets were created for analysis and therapy. The psychotherapy budget, currently 40,000,000 florins (approximately U.S. $20 million) is spread throughout the country by means of a distribution code for each region, managed by the Regional Institutes for Ambulatory Health (RIAGGs). The psychoanalytic budget is managed along similar lines, but the professionals and committees involved are analysts. This budget is currently 15 million florins (U.S. $8 million). Because of high overhead costs (salaries for the director, secretaries, and other administrators; rent, etc.), only a small part of this budget is actually used to pay for analytic sessions.

Patients contribute 20 florins (U.S. $10) to the cost of each session. They do not have to pay after they have contributed 900 florins (U.S. $450) in any year. This amounts to patients' paying a small user fee for about their first 45 sessions in a year. For further sessions that year, there is no charge to the patient.

Unemployed citizens contribute the same 20 florins per session, but they can apply for extra financial support by social security and would then not be expected to pay after having themselves contributed 180 florins (U.S. $90) in a year. That is, the unemployed pay a user fee for about their first nine sessions in any year, with the possibility of social security's paying the rest for that year. The patient needs to apply each year for this extra financial support.

The government attempted to create a plan in which therapists control the treatment system. Each year representatives of the insurance companies and the RIAGGs in each of the country's 10 regions meet to decide on a "production agreement." Each therapist is assigned a portion of the regional budget for his or her private practice. This translates into a fixed number of 45-minute sessions ("account hours") for each therapist, funded at a rate comparable to what salaried therapists would receive. No therapist is allowed to have more than six account hours per day, for a maximum of 36 sessions in a week. A therapist who works in a mental health facility for more than 28 hours per week is not allowed to do extra hours of private practice funded by the national insurance system. Thus, a therapist working in an agency with adults four days per week who has also been trained to work with children would not be reimbursed by the insurance system if he or she wanted to use those child therapy skills in a small private practice, no matter what the public need might be.

Therapists must be under 65 years of age. (This retirement policy would not appeal to all analysts, many of whom complete their lengthy professional training relatively late in life.) To become part of the newly organized system, therapists had to have conducted, in 1992 and 1993, a private practice of at least 15 account hours per week. Thus (as in Norway) recent regulations make it difficult or impossible for new therapists to enter the system. Unfortunately, young therapists just graduating cannot easily get jobs in the RIAGGs either as they currently have hiring freezes.

Psychotherapists must be certified and registered in the National Psychotherapy Registry if they want to be reimbursed by the health insurance plan. The government has been operating this Registry since 1986. It prevents therapists with no substantial training in assessment and therapy from being funded, a distinct advantage over some of the more seriously flawed systems, like the Canadian, which funds any medical doctor, even those having little or no formal training in psychodiagnostic and psychotherapeutic procedures, while denying funding to all registered psychologists, no matter how much doctoral and postdoctoral training they might have. Most registered psychotherapists in the Netherlands are psychologists, and there are some social workers and physicians on the Registry. Very few come from other disciplines. Psychiatrists do not have to be registered as therapists; they can bill the health insurance system for psychotherapy without demonstrating any specific training in this area.

A therapist cannot see a patient for more than 90 sessions under the psychotherapy budget. These sessions can be spread over several months or years. Patients needing further treatment must go to a RIAGG. They cannot have additional sessions with their independent practitioner for at least one year. After that year, they may see a private practitioner for another 90 sessions. When the 90 sessions run out, patients can continue to see their therapists by paying themselves. The government will not, however, sponsor another 90 sessions unless they interrupt their treatment for a least a year. The RIAGGs do not want patients to pay for therapy. They tell therapists that they should refer such long-term patients to RIAGGs or else see them free. One or two insurance companies provide some assistance for patients to continue treatment with their therapists beyond the 90 sessions. As usual, economically advantaged citizens have a better chance for continuity of care with a single, preferred therapist.

Until recently, in order to see a private therapist, a patient had to be referred by a GP, psychiatrist, or RIAGG. Now patients can apply for therapy directly, without referral. The therapist must diagnose the problem, decide on the type of treatment, and calculate the time required to execute the therapy. Each conclusion of the therapist must be tested by a regional commission of colleagues. If the commission refuses the treatment, the therapist has to communicate the bad news to the patient. The patient can appeal, but the procedures are very bureaucratic, with many time-consuming forms and meetings. The objective seems to be to control costs and to make it difficult to enter therapy. Psychiatrists are paid in a much more direct way. They do not face the maze of obstacles and bureaucratic impediments with which other psychotherapists (and their patients) struggle.

If a therapist does not use all his or her allotted sessions in any year, the unused sessions are given to other therapists who desire more account hours. If the therapist who lost the account hours can prove that he needs more hours for the next year, he can request them, but the chances of getting the lost hours back are not great. A similar redistribution is supposed to happen with the account hours taken from therapists who have reached the age of 65. There is some concern that, rather than being redistributed, these retracted funds may be used for other purposes, permanently reducing the psychological health care budget. There is talk that these freed-up funds might be used to permit some younger therapists to develop private practices.

Psychologists (and other Registered Psychotherapists) have escaped from the long-arm system. They have not achieved full parity with psychotherapists coming from a medical background, but they have, nonetheless, advanced beyond their Swiss colleagues who are still caught in the "delegated psychotherapy" system.

PLANS PROVIDING LITTLE OR NO COVERAGE

In addition to the reasonably equitable, the grossly discriminatory, and the in-between national health insurance plans, there are countries that provide little or no coverage for psychotherapy, and none for analysis.

Denmark

In Denmark (Paikin, 1992), where practically all social support and medical care is free, there is no provision for psychoanalysis. This intensive treatment is consequently out of reach of all but the very wealthy, of whom there are very few. What psychological and psychiatric help there is tends to be concentrated in psychiatric departments. There are few practicing psychiatrists. Even psychotherapy was, until recently, practically unknown in the public sector.

New Zealand

New Zealand is culturally similar to Australia. Consequently, one might expect that New Zealand would fund psychoanalytic treatment, at least on a discriminatory basis, as is done in neighboring Australia. Surprisingly, New Zealand turns out to be more like Denmark than like Australia in this regard (Muir, 1994, personal communication).

An interesting comparison of the Australian and New Zealand mental health care delivery systems showed a 44% lower cost per capita in Australia, despite the fact that there is much more readily available outpatient psychotherapy and psychoanalysis and insurance coverage for it in Australia than in New Zealand, which has a hospital-based system and little outpatient treatment. Over the time period studied, Australia spent $5.17 million per 100,000 population on mental health care whereas New Zealand spent $7 million per 100,000 (Andrews, 1989).

Hungary

In Hungary, most analysts are female psychologists (Harmatta and Szonyi, 1992). Psychoanalysis can be performed within the health care system only as a special exception. Analysts must generally conduct this work in private practice, as a second job, and private fees are very low. In contrast, the fee for membership in the International Psycho-Analytical Association, reduced by 20%, equals the monthly income of the typical psychologist. New health regulations are expected that may be more favorable to analytic practice, perhaps along the lines of development that we discussed in the neighboring Czech Republic. These advances will, however, likely be a long time coming.

England

Psychotherapy on an indefinite, once-weekly basis is available at some National Health Service clinics (Wallerstein, 1991). More intensive therapy must be financed privately by those who desire it and can afford it. All analyses take place outside the tax-supported health care system. Psychoanalysis is, consequently, limited mostly to London, where the requisite sophisticated, affluent population resides. The fee structure is typically less than half that of the United States, despite the fact that living costs in London are not significantly different from those in New York.

According to Tarnopolsky (1994, personal communication), the British Psycho-Analytical Society decided not to participate in the National Health Service, for fear of the consequent impact on the analytic process. As physicians were to be paid a salary related to size of practice rather than fee for service, there would have been considerable disincentive to perform intensive treatment. Long-term therapy may be practiced in some training facilities (e.g., the Tavistock Clinic) on a more frequent basis, such as three times a week.

In England, the independent profession of psychoanalytic child psychotherapist is well established. It used to be possible to treat children, in clinics, as frequently and as long as was necessary. With the economic recession and efforts to reduce expenditures, therapists have experienced increasing pressure to see people less frequently (Phillips, 1994, personal communication). While child and adolescent therapists in Germany are now recognized as an independent profession funded by the health insurance system, child therapists in private practice in England have never been eligible for such reimbursement.

Similar pressures to conduct shorter, less intensive treatments are being experienced in many other countries. Sometimes these deteriorations in health care are disguised with slogans or studies purporting to show that less is better, drugs are the treatment of choice, and so on. In Canada, where hospital services have historically been free of charge, some psychology departments are finding that in order to survive they must now charge user fees for some services. (Such fees are officially illegal, but some institutions have devised creative ways to circumvent these laws. The system itself has found equally ingenious ways of not seeing these developments.)

Spain

There is no coverage for psychoanalysis under the national health insurance plan (Sjodin, 1994).

Brazil

Psychoanalysis is not covered by the national health care plan (Sjodin, 1994).

Argentina

There is no coverage for psychoanalysis under national health insurance (Killam, 1994, personal communication).

CONCLUSION

Although it is beyond the scope of this chapter to examine the fate of psychoanalysis and psychotherapy under national health insurance schemes in every country, this overview of what has been happening in a variety of nations may suffice to provide some feel for the spectrum of contexts, ranging from the sublime to the unconscionable, in which patients and professionals thrive, or struggle to survive, around the globe. Considering the importance of these issues for citizens, governments, practitioners, and educators, it is surprising how little has been published on this topic. We have much to learn from increasing our awareness of systems, developments, and struggles in other countries, regardless of whether such situations are currently progressive or antiquated, regressive, and inequitable. We hope that this contribution will stimulate more discussion, writing, and related activism on these important matters.

REFERENCES

Abraham, J. (1994), The latest developments in the Netherlands for the practice of psychoanalysis under the national health care system. Presented at annual meeting of American Psychological Association, Los Angeles.

Andrews, G. (1989), Private and public psychiatry. *Amer. J. Psychiat.*, 146:881–886.

Balzert, C. (1994), The experience of psychoanalysts in Germany. Presented at annual meeting of American Psychological Association, Los Angeles.

Barron, J. W. & Sands, H. ed. (1996), *Impact of Managed Care on Psychodynamic Treatment*. Madison, CT: International Universities Press.

Birchard, K. (1994), States of health care—Global trends in health care reform: Sweden. *Can. Health Care Manager*, 1(3):16–18.

Condrau, G. (1994), Comment on the IFPS questionaire. *Internat. Forum Psychoanal.*, 3:21–24.

Coutts, J. (1994), Mental disorders plague one in 5. *The Globe and Mail*, Nov. 22, p. 1 and p. A7.

Cummings, N. A. & VandenBos, G. R. (1981), The twenty years Kaiser-Permanente experience with psychotherapy and medical utilization: Implications for national health policy and national health insurance. *Health Policy Quart.*, 1:159–175.

Danckward, J. F. & Gattig, E., with the collaboration of G. Bruns, C. Frank, U. von Goldacker, G. Junkers, E. Kaiser, C. Nedelmann & P. Schraivogel. (1995). Die Indikation zur hochfrequenten analytische Psychotherapy inder vertragsaerztlichen versorgung. [The indication for high-frequency analytic psychotherapy within the public health insurance system]. Unpublished manuscript

Fayek, A. (1994), The effect of health insurance on psychoanalysis in Canada. Presented at annual meeting of American Psychological Association, Los Angeles.

—— (1996), Working outside national health care: The impact on analytic practice and training. Presented at annual meeting of American Psychological Association, Toronto.

Freud, S. (1926), The question of lay analysis. *Standard Edition*, 20:183–258. London: Hogarth Press, 1959.

Gattig, E. (1996), *Report of the German Association. Psychoanal. in Eur.*, 47:Autumn, pp. 7–11.

Groen-Prakken, H. & de Nobel, L. (1992), The Netherlands. In: *Psychoanalysis International, Vol. 1*, ed. P. Kutter. Stuttgart-Bad Cannstatt: Frommann-Holzboog (dist. The Analytic Press), pp. 217–242.

Harmatta, J. & Szonyi, G. (1992), Hungary. In: *Psychoanalysis international, Vol. 1*, ed. P. Kutter. Stuttgart-Bad Cannstatt: Frommann Holzboog (dist. The Analytic Press), pp. 173–187.

Henseler, H. & Wegner, P. (1993), Psychoanalysen, die ihre zeit brauchen, [Psychoanalyses which take their time]. Opladen, Westdeutscher Verlag.

Jones, K. & Vischi, J. (1979), Impact of alcohol, drug abuse, and mental health treatment on medical care utilization: A review of the research literature. *Medical Care*, 17(12):1–82.

Mickleburgh, R. (1990), Doctor cleared of sexual impropriety. *The Globe and Mail*, Friday, Oct. 12, pp. A1, A8.

——— (1991), Mentally ill children face long wait. *The Globe and Mail*, Feb. 22, p. 2.

Moser, A. (1992), Switzerland. In: *Psychoanalysis International, Vol. 1*, ed. P. Kutter. Stuttgart-Bad Cannstatt: Frommann Holzboog (dist. The Analytic Press), pp. 278–313.

Mumford, E., Schlesinger, H. J., Glass, G. V., Patrick, C. & Cuerdon, B. A. (1984), A new look at evidence about reduced cost of medical utilization following mental health treatment. *Amer. J. Psychiat.*, 141:1145–1158.

Ontario Psychological Association. (1991), *Funding of Psychological Services Under the Ontario Health Insurance Plan*. February, 1991.

Paikin, H. (1992), Denmark. In: *Psychoanalysis International, Vol. l*, ed. P. Kutter. Stuttgart-Bad Cannstatt: Frommann-Holzboog (dist. The Analytic Press), pp. 50–53

Pawlak, K. & Sokolik, Z., with additions by A. Kokoszka & J. Pawlik. (1992), Poland. In: *Psychoanalysis International, Vol. l*, ed. P. Kutter. Stuttgart-Bad Cannstatt: Frommann-Holzboog (dist. The Analytic Press), pp. 243–250.

Sebek, M. (1993), Psychoanalysis in Czechoslovakia. *Psychoanal. Rev.*, 80:433–440.

Simon, B. (1992), "Incest—See under Oedipus complex": The history of an error in psychoanalysis. *J. Amer. Psychoanal. Assn.*, 40:955–988.

Sjodin, C. (1994), Psychoanalysis, socio-medical security systems and the healing tradition. *Internat. Forum Psychoanal.*, 3:5–16.

The Globe and Mail. (1991), 'Obvious errors' in ministry statement, psychologists receive apology. *The Globe and Mail*, Feb. 23, p. 3.

——— (1997), Doctor faces fraud charges for psychotherapy billings. *The Globe and Mail*, Dec. 5, p. A8.

Wallerstein, R. S. (1988), One psychoanalysis or many? *Internat. J. Psycho-Anal.*, 69:5–21.

——— (1991), The future of psychotherapy. *Bull. Menninger Clin.*, 55:421–443.

Willock, B. (1994), An examination of the incredible variety of national health insurance plans under which psychoanalysts practise around the world: the good, the bad, and the ugly. Presented at annual meeting of American Psychological Association, Los Angeles.

―――― (1995), Psychotherapy and psychoanalysis under national health insurance plans around the world: How do we stack up? What can we learn? What can we do? Presented at annual meeting of the Ontario Psychological Association, Toronto.

―――― & Cronan, K. (1988), Increasing accessibility to psychological services. Informal conversation hour, International Congress of Psychology, Sydney, Australia.

TWELVE

Psychoanalysis and Health Care in Australia

Health Care Budget Cuts Affect Psychoanalysis

RON SPIELMAN

Freud often wrote as if to an imaginary hostile reader (at worst) or a skeptical one (at best). Historically, there was good reason for him to anticipate a spectrum of responses in that range. It is an irony that it is only with the help of psychoanalysis itself that we can begin to understand *why* psychoanalysis arouses these complex responses.

If our critics are to be believed, we are charlatans (at worst) or merely misguided (at best). If Freud, when describing psychoanalytic issues, sensed this need to address people with an awareness of their inevitable negative responses, then we psychoanalysts, 100 years later, are still often forced onto the defensive when trying to assert the need for psychoanalytic thinking about clinical issues, psychoanalytic therapy, or even its relevance in one respect or another. This need to be aware of likely negative attitudes applies as much to psychoanalytic thinking within the broad field of health care as any other.

Australia is about as far from the wellspring of the psychoanalysis of Freud's Vienna as anything can be—both geographically and in terms of general lifestyle and living environment. We have been dubbed "The Lucky Country" by one of our better known intellectuals (Donald Horne, 1964)—and many would say we have few enough of these! Nevertheless, despite our fortunate climate, our never having had a military conflict on our land and our abundant natural resources, . . . we do get ill.

Australians—as far as one can generalize in these matters—are not known as being particularly introspective. We are largely action oriented, preferring sport and outdoor activities to intellectual and introspective pursuits.

161

So—do we have a need to think about *why* we get sick when we do? With this introduction, it may be a surprise to know that psychoanalytic treatment (either full psychoanalysis or psychoanalytic psychotherapy) has been available within the universal health insurance scheme that this country has enjoyed for the past 25 years—without restriction. That is, up to the time of writing this chapter for this volume. One of the editors (Harriette Kaley) was visiting Australia and invited this contribution in the week, in August 1996, just when, in the context of announcing severe cuts in many expenditure areas in the annual financial budget planning, the national government announced severe restrictions to the availability of long-term intensive treatments within the psychiatric component of the universal health insurance scheme. Knowing there was much to be learned by sharing between colleagues the experiences in countries where limitations are placed on health insurance coverage of psychoanalytic treatments, I eagerly responded to her invitation to contribute a chapter. There can be no doubt that the motivation for these restrictions, in Australia at least, was partly based on longstanding antipathy to psychoanalytic treatments and to the idea of the "worried well" receiving expensive useless treatments from psychiatrists who should really be spending their time treating the seriously mentally ill.

PSYCHOANALYSIS IN AUSTRALIA

The present situation needs to be understood in the context of the history of psychoanalysis in Australia. The first psychoanalyst was, as in so many countries, a refugee from wartime Europe: a Hungarian woman analyst, Clara Geroe. Dr. Geroe arrived in 1941, her coming to Australia having been orchestrated by Ernest Jones, then president of the International Psychoanalytical Association (Martin, 1996), who was responding to approaches from a small group of Melbourne psychiatrists who had become interested in Freud's writing and ideas. (Melbourne was then, as now, one of the two largest cities in Australia, with a population of 3.2 million.)

As elsewhere, from these small beginnings, analysis grew. In Australia, however, it grew slowly and to not a very great extent. No other psychoanalyst refugees migrated to our shores from war-torn Europe at that time. Dr. Geroe did everything: she psychoanalyzed, taught, and supervised a small number of candidates.[1]

From these beginnings (and their inevitable complications), together

---

[1] *Editors' note*: Readers may be familiar with the similar influence of the redoubtable European-trained woman analyst Frances Deri on the development of the first psychoanalytic institute in Los Angeles. See Farber and Green (1993).

with the addition of Australians who trained abroad (mainly in London) and a few later immigrants from overseas, the Australian Psychoanalytic Society was formed in 1971, initially as a Provisional Society of the I.P.A., and has grown to its present size of 65 members. These 65 members live and work mainly in three centers: Sydney (population 3.8 million), Melbourne (population 3.2 million) and Adelaide (population 1 million)—three capital cities of the states with the largest populations. But "large population" in Australia is very small by international standards. For example, Sydney, the largest metropolis, has, at the time of writing, 26 psychoanalysts and 7 candidates.

In each center, in the early days, the few analysts stimulated an interest in psychoanalytic thinking in the health care community with which they had some contacts, especially within the child treatment clinics. Thus, from the earliest days, there has been a growing interest in psychoanalytically oriented treatment, which has spread throughout much of the country. All states have organizations promoting psychoanalytically oriented psychotherapy, although there is far from homogeneity in this field. While the Australian Psychoanalytical Society has been strongly influenced by the British schools, more so by the Kleinians and the Independents, psychotherapy in general is even more "eclectic" and has quite a strong representation of self psychology, influenced by some psychotherapists who have themselves been influenced by their experiences in America and by American psychoanalyst visitors, who have been invited regularly to Australia by various psychotherapy groups.

The net result of all this has been quite a significant growth in the number of private practitioners offering a range of psychodynamically oriented psychotherapies—from full scale, five-day-per-week psychoanalysis with analysts trained according to International Psychoanalytical Association guidelines, to once-per-week psychotherapy of a variety of kinds, with formally and informally trained psychotherapists. Practitioners are both medically qualified (mostly psychiatrists and a few general practitioners) and a variety of nonmedical practitioners, who are mainly psychologists and social workers. It needs to be underscored that only medically trained practitioners' services are covered by the universal health insurance provisions. This means that only patients who are being seen by medically trained therapists receive rebates from the national health insurance ("Medicare") and until the time of this writing this was unrestricted in respect of the number of sessions covered. Thus, patients who otherwise might not have any possibility of being able to afford even a few treatment sessions have been able to undertake full psychoanalytic treatment for as many years as their disorders required. A lucky country indeed.

All has not been perfect in paradise, however. Needless to say, while this ready access to intensive psychoanalytic treatment may have been fortunate for a number of patients who could not otherwise have afforded it, this distinction between medical and nonmedical has resulted in significant consequences among the community of therapists. Fees charged by medically trained therapists (approx. US$100–110 per session) have been in line with those charged by general psychiatrists, albeit somewhat lower in respect of the frequent sessions involved, yet almost fully covered by the health insurance provisions. Fees paid by patients for all medical services provided by private medical practitioners in Australia are covered by Medicare, the universal health insurance scheme provided by the Australian government. These generous provisions provide 100% coverage of a so-called schedule fee, after the patient has incurred a "gap" (approximately US$275) in any calendar year, paid "out of pocket," between the fee charged by the medical practitioner and the fee for that item of service on the annually published fee schedule, which covers all medical and surgical services.

As will be appreciated, all the complex issues that flow from the presence of the third-party payor impinge in this situation. Many analysts charge slightly above the "schedule fee" in order that there be some patient contribution to the professional fee. This addition to the "gap" just mentioned is not covered by the 100% insurance coverage and results in a small amount of the fee which can be individualized according to a given patient's financial circumstances.

The services of nonmedical psychoanalysts and psychotherapists, however, have never been included in the provisions of the national health insurance scheme, and this has largely been so for nonmental health allied health practitioners in all fields allied to medicine (except for optometrists, who have recently become included, despite the protestations of ophthalmologists).

Nevertheless, as a general rule, medical therapists have usually sought to refer patients who conceivably *could* afford the relevant fees, to their nonmedical colleagues and sought to keep their own heavily subsidized availability for those patients who could not themselves afford such therapy. This is an informal practice that has developed in recognition of the fact that the psychoanalytic and psychotherapeutic training undertaken by medically and nonmedically qualified practitioners is the same, no matter what their basic health science degree might be. Of course, the quality of the personal relationships between practitioners in any mutually referring network is of considerable importance if these informal arrangements are to work well.

PSYCHOANALYTICALLY ORIENTED THERAPIES
AND THE HEALTH CARE SYSTEM

Australia is made up of six states and two smaller (in population) territories. Health care in Australia is funded primarily by two systems: capped grants to states, used to fund public hospitals and the public psychiatric service, and an uncapped, universal, federally funded health insurance scheme that subsidizes the payment of all services provided by the medical profession in private consulting rooms and private hospitals. All Australians have access to the generally excellent nonpsychiatric public hospital system at no personal cost, although waiting lists for elective surgery are lengthy.

Private health insurance is available for those who wish to have choice of doctor, immediate care for elective surgery, and better hotel facilities in private medical, surgical and psychiatric hospitals. As indicated earlier, the subsidies for medical services are generous, around 85% of the so-called schedule fee, with a small maximum gap for expensive procedures. When the universal health insurance provisions were first promulgated, the schedule fee was derived by ascertaining what was then a "common fee,"[2] although there are no variations in respect of regional considerations. More or less annual adjustments (increases) to the entire fee schedule are made through a combination of medico-political lobbying and governmental fiscal constraints. In recent years, the quite considerable past increases of up to 10% or more per year have been held to closer to 1 to 2% per year.

While most specialist physicians, surgeons, and psychiatrists charge close to the common fee (regrettably some others take the opportunity to add considerably to the common fee), a considerable proportion of general practitioners accept a reduction of approximately 15% in their fees by so-called bulk billing (directly billing Medicare and not the patient themselves). Together, these practices enable almost all patients to be managed in the private sector. Referrals of patients to specialists must be made by general practitioners, who thus act as gatekeepers to expensive consultant services. In the absence of managed care and other direct relationships between insurance organizations and practitioners, there are no present conflicts of interest in these practices, although there are indications that changes along such lines are on the way.

Australia's universal health scheme consumes about 8-9% of Gross Domestic Product. (Australian Bureau of Statistics, 1996). Frequently used medications, including psychotropic drugs, are also heavily subsidized through a Pharmaceutical Benefits Scheme. There have been almost no controls over this uncapped funding, and thus there is growing anxiety that the cost of this system will escalate. Accordingly, the amount contributed by patients has recently been increased appreciably, despite the political unpopularity of such measures.[3]

---

[2] *Editors' note*: Perhaps comparable to the "usual and customary fee" in the United States.
[3] This "uncapped" situation has changed radically in early 1998 with the introduction by the government of a scheme whereby the subsidy for the most commonly prescribed medications are pegged to the cheapest available generic equivalent for the given medication.

Uncontrolled cost increases have been due largely to a mixture of increasingly expensive technologies, increased utilization of new and expensive pharmaceutical agents, and the inevitable rises in salaries of all health professionals. The contribution to the considerable cost increases is minimally due to treatment for psychiatric disorder, and certainly in no sense a "blow out" due to unrestrained use of psychoanalytically oriented therapies. The medical community in Australia, claiming professional freedom in the clinical arena as justification, has been largely successful in resisting any attempts to impose even reasonable controls.

But psychiatry is a special case. Perhaps because psychiatry itself is subject to the worldwide stereotypes and misconceptions that mental illness seems to attract, governments have frequently targeted the mental health services to make at least token savings and institute token controls. However, in an already underfunded and "Cinderella" (unglamorous and having to do the type of work others decline to do!) part of the health care system, even token savings can be a significant proportion of existing funds. This has been the case on a number of occasions, and psychiatric services in the public sector—which is state funded—have been progressively plundered.

Public psychiatric services, historically poorly funded, have in recent years been subjected to massive cuts. As a result, the state psychiatric services have undergone the familiar deinstitutionalization that other countries have undertaken before us, with the same untoward consequences. Perhaps because, unlike in other countries, the private sector has been totally free from these false economies, at least some of the patients who might otherwise have gone completely without professional services have been able to receive treatment in the private sector. (This so-called cost-shifting from one bureaucracy to another is another cause of the uncontrolled escalation of costs in the federal sphere and another major threat to the health service economy itself.)

Thus, in Australia, as a result of a quite generous welfare system and the availability of private health care, displaced psychiatric patients are not as visible as they might be in some other countries. But not all psychiatric patients can—or even wish to—avail themselves of psychiatric help.

WHERE HAS PSYCHOANALYSIS CONTRIBUTED TO MENTAL HEALTH CARE SERVICES?

Perhaps more than any other form of treatment, psychoanalytically oriented therapy requires a considerable measure of commitment on the part of the patient. Therefore, it is only in certain compartments of the health care field that even a potentially receptive patient population might be available for interventions requiring thought rather than action.

Child Psychiatric Services

Psychodynamic therapy in the public sector has been largely confined to child and adolescent services and to some community health clinics. Of necessity, owing to the relatively small number of analysts in Australia, the opportunity to introduce a strong psychoanalytic influence throughout the health services has not been possible. It is fair to say, however, that it has largely been the case that individual analysts themselves have associated themselves with these services to create an environment wherein interest in and respect for psychoanalytically oriented approaches to treatment can be achieved.

There has never been an inpatient unit dedicated to psychoanalytic psychotherapies such as the (albeit few) well-known centers in America or England. But at least three or four child and adolescent treatment centers, in Sydney and Melbourne, have been strongly influenced by psychoanalysts and psychotherapists with a strong allegiance to psychoanalysis. A significant number of the present membership of the Australian Psychoanalytical Society, especially in Sydney, had their earliest exposure to psychoanalytic approaches and psychoanalytic treatment in such child treatment centers. Thus, a number of psychologists and social workers and a few psychiatrists were influenced sufficiently to undertake psychoanalytic training.

Child Protection Services

As a result of the quite strong presence of psychoanalytically informed thinking in one of the major Sydney teaching hospitals in the field of child health, one of the analysts (Dr. John Boots) has had considerable input into the provision of child protection services. These services are fraught with complex psychological, social, and legal issues and the psychoanalytically oriented supervision offered has certainly been of considerable benefit to the setting up and conduct of such services, at least in this particular service.

Early Intervention in Infant and Child Psychiatric Services

As with psychoanalytic communities elsewhere, there is a growing awareness among psychoanalysts and those working with psychoanalytic concepts that early intervention with mothers and babies who present with, say, sleep disturbance or other behavioral disorder in the child's early life can significantly help to overcome some of the developmental blocks that underlie these symptoms. Although by no means widespread in the health care system, these concepts are beginning to become integrated into some early intervention programs and are beginning to influence planning for further services.

Drug and Alcohol Services

An area in which I have had considerable input is that involving the addiction treatment services. Although characteristically an area strongly dominated by both medical model and self-help-philosophy thinking, there has been the opportunity to influence at least one geographical area service to take account of underlying psychodynamic issues contributing to personality disorder and family dysfunction—and the notion that drug use of any kind is an attempt at "self medicating" unbearable psychic dysphorias of a variety of kinds.

Although only of anecdotal value, it is worth recording that, in an area of the health service characterized by high burnout rates and marked staff turnover rates, the team of counselors receiving psychoanalytic supervision—for some 20 years now!—has remained largely intact, with only minimal turnover. Many clients have been contained in long-term psychotherapeutic relationships, with notable benefit. This is one of the few areas of public sector mental health services where long-term therapy has been able to survive the relentless economic restrictions on service provision that have eroded the mental health services in this country over the years.

Psychoanalysis and Outpatient Treatment Services

As already outlined, the major contribution of psychoanalytically trained health professionals is in the provision of treatment for voluntary, ambulant patients able and willing to attend the private consulting rooms of their therapists. Referral to nonmedical therapists is almost solely on the basis of their own established referral networks, and would only rarely involve referral from the public sector. While this is also largely the case with medically qualified therapists, there would be an appreciable number of referrals from inpatient units where a hospital-based doctor may have had favorable contact with psychoanalytic approaches, say during training. Nevertheless, the bulk of psychoanalytically oriented therapy in Australia is conducted by private practitioners, with medically qualified therapists having their work heavily subsidized by the (until now) universal health insurance system.

MANAGED CARE IN AUSTRALIA

There has—as yet!—been no influence by privately owned managed care organizations in Australia, although the concept has been under discussion for many years. The concept has had no support from the organized medical profession, and whatever inroads have been made have been made in the public hospital system. There has been some overt acknowledgment by the government's health department officers that managed care concepts are difficult to apply in the field of psychiatric services. A national research project is underway to attempt to establish costing guidelines for psychiatric illness, comparable to the concept of "diagnostic related groups" (DRGs), which have been developed for medical and surgical illnesses (Mental Health Classification and Service Costs Project of the Australian Health Ministers' Advisory Committee, 1995). Thus far, the consensus seems to be that DRGs do not as readily apply in mental health fields as in physical medicine.[4]

THE SITUATION AS OF OCTOBER 1996

Although there have been many threats to the participation of psychoanalytically oriented practitioners in the field of mental health service delivery over the past years, an approach largely constituting seeking direct contact with and education of those bureaucrats responsible for the decisions has been successful, in most instances, at keeping the threats at bay. Successive Federal Health Ministers have each made moves to curtail aspects of psychoanalytically oriented treatment. There is general agreement that they have been motivated by preconceptions over and above any simple consideration of the costs involved. Nevertheless, to their credit, each has responded to the efforts of the psychoanalytic profession, especially through working parties of the Australian Psychoanalytical Society, to educate the relevant bureaucrats, who, in turn, have persuaded their political masters to withhold their intentions. It has always been within the ambit of any Health Minister to act as he or she pleases in this regard and to make relevant decisions without the need to listen to expert advice.

Regrettably, this long-feared eventuality took place in August, 1996. The then Federal Health Minister, Dr. Michael Wooldridge, a medically qualified member of a newly elected Conservative Government which had been out of office for some 13 years, swept in a number of ostensibly cost-cutting and restructuring measures, including the curtailment of full insurance (subsidy) for psychiatric treatment to 50 sessions in any given year. Beyond this figure, the rebate received by patients was cut to 50% of the usual fee for any further sessions that may be undertaken.

In response to the protests of the psychiatric profession in Australia at

---

[4] *Editors' note*: The current emergence of managed care kinds of approaches to health services in Australia appears to come not from the private sector, as in the United States, but from the government.

this measure, the Minister himself retorted in public, that overseas health administrators, especially in the USA, "will fall about laughing." The implication was that Australian psychiatrists had been getting away with heavily subsidized, unsubstantiated long-term psychiatric treatments for too long. Even so, this laughter is short sighted and probably driven by the unconscious hostile forces identified 80 to 90 years ago by Freud, whenever the need to painstakingly uncover underlying causes of illness is broached.

As is abundantly clear now from a multitude of studies, there are demonstrable cost-benefits and cost-offsets from the availability of psychodynamic treatments for a wide range of conditions (Roth and Fonagy, 1996; Gabbard et al., 1997).

Considerable efforts were made, both by individuals and by professional organizations, to inform the Minister that obliging psychiatrists to curtail longer term therapies (or else suffer a significant reduction in income) would result only in their replacing these therapy hours with hours seeing more patients on fewer occasions. Even though part of the intended "restructuring" involves an increased capacity to see "new" patients and the psychiatrist's acting as consultant rather than therapist, the health system does not have the capacity to take up the treatments that the "consultant psychiatrist" may recommend—and that, under the previous arrangements, they conducted themselves.

Fears that severely depressed and suicidal patients who have been contained in psychodynamic treatment may in fact commit suicide were denounced by the Health Minister as "shroud waving" on the part of the profession. Expressed concerns for the children and partners of mentally disordered patients undergoing longer term treatment fell on deaf ears, and all related efforts to convey the short-sighted nature of this measure were dismissed as self-serving on the part of the psychiatrists involved. Efforts by the Royal Australian and New Zealand College of Psychiatrists to engage in dialogue (let alone negotiations) with the new Health Minister were rebuffed, and the restrictions so long averted were put into place.

THE SITUATION AS OF DECEMBER 1996

Eventually, the Royal Australian and New Zealand College of Psychiatrists (hereinafter referred to as "The College"), the Australian and New Zealand counterpart of the American Psychiatric Association, was able to secure from the Health Minister an agreement to establish a working party with government health department officials and health insurance (Medicare) officers to explore the expected consequences of the government's cost-cutting measures, and, if necessary, make appropriate recommendations for the Minister's consideration. A deadline of early December 1996 was imposed, so that any potential recommendations could be implemented in May 1997, when it was anticipated further budgetary measures would be taking place.

Intense work was undertaken by College members—particularly members within the College's Section of Psychotherapy—and by members of the Australian Psychoanalytical Society (both medical and nonmedical) to prepare submissions for the working party. As the government only belatedly was prepared to consult with even the College, the psychoanalytic input to the working party was through the Section of Psychotherapy of the College, which appointed me to represent the Section of Psychotherapy on the College delegation to the working party.

Another stream of intense activity that sprang up during the last months of 1996 was the establishment of an organization representing patients affected by the financial restrictions on rebates. This organization was called M.I.N.D.—Mental Illness Network against Discrimination. Psychiatrists involved in psychotherapeutic treatment were, in the past, loath, for reasons to do with transference and countertransference, to seek to activate their patients in the service of lobbying. This reluctance is in stark contrast to psychiatrist colleagues who treat schizophrenic and depressed patients. These psychiatrists appear only too happy for such patients to become involved in self-help and lobby groups, and some such psychiatrists themselves work actively with patient and care groups. Perhaps there is something to be learned from this. Nevertheless, on this occasion, psychiatrists undertaking long-term intensive psychotherapeutic treatment did provide support to M.I.N.D. in various ways, both formally and informally. Even so, it became apparent that the participation of both patients and psychiatrists in this area fraught with transference and countertransference acting-out potential, had stimulated many such instances which needed to be analyzed in the course of ongoing analyses and psychotherapies.

Thus, alongside the efforts of professionals through the formal channels provided by the working party, a degree of influence *was* achieved by patients, through their own efforts, by having the government appreciate that considerable suffering would result from the withdrawal of access to needed intensive psychotherapeutic treatments. The voice of patients who had suffered from sexual abuses appeared to be especially strong.

The working party met on three occasions and argued the pros and cons of efficacy of psychotherapeutic treatments and the cost–benefit and equity issues of expensive long-term treatments by psychiatrists who might be better deployed as consultants to general practitioners and other health professionals. There was evident suspicion that psychiatrists were concerned merely about preserving their incomes and their preferred way of working with patients; further evidence was provided from health insurance statistics that there were indeed some few psychiatrists earning what appeared to be inordinately large incomes through Medicare funding. Nonetheless, an atmosphere of goodwill and understanding was established sufficient to permit the consideration of some possible relaxation of the restrictions that had been put into place on November 1, 1996.

The government, through the Minister's delegate to the working party, was prepared to consider provisions that would potentially permit extended funding (beyond the now-current post-50 sessions step-down to 50% funding) for patients, within a limited set of diagnostic categories, who were sufficiently distressed and disabled and who had failed previous attempts at treatment and were being treated by psychiatrists with some yet-to-be-agreed form of accreditation to conduct the more intensive treatments.

It was appreciated that the Health Minister was constrained by broad government concerns about budgetary "blow-outs" and was subject to his own ministerial colleagues' pressures to achieve substantial cuts within his own portfolio. Thus, it was with considerable relief and appreciation that the College representatives met with the Minister and his advisors; he agreed in principle to the limited relaxations of the earlier blanket restrictions. Final details of what changes could be made were negotiated between the Minister's representative and the Secretary of the College.

THE NEW ARRANGEMENTS

As of January 1, 1997, patients suffering either from the severe psychiatric sequelae of sexual and/or physical abuse, from borderline personality disorder, or from eating disorder—provided that they scored 50 or less on the Global Assessment of Function scale—would be entitled to up to 160 subsidized sessions (in a given year) as previously, before a step-down to 50% funding then takes place. The question of how "accreditation" of psychiatrists who may utilize these new provisions for their patients is to be achieved has yet to be determined. Both the College and the Australian Psychoanalytical Society have established subcommittees to grapple with this potentially divisive issue in a way that will satisfy the Government. The Government agreed that the working party should meet again in the second half of 1997 to review what effect the changes caused in the patterns of utilization of the new "Item Numbers" on the schedule that pertain to the psychiatric patients being seen more than 50 times per year.

Needless to say, there have been considerable disruptions to the course of existing analyses and therapies, as psychiatrists and patients together grapple with the issues of qualifying or not qualifying under the new conditions. There remains much working through to be done!

POSTSCRIPT

The body of this chapter was written in December, 1996. In August 1997, as agreed, representatives of the College again met with officers of the government's Department of Health and Family Services and with officers of the Health Insurance Commission to review the utilization data available and to negotiate any necessary changes.

The data provided by health department officers indicated that a very considerable reduction in utilization of intensive psychiatric treatment at the fully funded level had been achieved, with considerable cost savings. Clinical experience reported by College Fellows, however, showed that patients with severe personality disorder of aetiologies other than overt physical or sexual abuse were being denied the funding available to those with similarly disabling severe personality disorder, but of defined etiology. In addition, patients needing to claim rebates under the new Item were, when submitting claims, automatically identified as those having suffered the "required" form of abuse.

It was agreed by the Government officers that this procedure was discriminatory and that all severe disabling personality disorders—of whatever etiology—should be eligible for the same level of funding. It was also agreed that children and adolescents needing intensive psychiatric treatment did not fit easily under the criteria applicable to adult patients and that a broadening of the criteria was appropriate.

While the *status quo ante* had not been restored by any means, the College representatives felt that the government representatives had moved as far as was politically possible in ensuring that severely disabled personality disordered patients—and especially disturbed children and adolescents—could still gain access to the intensive treatment services which they needed.

REFERENCES

Australian Bureau of Statistics (1996), Government Printing Office, Canberra.

Farber, S. & Green, M. (1993), *Psychoanalysis on the Couch*. New York: William Morrow.

Gabbard, G. O., Lazar, S. G., Hornberger, J. & Spiegel, D. (1997), The economic impact of psychotherapy: A review. *Amer. J. Psychiat.*, 154:147–155.

Horne, D. (1964), *The Lucky Country*. Ringwood, Victoria, Aust.: Penguin Books.

Martin, R. T. (1996), Some observations on the history and developments of psychoanalysis in Australia. Scientific proceedings of the Australian Psychoanalytical Society, No. 25.

Mental Health Classification and Services Costs Project of the Australian Health Ministers' Advisory Committee, 1995.

Roth, A. & Fonagy, P. (1996) *What Works for Whom?* New York: Guilford.

PART IV

Current Issues and Special Populations

THIRTEEN

Who Is in Psychoanalysis Now?

Empirical Data and Reflections On Some Common Misperceptions

NORMAN DOIDGE

This chapter reviews some of the empirical data on who is currently in psychoanalysis in the Canadian Province of Ontario, according to demographics, previous treatment history, childhood trauma, and DSM-III-R diagnoses. In Ontario, the province in which we (Doidge et al., 1994) conducted our study, psychoanalysis by a medical doctor is covered by the Ontario Health Insurance Plan after a review of the data, some causes of common misconceptions about psychoanalytic patients are discussed.

EMPIRICAL STUDIES OF PSYCHIATRIC MORBIDITY, CHILDHOOD TRAUMA, AND PREVIOUS TREATMENT ATTEMPTS IN PSYCHOANALYTIC PATIENTS IN ONTARIO

Psychoanalysis is generally the most intensive form of psychoanalytic psychotherapy in terms of dose, which one can define as the number of sessions times the duration of treatment. Its indications are quite specific (American Psychiatric Association, 1985), and a patient's motivation to complete as intensive a treatment as psychoanalysis has to be quite high, even if one considers only the time a patient must devote to it. It seems reasonable to assume that analytic patients, as a group, will share some specific characteristics.

The Survey of Psychoanalysis in Ontario (Doidge et al., 1994) was a survey of practice of all psychoanalysts in Ontario (n = 174) accredited by the International Psychoanalytic Association. Ontario is Canada's most populous province, with a population of 9.9 million. The survey was sent out in May of 1992. The survey questionnaire asked about analyst demographics and patterns of practice, analysand demographics, previous treatment history and history of childhood traumata, and indications for analysis. The section on indications used the approach outlined in the American Psychiatric Association Manual of Peer Review Guidelines for Psychoanalysis (1985). We defined sexual abuse as "the involvement of dependent, developmentally immature children in sexual activity that they do not fully comprehend and without consideration for their stage of psycho-social sexual development." This definition was taken from Levine (1990). We gave clinicians the option of saying Yes, No, or Not sure in response to questions about sexual abuse; thus, only cases in which the clinician was certain the abuse had occurred were included. Respondents were asked to refer to a list of DSM-III-R criteria included in the questionnaire in making diagnoses. The questionnaire packages were mailed with an anonymous stamped, addressed return envelope. One hundred and seventeen psychoanalysts returned the questionnaires, giving a response rate of 67%. Of the 117 respondent analysts, six were Ph.D.s, and the rest were M.D.s, virtually all with psychiatric training. Fourteen of the analysts were training analysts, 16 were trainees, and three were child analysts. The mean number of psychoanalytic patients in treatment with each analyst was 4.96 (SD = 2.78; mode = 3.0; median = 5.0; range = 14.0). The mean length of the analyses completed by the analysts was 4.90 years (SD = 1.87; mode = 5.0; median = 5.0; range = 5.5). Forms were received for 580 patients, representing two thirds of all analytic patients in Ontario.

Fifty-nine percent of those receiving psychoanalysis were women, and 41% men. The vast majority of patients (82%) had attempted previous treatments, including use of medication and briefer forms of therapy, and resorted to analysis when previous treatments did not resolve existing symptoms.

The levels of childhood trauma reported in this group of patients were as follows: Twenty-three percent had suffered traumatic separation in childhood; 23% had been sexually abused; 22.2% had been physically abused; 21.3% had parents or siblings die in childhood or during the teen years, and a significant number suffered some other kind of overwhelming point trauma. These group findings are consistent with the emphasis on the role of trauma in the development of many of the neuroses reported in psychoanalytic case histories. Nonetheless, these high rates of trauma do not mean that all patients with character neuroses have had childhood traumas. Moreover, the questionnaire asked about many kinds of strain traumas—lower level traumas that have an effect by virtue of their chronicity.

Patients presented with a mode of two psychiatric disorders and a mean of approximately four current psychiatric diagnoses. As expected, character diagnoses were prevalent, with a mean of one DSM-III-R personality disorder per patient. While this study was limited by the survey methodology, its findings are consistent with the prevalence of personality disorders in psychoanalytic patients in other studies using structured interviews (see Doidge et al., 1994, for a discussion of related studies). The Axis I disorders found in these patients are listed in Table 1 and the personality disorders found in these patients are listed in Table 2.

The most common Axis I diagnoses made were of mood (48% had dysthymia), anxiety, and sexual dysfunction disorders. Dysthymia has been found to have a prevalence of 36% in general outpatient populations (Markowitz et al., 1992). As noted in the text of DSM-III-R, dysthymia is frequently associated with personality disorders and has a poor prognosis (Wells, et al., 1992). We noted that many of the diagnoses seen in analytic patients, such as sexual dysfunction disorders, dissociative disorders, sleep disorders, and posttraumatic stress disorders, are not specifically asked about

Table 1.
DSM-III-R Axis I Disorders In Psychoanalytic Patients

	N	Total %	Female N	Prev*	Male N	Prev**
Substance Dependence or Abuse	69	11.9	35	10.2	34	14.4
Psychotic Disorder Present	18	3.1	11	3.2	7	3.0
Mood Disorder Present	376	64.8	231	67.2	145	61.4
Anxiety Disorder Present	284	48.9	166	48.3	118	50.0
Somatoform Disorder	135	23.3	77	22.4	58	24.6
Dissociative Disorder	56	9.7	44	12.8	12	5.1
Sexual Disorder	54	9.3	22	6.4	32	13.6
Sexual Dysfunction	252	43.4	141	41.0	111	47.0
Sleep Disorder	89	15.3	60	17.4	29	12.3
Impulse Disorder	27	4.7	12	3.5	15	6.4
Adjustment Disorder	42	7.2	26	7.6	16	6.8
Adult Disorder Not listed	19	3.3	13	3.8	6	2.5
Psychological Factors Affecting Physical Disease	118	20.3	80	23.3	38	16.1
Eating Disorders***	17	2.9	13	3.8	4	1.7
Gender Identity Disorders***	11	1.9	4	1.2	7	3.0

*number of women with the diagnosis divided by the number of women in the sample (344)
**number of men with the diagnosis divided by the number of men in the sample (236)
***If eating disorders and gender identity disorders are included in the overall totals of DSM disorders, the mean number of Axis I disorders rises to 3.25 (SD = 2.53; median = 3.0; mode = 2.0; range = 17.0).
Source: Doidge et al. (1994). Reproduced by permission of the publisher

Table 2.
DSM-III-R Personality Disorders By Descending Order
in Psychoanalytic Patients

Cluster		Total N	%	Female N	%*	Pre**	Male N	%***	Prev****
Narcissistic	B	108	18.6	51	47.2	14.8	57	52.8	24.2
Self-Defeating		87	15.0	60	69.0	17.4	27	31.0	11.4
Personality NOS		84	14.5	55	65.5	15.9	29	34.5	12.3
Obsessive Com.	C	68	11.7	24	35.3	6.9	44	64.7	18.6
Dependent	C	44	7.6	25	56.8	7.3	19	43.2	8.1
Histrionic	B	43	7.4	39	90.7	11.3	4	9.3	1.7
Borderline	B	41	7.1	31	75.6	9.0	10	24.4	4.2
Avoidant	C	28	4.8	13	46.4	3.8	15	53.6	6.4
Passive-Aggre	C	27	4.7	7	25.9	2.0	20	74.1	8.5
Schizoid	A	15	2.6	5	33.3	1.5	10	66.7	4.2
Paranoid	A	11	1.9	4	36.4	1.2	7	63.6	3.0
Antisocial	B	3	0.5	0	0	0	3	100.0	1.3
Schizotypal	A	0							
No Pers Disorder		166	28.6	107	64.5	31.1	59	35.5	25.0

*number of women with diagnosis divided by number of individuals with that diagnosis
**number of women with the diagnosis divided by the number of women in the sample
(344)
*** number of men with the diagnosis divided by the number of individuals with the diagnosis
****number of men with the diagnosis divided by the number of men in the sample (236)
Source: Doidge et al. (1994). Reproduced by permission of the publisher.

in the current Structured Clinical Interviews for DSM-III-R (SCID), and
any researchers who wish to make use of such interviews for studying psychoanalytic patients would be well advised to modify the SCID accordingly; similarly, anyone interpreting studies of psychoanalytic patients
employing the SCID will have to take this into account.

The high number of mood and anxiety disorders is consistent with
the Menninger study (Wallerstein, 1986), which found that 88% of patients in psychoanalysis or psychoanalytic psychotherapy had anxiety, depression, or both. The well-known Penn Psychotherapy Study by Luborsky
et al. (1988) found that the most common Axis I diagnoses in patients in
psychoanalytic psychotherapy were dysthymia and anxiety disorders. Preliminary data from a study that is being conducted by Doidge and colleagues on psychoanalytic patients in all 50 United States shows similar
rates for diagnoses for patients in psychoanalysis (Doidge, 1994).

Recent SCID studies of the symptoms of applicants for psychoanalysis in New York show that 32% of these patients have mood disorders, 32%
have anxiety disorders, and 12% have substance abuse disorders (Hyler et
al., 1992; Oldham et al., 1995).

The Ontario findings are consistent with the Guidelines for Psycho-analytic Peer Review in the American Psychiatric Association's Manual of Peer Review of Psychoanalysis. The Manual notes that information about the Axis I or Axis II diagnosis is not sufficient for determining that analysis is indicated. The Manual requires that a patient's difficulties be based on both chronic intrapsychic conflict and developmental inhibition or arrest. Other, less intensive treatments may not be sufficient to resolve the patient's problems. The patients in psychoanalysis in Ontario showed a number of indicators of chronicity, including childhood traumata, previous treatment, and Axis II pathology. The Manual also emphasizes that, within diagnostic categories, there are patients for whom analysis is optimally, relatively or heroically indicated, or contraindicated. Ratings of these specific indicators from the Manual of Peer Review for the Ontario population of patients in psychoanalysis will be reported in a future publication, but preliminary data analysis shows that these indicators were adhered to in the overwhelming majority of cases.

We interpreted the high number of attempts at briefer or less intensive treatments as an important finding. Briefer treatments have a place, but are not the solution for every patient's needs.

In terms of personality disorders, psychoanalysis in Canada appears to be largely a treatment for Cluster B (the dramatic cluster) and C (the anxious-fearful cluster) of personality disorders. Narcissistic and self-defeating (masochistic) personality disorders are the commonest disorders. If one keeps in mind that the DSM-III-R describes only the thick-skinned, grandiose narcissist, and that many thin-skinned, rejection-sensitive narcissists might qualify for other diagnostic categories (for example, the avoidant personality disorder for those who, to avoid being rejected, avoid relationships altogether; and histrionic personality disorder for those who often have to be the center of attention) the extent of narcissistic difficulties is more impressive still.

The extremely common, self-defeating personality disorder was replaced in DSM-IV, against the objection of many psychoanalysts, with a disorder, which is in the appendix for further study, called depressive personality disorder. At times the terms depressive character, masochistic character, and self-defeating character have been used to describe a similar constellation. It may be anticipated that psychoanalytic patients with masochistic features will in the future often receive the diagnosis of depressive personality disorder or personality disorder NOS, until masochistic character phenomena are again described in their own right.

One of the reasons that psychoanalysts may diagnose narcissistic and self-defeating or masochistic personality disorders more frequently than researchers do is that researchers do not detect these disorders on structured interviews. While there is much agreement that standardized criteria and structured interviews are helpful for assessing Axis I diagnoses, the current structured clinical interviews for Axis II, often based on a two to three hour interview with the patient, have poor agreement with each other beyond chance (median kappa = 0.25) (Perry, 1992). Clinical judgment, over a significant period of time, using standardized criteria, remains essential in diagnosing the personality conditions that psychoanalysts treat (Spitzer, 1983). To make a personality diagnosis, psychoanalysts find it important to assess the type of transference that emerges over time (Greenson, 1967; Kohut, 1971; Kernberg, 1984) when socially undesirable, embarrassing, repressed or split-off aspects of the personality are being assessed. One study, which compared the use of structured clinical interviews with longitudinal evaluation of clinical data, showed that the structured interviews were effective in discriminating behaviorally defined diagnoses but not others, such as the narcissistic and self-defeating disorders, which require inference about intentions (Skodol et al., 1991). The features of these disorders (egocentrism, contempt, selfishness, narcissistic vulnerability, masochistic tendencies) are profoundly shame laden and difficult for patients to acknowledge to people they hardly know, and it is no surprise that such characteristics are not easily disclosed to strangers.

OTHER CATEGORIES RELEVANT TO PSYCHOANALYTIC PATIENTS

There are other situations, not highlighted in the aforementioned tables, for which patients frequently seek psychoanalysis. An important diagnostic category are the V codes, which include problems related to abuse and neglect. This category might include patients who had severe childhood traumata, but who do not meet adult PTSD criteria, and yet have subtle disturbances. Another important V code is bereavement (V.6282), which might be one place under which "frozen" responses to early parent loss that extend into adulthood might be subsumed. Some homosexuals seek psychoanalysis, hoping either to deal with painful experiences relating to growing up homosexual, to improve their adaptation to their sexual orientation, or, in some cases, to change their sexual orientation. What is usually called homosexuality is probably best described as "the homosexualities" since it represents a complex phenomenon. According to MacIntosh (1994), 23% of 1215 homosexual patients (in treatment with 285 analysts) changed to a heterosexual sexual orientation in the course of psychoanalysis, even though 97.6% of the psychoanalysts rejected the idea that a homosexual patient in analysis can and should change to heterosexuality. The majority of homosexual patients did not change their sexual orientation but gained a number of benefits from psychoanalysis.

The findings of Doidge et al. (1994) in Ontario are consistent with the findings of the Task Force Report of the American Psychiatric Association (1989), which represents a compilation of expert opinion. This document lists, by disorder, the conditions for which psychoanalysis and psychodynamic psychotherapy may be the treatment of choice or a second-line treatment, depending on clinical conditions. A summary is produced in Table 3.

Table 4 is a collation by Dr. Glen Gabbard, taken from Treatments of Psychiatric Disorders: The DSM-IV Edition, American Psychiatric Press, (1995) edited by Glen O. Gabbard. It is an update of the 1989 Task Force Report. That text represents an assembly of expert opinions, based on literature reviews, and is to be used as a guideline and not a "cookbook" approach to treatments. Table 4 lists all the disorders for which psychoanalytic

Table 3.
American Psychiatric Association Task Force Report on Treatments,
DSM-III Disorders which respond to Psychoanalysis or
Psychoanalytic Psychotherapy

According to the Task Force Report on Treatments of the American Psychiatric Association (American Psychiatric Association, 1989) psychoanalysis, or psychodynamic psychotherapy, *when indicated,* are effective treatments for a number of disorders in adults including:

1) the character or personality disorders including the *avoidant, dependent, self-defeating, obsessional, passive aggressive,* some *paranoid,* some *schizoid, histrionic, narcissistic,* some *borderline* personality disorders, as well as *personality disorders not otherwise specified.* (But not the antisocial personality disorder)
2) substance abuse disorders
3) eating disorders
4) anxiety disorders, including post-traumatic disorders
5) mild to moderate mood disorders, i.e. depressions and dysthymia
6) sexual function and arousal disorders
7) sexual disorders, such as fetishism, courtship disorders, paraphilias (perversions such as sadism and masochism)
8) with modifications, some dissociative disorders, including multiple personality disorder
9) impulse disorders
10) psychological factors affecting physical disease, some somatoform disorders and sleep disorders

As well, a modified form of psychoanalytic psychotherapy, called supportive psychoanalytic psychotherapy, is useful in some psychotic disorders, crisis intervention and adjustment disorders.

A number of childhood disorders are treated in child analysis.

psychotherapy or psychoanalysis are indicated in the fourth edition. As can be seen, there are few changes from the earlier edition in terms of recommendations for psychoanalysis and psychoanalytic therapy. In fact, there are few changes since the compilation of Knight (1941). This stability in recommendations for psychoanalysis can be taken as a sign that the clinical consensus of practitioners has been consistent.

Table 4. Treatments of Psychiatric Disorders: the DSM-IV Edition, Edited by Glen Gabbard. (Table 4. was compiled by Dr. Gabbard.)

I. DISORDERS OF CHILDHOOD AND ADOLESCENCE
  A. Anxiety disorders of childhood and adolescence
  B. Post traumatic stress disorder
  C. Conduct disorders with high level of ego organization
  D. Childhood schizophrenia may require dynamically informed supportive psychotherapy.
  E. Some cases of obsessive-compulsive disorder may require psychodynamic therapy to improve relationships, self-esteem, and intrapsychic conflicts even though behaviour therapy and medication are generally considered treatments of choice.
  F. Depression in childhood and adolescence (Fonagy's study showed that psychoanalysis was effective in this disorder.)

II. SUBSTANCE USE
  A. Chronic hallucinogen abuse
  B. Cocaine abuse
  C. Chronic substance abusers
  D. Some alcoholics who cannot use traditional 12-steps methods

III. SCHIZOPHRENIA AND PSYCHOTIC DISORDERS
  Wayne Fenton and Stephen Cole, editors of the chapter wrote: "A primary focus on the insight-oriented tasks associated with investigative psychotherapy should likely be reserved for selected patients once clinical stability has been securely established. These patients are likely to have had good premorbid functioning, intermittent and less severe forms of schizophrenia, minimal residual deficits, and retention of the capacity for self-observation, curiosity, frustration tolerance, and humour" (p. 992).

IV. MOOD DISORDERS
  Glen Gabbard, who wrote the chapter in the DSM-IV volume on mood disorders has written: "Most therapists would agree, however, that those modalities are not indicated as the exclusive treatment for acute-phase patients with major depression. These modalities are certainly indicated for some patients who have failed to respond fully to pharmacotherapy or reeducative psychotherapies. A reanalysis of the data from the National Institute of Mental Health (NIMH) Treatment of Depression Collaborative Research Project (Blatt et al., in press) suggested that highly perfectionistic and self-critical patients are not likely to respond to either brief pharmacological or psychological treatments. This subgroup of depressed persons may be particularly

suited to more extended psychodynamic approaches. Also, when patients have significant Axis II pathology in addition to major depressive episodes, extended psychodynamic psychotherapy or psychoanalysis will generally be considered the treatment of choice. The clinician may need to wait for an acute episode to resolve before these characterological features become apparent. At that point, continued interpersonal problems, chronically low self-esteem, and other conflicted areas can be more completely assessed" (p. 1207). In addition, only about 40% to 45% of dysthymic patients are likely to respond to antidepressants, so the remainder may need psychoanalysis or extended dynamic psychotherapy.

V. ANXIETY DISORDERS, DISSOCIATIVE DISORDERS & ADJUSTMENT DISORDERS
   A. Adjustment disorders
   B. Depersonalization disorder
   C. Dissociative identity disorder (MPD)
   D. Acute stress disorder
   E. Panic disorder/agoraphobia—may be indicated for patients who only respond partially to pharmacotherapy or cognitive-behavioral based treatments
   F. Generalized anxiety disorder—indicated for some patients, but generally viewed as complementary to other forms of treatment
   G. Phobias—indicated for some cases of social phobia
   H. Dissociative amnesia and dissociative fugue

VI. SOMATOFORM DISORDERS
   A. Pain disorders—indicated in some cases

VII. SEXUAL DISORDERS
   A. Female sexual arousal disorder—indicated in some cases or as part of a multi-modal approach
   B. Male erectile disorder—indicated in some cases or as part of a multi-modal approach
   C. Sexual pain disorders—may be useful as an adjunct to behavioral approaches
   D. Transvestism
   E. Hypoactive sexual desire and sexual aversions—useful in some cases.

VIII. EATING DISORDERS
   A. Anorexia nervosa

IX. PERSONALITY DISORDERS
   A. Borderline personality disorder
   B. Dependent personality disorder
   C. Avoidant personality disorder
   D. Histrionic personality disorder
   E. Narcissistic personality disorder
   F. Obsessive-compulsive personality disorder
   G. Paranoid personality disorder
   H. Schizoid and schizotypal personality disorders—in some cases

X. DISORDERS OF IMPULSE CONTROL NOT OTHERWISE SPECIFIED
   A. Intermittent explosive disorder

DISCUSSION

An examination of the foregoing data suggests that the assertion that patients in analysis are the worried and the well is based on misinformation about the nature of the majority of patients undergoing psychoanalysis.

Misperceptions of Psychoanalytic Patients

What are some of the likely causes of these misperceptions? I suggest the following list, which is by no means exhaustive.

1) *The psychoanalytic situation is threatening to those who are outside of it.* It is easy to forget that, before Freud, psychiatrists, medical doctors, and other mental health practitioners seldom if ever talked to their patients for the length of time that Freud did. Extensive immersion in the patient's world leads to a relationship of extraordinary emotional intimacy, an unearthing of family problems, or even of the ambivalence that exists in ordinary, good family life. This new circumstance easily becomes threatening to family members, lovers, and friends of the patients. The analyst's privileged access to the patient's inner life is most easily misinterpreted by those who have not experienced therapy or analysis or who have not faced their own mixed or warded-off feelings.

2) *The reports of the presenting problems patients who get better are often, understandably, airbrushed for the sake of discretion.* The characterization of psychoanalytic patients as not requiring treatment stems in part from the fact that patients who have suffered from personality difficulties, developmental problems, or chronic sexual, mood, or anxiety problems related to unconscious fantasies, or development, are often ashamed to parade their past difficulties in front of others. They often are more comfortable saying, "My analysis was very helpful" or speaking in vague ways about the nonspecific benefits to self-esteem. Psychoanalysis often works by exposing warded off, shameful, guilt-inducing material. Thus, unlike other therapies that speak of very general mechanisms (such as behavior therapy), there is a tendency in analysands to keep the understandably private details of what emerged in analysis out of their anecdotal discussions of their treatment. As well, psychoanalysis often shows the relation between symptoms and personality; thus, for an analytic patient to admit to a particular group of symptoms is to admit to a kind of personality problem; it is the individual, idiosyncratic patient who is treated, not the general disorder. In contrast, biological treatment for major depression allows those patients to view themselves as having a difficulty that in no way is their "fault". Their difficulties are shared with others. One suspects it is for this reason that there have not been self-support groups for psychoanalytic patients in which they speak publicly of their shared difficulties.

Common sense suggests that people would not be willing to spend the vast amount of time required for psychoanalytic treatment unless they were significantly troubled in some portion of their lives.

3) *Third parties have a short-term interest in depicting psychoanalytic patients as not requiring treatment—for the time being.* In jurisdictions where insurance coverage changes frequently, such as is the case in the United States at this time, where patients change jobs and hence change insurance companies every few years, the insurer does not have an interest in the patient's long-term well-being or long-term preventive care. There is a tendency for individual insurance companies, or HMO's to recommend the shortest term, least costly form of treatment to patients during the time that they are covered by the company. Because of the frequency of job changes, these companies know that they will not be paying for the long-term effects of partially treated conditions in the employees they currently cover—the next insurance company will pick up the tab, as it were. In jurisdictions where insurance covers one for life, or long periods, the insurer has an interest in determining whether multiple short-term treatments, and partially treated conditions, will end up both costing the system more money and resulting in patient dissatisfaction. Moreover, in jurisdictions where the insurance agreement is not between the insurance company and the patient but between the insurance company and the employer, individual patient dissatisfaction is not a compelling factor in determining coverage; all that matters is employer dissatisfaction. Add to this that psychoanalysis—like many forms of treatment—applies only to a fairly small patient population at any given time, and the power of psychoanalytic patients as "consumers" becomes far from impressive.

4) *Analysts frequently prefer to think in etiological, as opposed to nosological terms.* Analysts have many motives for not using psychiatric terms with their patients. In general, they prefer to think etiologically about symptomatology. Patients often fear being stigmatized by psychiatric diagnoses, even if they have those disorders. Until very recently, analysts, like many psychiatrists, would, for purposes of patient confidentiality, attempt to give the least descriptive, vaguest diagnosis within reason, because they were concerned that this kind of information could be used against patients for insurance purposes or in court battles. One should remember that, in many jurisdictions, insurance coverage is discriminatory against those with illnesses. Such people may not get coverage or may only get it at very high rates. But there are additional reasons that psychiatric diagnoses have not been favored. Some psychologists, and lay analysts, have been trained in other diagnostic systems. Analysts who are psychiatrists of an older generation may not have kept up with the *Diagnostic and Statistical Manual* and are at times misinformed about how comprehensive it can be for noting areas of difficulty.

Theoretical developments have also led some analysts to be unenthu-siastic about using psychiatric diagnoses for their patients. Freud's earliest cases were of patients with symptom neuroses, and he was at pains to vouchsafe their good character, so that they would not be thought to suffer from a kind of organic taint. Nonetheless, it gradually became ap-parent to Freud and other psychoanalysts that there was a complex rela-tionship between character and symptom and that analytic patients had character difficulties as well as symptom difficulties. Any number of papers demonstrate the great shift of attention moving from the study of symp-toms to the study of character. Marmor (1953), for instance, speaking of hysteria, pointed out that the very suggestibility or plasticity that quickly gave rise to symptoms could lead to their quick removal. While the symp-toms themselves could be changed, however, the suggestibility, which is now widely seen as part of the underlying hysterical character structure, turns out to be extremely difficult to alter. Thus psychoanalysts began to be interested in the relationship of symptoms to character.

Given the fluidity of symptoms, many analysts became less interested in the initial diagnostic presentation of symptoms and more interested in etiology. Michels (1987) argued that

> what is diagnosed is the disease, not the person who suffers from it. A central purpose of diagnosis is to identify the disorder. . . . If we are interested in what makes a group of patients similar, we will be interested in diagnostic issues. If we are interested in what makes each member of a group different from the others, diagnosis will be of less importance [p. 698].

A fear that hard-won analytic insights, such as the role of defensive dis-guise of core issues, individual psychology, and fantasy, might be trimmed on the Procrustean bed of diagnosis led to a wariness of the *DSM* process. Yet, as Michel's statement intimates, the attitude of most analysts toward diagnosis was not either for or against but, rather, was a vacillation depending on the problems one is dealing with.

These debates were occurring at the very historical moment that bio-logical psychiatry was on the rise and held out much promise. There was strong pressure within departments of psychiatry to divide themselves into research-oriented clinical divisions that addressed various symptoms or disorders, and in the 1970s, Mood, Anxiety, and Sexual Disorder divisions and the like became increasingly commonplace, replacing the older divi-sions of outpatient verses inpatient departments. In general, psychoana-lysts became identified with that part of outpatient departments which treated "personality disorders." This division of mental illness between analysts and biologists was never formal and never complete, but anyone who lived through this period was aware of how frequently the older, retiring inpatient analysts were replaced in most departments by younger biological researchers.

At times, a cursory reading of what psychoanalysts were saying at the time seemed to support this distribution of what was now called "Axis II" (Personality Disorders) to the psychoanalysts. Yet a close reading of the following shows that this simply was not the case, at least for Auchincloss and Michels (1983), who wrote:

> Psychoanalysis is indicated when the patient suffers from persistent maladaptive character traits or when the recurrence and stability of the symptoms suggest that they are embedded in underlying character pathology that cannot be disregarded in the treatment. In other words, psychoanalysis (as a technique) and character analysis have become synonymous [p. 2].

In short, that analytic technique was increasingly focused on character did not necessarily mean that analytic patients did not have symptoms that could be measured. For instance it is frequently observed (particularly by the Kleinians) that many narcissistic patients actually develop depressive-type reactions as they mature and develop the capacity for concern. Still, psychodynamic psychiatrists frequently focus on what they think causes the symptoms, and when later editions of *DSM* came out, it is fair to say there was no rush to study updated *DSM* disorders in analytic patients.

5) *A conflation of mental health professionals in analysis with patients in analysis in general.* A study (Norcross, Strausser, and Faltus, 1988) of the type of therapy psychiatrists, psychologists, and social workers *choose for themselves* when they seek treatment showed that the majority undertook a psychoanalytic form of treatment: 41% undertook psychoanalysis, and 18% undertook psychoanalytic psychotherapy. This is a fairly impressive endorsement. It may, however, give those mental health professionals who themselves are not well disposed to psychoanalysis a biased sample of who is in analysis. In the absence of familiarity with the empirical data on psychoanalytic patients, there is a tendency to generalize from their fairly high-achieving colleagues in analysis about the nature of all analytic patients. Those of us who have worked in psychoanalytic clinics or seen many psychoanalytic patients, or who are familiar with case histories or the empirical data, do not have such a rosy picture of the health of patients in analysis.

THE RHETORICAL DEVALUATON OF PSYCHOANALYTIC PATIENTS

The rhetorical devaluation of psychoanalytic patients has been fairly consistent. It has been based on three assertions—unproven—that come up again and again: a) psychoanalytic patients are depicted as "the worried well" rather than people with significant problems (Sharfstein, 1978); b) psychoanalysis is only for the wealthy and those who do not need to make major sacrifices of time and money (even when coinsured) to undertake their treatments; and c) the analytic process is "narcissistic," or self-indulgent "navel gazing." Thus, for instance, even the treatment of a narcissistic disorder is seen not so much as modifying narcissism but, rather, as promoting it. The idea that treatment often requires that patients face warded-off painful truths about themselves and their experience, and that treatment is in fact at times quite painful, is not acknowledged.

These descriptions delegitimize psychoanalysis by stigmatizing it as frivolous, elitist, and indulgent. Occasionally, assertions are made, often by the same critics, that it is also not effective, that it is frivolous and wasteful. A review of the extensive empirical evidence in support of psychoanalytic efficacy is not within the purview of this chapter but can be found elsewhere (Doidge, 1997). While such negative perceptions tend to be highly selective and anecdotal, it is worth reviewing their sources. Indeed, some of them came about and have been maintained by an incomplete acquaintance with the history of psychoanalysis and psychoanalytic writings.

THE TREATMENT FOR THE WORRIED WELL?

One of the origins of the charge that psychoanalytic patients are merely the worried well comes from citing specific passages out of context from Freud's works. Freud emphasized many times that his patients did not have the taint of organic degeneracy. Degeneracy, before the turn of the century, was often linked to a kind of moral degeneracy, and there was a lot of stigma attached to that label. As analysts know, some of the first psychoanalytic patients, such as Anna O or Elizabeth von R, were seriously disturbed and frequently nonfunctional women suffering from conversion hysteria. Freud (1910) was at pains to emphasize that these women were not "degenerates"; at the time, the major competing theories explaining hysteria were those of Janet, who theorized that hysterics had constitutional difficulties related to degeneracy making it difficult for them to synthesize their thoughts (cited in Auchincloss and Michels, 1983). Thus Freud (1910) emphasized that the patients in analysis were not only free of degeneracy, but also often were intelligent (think of Elizabeth von R), often interesting, and morally decent. In fact, it was often their moral sentiments that gave rise, in part, to their symptoms. These flattering pictures have frequently been taken out of context to support the notion that psychoanalysis was somehow confined to the refined and that these people did not really suffer in significant ways.

Psychoanalysis, like many new treatments, was first known about by intellectuals, as Freud wrote books for both medical and nonmedical intelligent readers. Of course, even if psychoanalysis were exclusively a treatment for people who are intelligent and of some kind of delicate neurotic sensibility—which it is not—that would not invalidate it, except in a society that thought suffering intelligence ought in some way to be less deserving of succor than suffering ignorance.

The claim that psychoanalytic patients are the worried well has undoubtedly harmed psychoanalysis. Just before the Province of Manitoba deinsured psychoanalysis from the provincial health scheme, Manitoba's Chief Medical Assessor endorsed the notion that the typical analytic patient is a "paragon of mental health." He was alluding to the ego strengths of some analytic patients (Manitoba Government Memo, 1991, quoting a text by Maxmen), as though these strengths somehow negated the coexistence of psychopathology. That psychoanalytic patients must have certain strengths to undergo the rigors of psychoanalytic regression is not to be disputed. But just as one can have a healthy heart and still develop a serious infection, one can have certain psychological strengths alongside significant psychological weaknesses. The origin of the charge is, of course, that textbooks on psychiatry and psychoanalysis emphasize that psychoanalytic patients have to have sufficient reality testing to endure regression and sufficient ego functions to be analyzable. To do as the Manitoba government did, however—move from alluding to specific ego strengths to describing these patients as "paragons of mental health"—is to make a unwarranted leap that does not follow logically.

Members of the New Democratic Party, which formed the socialist government that delisted psychoanalysis from the provincial insurance plan in Manitoba, won victory in Ontario and made the same attempt to delist psychoanalysis in Ontario in 1991. They began the campaign by repeating the same slogans. Psychoanalysis was listed with a number of "cosmetic" procedures (including tattoo removal) deemed unworthy of coverage. Some biological psychiatrists were said to have lent their support to the campaign, behind the scenes. A colorful democratic debate ensued, in which a number of patients in Ontario began to fight to have their treatment continue. In one encounter, a patient approached the Minister of Health and asked her, "Why are you stopping my treatment?" The Minister, a forthright woman, answered, "Why don't you try Prozac instead? It worked for me." The patient responded, "I did. And it didn't work for me. But my analysis is working."

The campaign to deinsure psychoanalysis failed at that time because sufficient data were available to persuade patients, allied health professionals, government officials, and bureaucrats that the anecdotal charges were, in fact, only anecdotal and that there was significant empirical evidence showing that patients in analysis had significant problems. It also succeeded because, in the end, the government listened.

ARE PSYCHOANALYTIC PATIENTS WELL HEELED?

Frequently it is assumed that Freud's patients were all rich. In fact, this assumption is not true. Before Freud became famous, his patients appear to have been fairly educated but from a wide range of circumstances. Treatments were short—often a number of weeks—and affordable. He also treated a number of patients at no cost for some time. Once Freud's fame grew, children of the more well-to-do, who could not get relief in their home town, city or country and who could afford to travel to see him, did seek out his assistance, as they would have used their resources to seek out any physician to help them.

In Ontario, we found that the mean income for analytic patients was equivalent to a starting teacher's salary; these patients were firmly in the middle and by no means upper classes (Doidge et al., 1994). The idea that analysis is for the upper middle classes is likely perpetuated, in part, by the fact that educated people are drawn to it when they have difficulties and are most likely to write about their analytic experiences; mental health professionals not in analysis generalize from their mental health professional colleagues who undertake it for professional reasons.

The study in Ontario parallels similar work done in Germany, which showed that patients in analysis often are not well off at all. In the Federal Republic of Germany, where analysis and therapy are also funded by large insurance companies, Rudolph (1990), comparing patients who received psychoanalytic therapy with those who did not, found that

> the patients in psychoanalytic practice are not the type of upper-class patients whom we had assumed we would find. Although they are young and well educated, only 12% live in economically secure situations and work at a high vocational level. Approximately half of them live alone without a steady partner and without a secure vocational orientation [p.187].

In short, in Germany, therapy was being directed toward young people with interpersonal difficulties that prevented them from being full contributors to society.

Jones, Hall and Parke (1990) in the United States, in a series of studies, challenged the notion that psychodynamic psychotherapies are ineffective with people who are "economically disadvantaged or members of minority groups." On the basis of an analysis of previous research and a series of their own studies, they showed that "socioeconomic status and culture are highly unreliable predictors of therapy outcomes. Demographic categories are not psychological variables. . . ." (p. 98). Thus, it appears, while psychoanalysis and related treatments may have initially been used by those who were educated enough to know about it, or afford it, in this it is no way different from any other new medical treatment. In situations where psychoanalysis has been made available to others than the most fortunate, it is useful.

IS PSYCHOANALYSIS A NARCISSISTIC OR ANTINARCISSISTIC UNDERTAKING?

The idea that psychoanalysis promotes a kind of narcissism is a more recent allegation. Although Freud had what is at times called a hedonistic theory of the drives—meaning that the drives seek pleasure—he was very clear that being human meant having moral conflicts. In other words, he never embraced a hedonistic, selfish expression of warded-off drives and often helped patients make their "selfish" desires conscious, not simply to act on them but to reign them in with conscious control (Freud, 1910). If anything, Freud's early patients often—at least as he described them—developed symptoms because of their moral qualms about unconscious urges. Far from being selfish they were struggling to overcome selfishness, and struggling to be good.

Psychoanalysis might be taken to promote narcissism in another way that is quite unfair. Freud was part of the movement of thinkers who felt that religious ideas are often illusions more readily explained as the product of men's minds, a view that religious thinkers may regard as hubristic. But Freud's (1927) image of man without religion is by no means the image of a ruler of the universe; he is not even ruler of himself and clings to religion not because he is great but, rather, because he is so inadequate in the face of the forces of nature, death and loss.

When psychoanalysis is described as narcissistic, what is usually meant is that psychoanalysis promotes the narcissism of individual psychoanalytic patients. Freud (1914) thought that narcissism was an early form of development, that, if not modified by later development, became a form of pathology. Narcissism for Freud was not to be promoted and was not susceptible to analysis. In recent years, psychoanalysts have largely been of two views about how to handle the narcissistic disorders. One stream

(Kernberg, 1984) continues Freud's largely negative view of adult narcissism and sees it as a clearly pathological defense against self-hatred caused by either indulgence or deprivation. Another stream, self psychology (Kohut, 1971), sees it as having arcahic forms that feed into pathological forms if the child is reared in a nonempathic environment; but it also speaks of healthier forms of narcissism as well. Self psychology sees the narcissistic disorders as disorders, but ones that can be modified by empathic interventions in the analyses that do not so much attack the patient's narcissism head on but, rather, create an environment where the patient slowly outgrows it by modifying it. When self psychology is practised inexpertly, it is possible to see how some would argue that it amounts to nothing more than coddling narcissistic patients. Such a characterization leaves out the consideration that narcissistic patients are hypersensitive to slights and do not generally respond well to "frontal attacks" on their narcissism. Still, there is some truth to Kohut's belief that Freud was critical of narcissism.

It also seems that more and more patients with narcissistic difficulties are being seen in psychoanalytic clinics in recent years. It is not clear whether these conditions have existed all along but were not described or are now emerging in greater numbers. (Since previous generations had many fine phenomenologists, I favor the notion that they were beginning to be seen in clinical practice in greater numbers.) Whereas Freud's patients did not seem to talk so much about pride or issues of self-esteem, these patients seem preoccupied with feeling either inadequate or empty, or in appearing superior, as an attempt to ward off such feelings. One may be tempted to joke about these matters: a patient goes to an analyst saying that he thinks he is suffering from an inferiority complex, to which the clinician answers, "I have good news. You do not have a neurosis. You are inferior." Narcissistic patients are not, however, to be thought of as mediocre or inferior, as their sense of inferiority does not necessarily correlate with a lack of talent or even achievement. In the 1950s and 1960s these conditions were not always classified as narcissistic; rather, the term character disorders was used to describe patients who had these kinds of interpersonal difficulties, or difficulties with their character. Gitelson (1963), writing on the problem of the emerging character disorders as he was seeing them, said:

> This brings me to my final statement in this theoretical consideration of the problem of the "neuroses" and "disorders" of character: why are they more prevalent today than the psychoneuroses; why do most of our nonpsychotic patients come to us with complaints of interpersonal unhappiness, feelings of inadequacy and incompleteness, vague tension and anxiety, psychosomatic symptoms, and emptiness in the presence of apprarent surfeit? [p. 77].

Gitelson went on to attempt to relate the new disorders to the gradual loss of fixed cultural forms in an age of rapid change—an age character- ized by the questioning of established faith, abandonment of traditions, and repudiation of long-held values. He described the ways in which these changes had influenced families in which the patients were raised:

> I think that all this is reflected in the psychological climate of the families from which we and our patients come. The sexual status of the parents has become unclear; their hierar- chical differentiation and function uncertain. The chief con- sequence is that repression is no longer the primary and central mechanism of defense and adaptation. For this is dependent for its effective operation on definite structure in the personalities of the formative people, and an established hierarchy of relationships among them in the operations of the family. In the absence of a model towards which to as- pire, object relations become relative and conditional; iden- tifications are impaired and conflictual. While the instincts and the mechanisms of defense retain their intrinsic quali- ties, whatever I have said about them in the context of the classical conceptions of character and neuroses becomes, operationally, a matter of "more or less," contingent on the new factors which now surround them. The secondary "ad- justment" value of such defenses as identification with the aggressor, altruistic surrender, ego restriction, denial, isola- tion, and reaction formation makes them more important than outright repression. In effect, what has become impor- tant is not repression of the content of the unconscious but the successful deployment of defenses, in the guise of adap- tation, but enlisted in the service of social accommodation. Personality thus, to a large extent, has returned to its origi- nal Latin meaning in the word "persona," a "mask." This is the essence of the "crisis of identity" to which Erikson has devoted his attention. It is also near the heart of the problem of the neurosis of character, in our time [p. 78].

I take Gitelson to mean that, in an age of relativism, the family is in flux, and so are the parents; and their roles, and moral conflicts, hence, are relative and in flux, not definite. I would add that people probably feel that there is less of a need to repress immoral inclinations, as the world around us argues that there is less reason to be certain that those inclina- tions are immoral. One accommodates, as it were, to a regime that is con- stantly changing and uncertain about itself and its goals. This accommodation requires different defenses, and evolves into a series of accommodations. Hence the self is a series of masks, and even its deeper identifications are partial and in flux. With no certain goals, there can be no marshaling of the self, or external ideal or cause to discipline or master it; without self-mastery there is no self-confidence, but a sense of an incoherent structure of yearnings without confidence. Insofar as the self is nothing but a series of accommodations, it takes itself to be craven, opportunistic, and empty.

Gitelson's observations are consistent with the high rates of narcissistic complaints seen in the Canadian study. The philosophical relativism to which he alludes has led to a more widespread cultural relativism; the family in flux has led to widespread family breakdown. The new patients that Gitelson describes may suffer just as much torment as the patients Freud described, but they are less likely to win our sympathy on first glance. If Freud's patients were more sure of themselves and more sure of what was right and wrong, these new patients are sure of neither, and hence their struggles seem, to an outside observer, less noble. While psychoanalysts may disagree as to whether the emptiness and inadequacy these patients report is defensive, or the product of a developmental inhibition or neglect, or a psychological deficit, it is clear that these difficulties are in a certain sense more difficult to describe.

Now, clearly such patients could more easily be depicted as selfish and self-indulgent. But it is important to keep in mind that—for Gitelson at least—to a large degree their lack of an identity and, implicitly, a sense of direction (and note that lack of direction also means a lack of moral compass) have come about because they have been born into a situation where not just specific ideals, but ideals in general have been called radically into question. This is not to imply that the only path toward pathological narcissism is through the breakdown of structures that Gitelson describes; history is replete with examples of pathological narcissism. Gitelson's account, however, implies that the breakdown he describes has led to a growth industry, if you will, of a certain type of narcissism of diffuse complaints.

SUMMARY

Data are presented from a Canadian study showing the previous treatment histories and psychiatric diagnoses of patients in psychoanalysis. These patients have high rates of having tried less intensive forms of treatment (82%) before beginning analysis. They have high rates of psychiatric disorders and a pattern of Axis I/Axis II comorbidity. Anecdotal claims are still often made about patients in analyses, but clearly they are at variance with the data when it has been examined.

REFERERENCES

American Psychiatric Association (1985), *Manual of Psychiatric Peer Review* (3rd ed.). Washington, DC: American Psychiatric Association.

—— (1989), *Treatments of Psychiatric Disorders*. Washington, DC: American Psychiatric Association.

Auchincloss, E. & Michels, R. (1983), Psychoanalytic theory of character. In: *Current Perspectives on Personality Disorders,* ed. J. Frosch. Washington, DC: American Psychiatric Press, pp. 2–17.

Doidge, N. (1994), Changing defenses over the course of psychoanalysis: preliminary data. Presented at meeting of the American Psychoanalytic Association, New York City.

—— (1997), Empirical evidence for the efficacy of psychoanalytic psychotherapies and psychoanlysis: an overview. *Psychoanal. Inq.,* Sup., pp 102–150.

—— Simon, B., Gillies, L. A. & Ruskin, R. (1994), Characteristics of psychoanalytic patients under a nationalized health plan: DSM-III-R diagnoses, previous treatment and childhood traumata. *Amer. J. Psychiat.,* 151: 586–590.

Fenton, W. S. & Cole, S. A. (1995), Psychosocial therapies of schizophrenia: individual, group, and family. In: *Treatments of Psychiatric Disorders: The DSM-IV Edition,* ed. G. Gabbard, Washington, DC: American Psychiatric Press, pp. 987–1089.

Freud, S. (1910), Five lectures on psycho-analysis. *Standard Edition,* 11:3–55. London: Hogarth Press, 1957.

—— (1913), On beginning the treatment. *Standard Edition,* 12:121–144. London: Hogarth Press, 1958.

—— (1914), On narcissism. *Standard Edition,* 14:73–102. London: Hogarth Press, 1957.

—— (1927), The future of an illusion. *Standard Edition,* 21:3–56. London: Hogarth Press, 1961.

Gabbard, G., ed. (1995), *Treatments of Psychiatric Disorders: The DSM-IV Edition*. Washington DC: American Psychiatric Press.

—— Psychodynamic psychotherapies. In :*Treatments of Psychiatric Disorders: The DSM-IV Edition,* ed. G. Gabbard. Washington, DC: American Psychiatric Press, 1995, pp. 1205–1220.

Gitelson, M. (1963), On the problem of character neurosis. In: *Essential Papers on Character Neurosis and Treatment,* ed. R. Lax. New York: New York University Press, 1989, pp. 65-78.

Greenson R. (1967), *The Technique and Practice of Psychoanalysis*. New York: International Universities Press.

Hyler, S. E., Skodol, A. E., Oldham, J. M., Kellman, H. D. & Doidge, N. (1992), Validity of the Personality Diagnostic Questionnaire-Revised: a replication in an outpatient sample. *Comprehen. Psychiat.,* 33: 73–76.

Jones, E., Hall, S. & Parke, L. (1990), The process of change: The Berkeley Psychotherapy Research Group. In: *Psychotherapy Research,* ed. L. E. Beutler

& M. Crago. Washington, DC: American Psychological Association, pp. 98–106.

Kernberg, O. (1984), *Severe Personality Disorders*. New Haven, CT: Yale University Press.

Knight, R. (1941), Evaluation of the results of psychoanalytic therapy. *Amer. J. Psychiat.*, 98:434–446.

Kohut, H. (1971), *The Analysis of the Self*. New York: International Universities Press.

Levine H. B. ed. (1990), *Adult Analysis and Childhood Sexual Abuse*. Hillsdale, NJ: The Analytic Press.

Luborsky, L., Crits-Christoph, P., Mintz, J. & Auerbach, A. (1988), *Who Will Benefit from Psychotherapy?* New York: Basic Books.

MacIntosh, H. (1994), Analyzing homosexual patients. *J. Amer. Psychoanal. Assn.*, 42:1183–1205.

Manitoba Provincial Goverment Memo, (1991), August 13.

Markowitz, J. C., Moran, M. E., Kocsis, J. H. & Frances, A. J. (1992), Prevalence and comorbidity of dysthymic disorder among psychiatric outpatients. *J. Affect. Disord.*, 24:63–71.

Marmor, J. (1953), Orality in the hysterical personality. *J. Amer. Psychoanal. Assn.*, 1:656–671.

Michels, R. (1987), Panel. Psychoanalytic contributions to psychiatric nosology, M. L. Peltz, reporter. *J. Amer. Psychoanal. Assn.*, 35:3:693–711.

Norcross, J., Strausser, D. & Faltus, F. (1988), The therapist's therapist. *Amer. J. Psychother.*, 42: 53–66.

Norcross, J., Prochaska, J. & Gallagher, K. (1989) Clinical psychologists in the 1980's: Theory, research and practice. *Clin. Psychol.*, 42:45–53.

Oldham, J. M., Skodol, A. E., Kellman, D. H., Hyler, S. E., Doidge, N.R. Rosnick, L. & Gallaher, P. E. (1995), Comorbidity of Axis I and II disorders. *Amer. J. Psychiat.*, 152:571–578.

Perry, J. C. (1992), Problems and considerations in the valid assessment of personality disorders. *Amer. J. Psychiat.*, 149:1645–1653.

Rudolph, G. (1990), Free university of Berlin: Berlin psychotherapy study. In: *Psychotherapy Research*, ed. L. E. Beutler & M. Crago. Washington, DC: American Psychological Assocation, pp. 185–193.

Sharfstein S. S. (1978), Third-party payers: To pay or not to pay. *Amer. J. Psychiat.*, 135: 1185–1188.

Skodol, A. E., Rosnick, L., Kellman, D. H., Oldham, J. M. & Hyler, S. (1991), Development of a procedure for validating structured assessments of Axis II, In: *Personality Disorders: New Perspectives on Diagnostic Validity*, ed. J. M. Oldham. Washington, DC: American Psychiatric Press, pp. 47–70.

Spitzer, R. L. (1983), Psychiatric diagnosis: Are clinicians still necessary? *Comprehen. Psychiat.*, 4:399–411.

Wallerstein R. (1986), *Forty-Two Lives in Treatment*. New York: Guilford Press.

Wells, K. B., Burnam, A., Rogers, W., Hays, R. & Camp, P. (1992) The course of depression in adult outpatients. *Arch. Gen. Psychiat.*, 49:788–794.

FOURTEEN

Psychoanalytic Approaches to the AIDS Epidemic

MARK J. BLECHNER

AIDS has changed all of us, as mental health professionals, as individuals, and as a society. Twenty years ago none of us thought we would see hundreds of thousands of relatively young people dying of a communicable disease. AIDS has really humbled us. Through most of modern Western history, there have been serious sexually transmitted diseases that were incurable. Many of us who came of age in the postpenicillin generation enjoyed a very brief, unusual window in the history of time, a time when it seemed that there were no fatal sexually transmitted diseases, indeed, that there would be no more to fear. We became arrogant in our faith in modern medicine. AIDS shocked us out of our arrogance. It returned the specter of incurable, sexually transmitted disease to us and reminded us that nature is a formidable and clever adversary to human medicine and will probably always stay one step ahead of mankind. Besides the terrible losses that we all have had to face, AIDS has forced psychological changes in all of us. It has forced us to rethink our relation to sickness and health, mortality, sexuality, drug use, and what we consider valuable in life.

Earlier versions of portions of this chapter appeared in *Hope and Mortality* (The Analytic Press, 1997) and in *Contemporary Psychoanalysis,* 33:89–108, and 29:61–80.

HISTORICAL OVERVIEW

In the earliest years, AIDS was a mystery. In 1980, the "epidemic" did not exist as a recognized entity. Still, at that time, I personally knew one man, James Allen, who was in his late 20s and was having unusual medical problems. He was first diagnosed with shingles, then with Hodgkin's disease, but his medical progress did not fit the diagnoses. By 1981, we knew the rumors of some horrible disease that was striking mainly gay men, but no one knew how it was caused, whether it was contagious, or much of anything else—only that young men were becoming very sick and dying quickly. James now knew that he had this disease, whatever it was. The last time I saw him was at the opera; he was walking feebly with a cane. He said, "Next year at this time, I will be the late James Allen." He was right. I still remember the shock of seeing a friend, so young and with so much promise, yet so debilitated and resigned to death. Now I have seen the same thing happen, over and over, with patients, colleagues, and friends, and the cumulative effect is one of numbing shock and despair.

At first, the disease was thought to be restricted to gay men and was dubbed GRID (Gay-Related Immune Disorder). Colloquially, some people referred to Kaposi's sarcoma as the "gay cancer." In early 1983, I heard a man at a party bragging cheerfully that he had had the gay cancer and was cured of it. He was wrong. This man's bravado was an example of reaction formation, a reversal of the terror that was the most common emotion at the time in gay men. No one knew who would next get the illness. No organism had been identified as causative, and no marker had been identified that would predict who was contagious or who would next be stricken. Physicians and psychotherapists alike had no idea whether one could get the illness just by being with a patient who had AIDS.

In this period of mystery and terror, irrational ideas were rampant and caused much havoc. Psychoanalysis is the field that established the irrational and the unconscious as areas worthy of study. So what can we learn from psychoanalysis about the irrational thinking that is aroused by AIDS? Freud, Sullivan, and others have taught us how all aspects of human psychology—memory, perception, thinking and reasoning—can be altered by intense emotional concerns. To understand HIV and the irrational attitudes connected with it, one ought to invoke two of the great concepts of psychoanalysis: Freud's (1900) concept of wish-fulfillment, and Sullivan's (1953) notion of the not-me. Both concepts were intended to describe the processes of individual psychology, but both can be expanded to describe the group psychological processes of distortion and myth making that we have seen rampant in the AIDS epidemic and that still continue today.

Freud (1900, 1901) postulated that, when we are under great emotional stress, our reasoning can be rendered illogical by the same mechanisms that usually make our dreams so strange. Our waking thoughts can be distorted by primary processes and ego defenses, like displacement, repression, denial, and reaction formation. I think that the great fear and panic invoked by the AIDS epidemic have led to those kinds of distorted thinking. But the distortions have been not only on the level of individual psychology, but also on the level of large groups and ultimately all of society. Over and over during the AIDS epidemic, we have seen the distortions of individuals coalescing into distorted group beliefs, which we also call myths. Because these myths fulfill such a strong psychological need, they are very hard to dispel.

And what are the AIDS myths that have been produced? There have been many, but a common theme of the myths is that the AIDS epidemic affects people who are "not-me," to use Sullivan's term. In the beginning of the epidemic, when few facts were available, everyone wanted to project the danger of the epidemic onto someone else, and the most convenient targets were groups that are hated or looked down on. For instance, at the beginning, there was a rumor among white gay men that the only people getting AIDS were those who were sleeping with black men. Meanwhile, as Washington (1995) has documented, black men thought the opposite, that AIDS was a disease of white gay men, and black men could be safe as long as they slept only with each other. Of course, both groups were wrong. The same phenomenon is repeating today in many parts of the world; in Cambodia, for example, a poll showed that most hospital nurses believe that AIDS is a disease of foreigners, and that it cannot be passed between Cambodians (Shenon, 1996).

In 1983, things changed dramatically. A virus was finally isolated that was presumed to cause AIDS, which was eventually called HIV (human immunodeficiency virus). Soon thereafter, there emerged a blood test for antibodies to the virus. Now there was a name for what was happening, and a biological marker for the presumed cause of the illness. It was recognized that the illness was contagious through sexual contact or exchange of blood products and that those who had already acquired the virus but were asymptomatic could be identified.

The psychological effect of this medical discovery was of tremendous importance. What had previously been blind terror now became more concrete. Those who were ill had some idea of what was going on, although much was still unknown. Those who were HIV-negative could find out and react to that news (with relief, guilt, or other emotions). A class of psychopathology, the "worried well," became more precise, now that it could be determined who was well in a biological sense. And in those days, with more concreteness to the horror, there was concomitantly more hope, as well. Science had developed vaccines against other viral diseases. Surely, people thought, science would find a way to cure or prevent AIDS. People spoke of a cure around the corner, and, on April 23, 1984, Margaret Heckler, then Secretary of Health and Human Services, even made an official government announcement to that effect. Such events often crossed the border into denial; there was a pervasive belief among white American heterosexuals that the illness was restricted primarily to "risk groups"—gay men, IV drug users, hemophiliacs, and Haitians. This belief was maintained despite the fact that in Africa the epidemic was affecting heterosexuals for the most part, but that incidence was explained away vaguely as resulting from open chancre sores caused by other sexually transmitted diseases, or perhaps female circumcision, or some other exotic practices—anything to prove that the African is "not-me." Denial is a strong defense, and it finds ways to produce all sorts of flimsy data that seem to acquire merit through the wish that they be true. There was a continual attempt to ascribe AIDS to the "other," the "not-me." Gay men in their 20s originally thought that they were safe as long as they avoided sex with people over 30. The subsequent upsurge in HIV-infection in young people proved how wrong and tragic such misconceptions are.

"Risk groups," the term used by epidemiologists, was itself very misleading. It implied that those who were not members of the risk groups were not at risk of contracting HIV. Perhaps "highest risk" groups would have been more accurate and would have allowed for less denial. But the damage has been done, and the epidemic has spread among heterosexuals, who were once not included in the risk groups (see Blechner, 1986). In the 1990s, women became the fastest-growing group affected by AIDS in the United States; their numbers were increasing by 45% each year (HIV Center, 1991).

Over time, our understanding of the nature and epidemiology of the disease has changed, and with it our assessment of fears of it. Yesterday's irrationality has more than once become today's reality, and vice versa. In the mid 1980s, when it was thought that only 30% of seropositive persons would progress to AIDS, the belief that one was facing certain death from HIV infection was considered irrational. Since then, the estimate has been gradually moved upward, so that some clinicians felt that with time, nearly all HIV-infected individuals would contract the disease. This dire outlook was somewhat tempered when a certain group of people, the "nonprogressors," seemed not to become symptomatic despite HIV infection (Pantaleo et al., 1995) and when it was discovered, in 1996, that a genetic anomaly produced a natural resistance to the HIV virus in about one person in 100 (among Caucasians).

In addition, there is more hope than ever that a medical solution will be found and that AIDS will shift from being a terminal illness to being a chronic, manageable one, like diabetes, or even a totally curable or preventable one. Also, we now know that the human-immunodeficiency virus is transmitted only through the transfer of blood products or bodily fluids directly into the bloodstream or through mucous membranes, and so fears of casual contact are unfounded. There is no danger that a psychotherapist who chooses to work with AIDS patients will get AIDS from them.

The level of irrationality about AIDS produces the most bizarre belief systems. Think about the following question: What do you believe is the risk that two gay men who are HIV-negative can transmit the HIV virus to one another during anal intercourse? Herek and Capitanio (1993) studied this question. They found that about half their subjects believed there was a strong chance of HIV transmission between two uninfected homosexual men. Of course, the correct answer is 0. But their study shows how many people irrationally connect HIV transmission with specific behaviors, if anal intercourse is one of the most efficient ways of spreading the HIV virus, then any act of anal intercourse is thought to cause AIDS. This notion is not so different from the principle of von Domarus (1944), which has been applied to schizophrenic reasoning, that things merely associated with one another have a causal or inclusive relationship. For example, a schizophrenic may think, "If my mother's name is Mary, and Mary is the mother of God, then I am God." You may think that only schizophrenics think like this, but, as Freud and Jung have shown us, when we are under great emotional pressure, we are all capable of reasoning like madmen.

One would like to think that after a decade and a half of AIDS, we would see the most severe forms of irrationality, fear, and ignorance disappearing. But we do not. In 1995, a group of gay political leaders were to meet with President Clinton at the White House. Secret service members who frisked them wore rubber gloves as a precaution against contracting AIDS. What was their reasoning? The same von Domarus principle seems to have been at work. Many gay people have AIDS. Therefore, all gay people have AIDS. Doctors use rubber gloves when examining AIDS patients where there are bodily fluids. So rubber gloves will prevent me from getting AIDS by frisking gay men. Of course, the fact is that you cannot get AIDS by frisking anyone, with or without gloves. But if such ignorance exists at the top levels of American government, what can we expect of those with less education and less public responsibility?

Irrational beliefs and prejudice also limit research into the issues of drug use and sexuality that are crucial to AIDS transmission. June Osborn (1992), chair of the National Commission on AIDS, said that "even our most basic efforts to better understand and respond to this new plague have been hampered. Efforts have been made to constrain or forbid behavioral research." Even though we know that clean needles dramatically reduce the spread of HIV among IV drug users (Hausman, 1993; Karel, 1993), most states do not allow ready access to such clean needles, because of a fear that it will encourage drug use. Even though anal intercourse is known to be the most efficient means of transmitting HIV sexually, the government has refused funding for literature that would explicitly mention anal intercourse, for fear that it will encourage such behavior. The unconscious ideas here are that if you talk about a behavior, you encourage it. Not talking or thinking about it causes the behavior to be less present. Both ideas are false and dangerous. Needle exchange programs do not cause more people to be drug addicts, and safer sex education does not increase the rate of anal intercourse. But while such programs are discouraged in Congress AIDS has been spreading relentlessly.

The press has shown many of the same psychological defenses and prejudices in its coverage of AIDS news—a combination of denial and dissociation of the not-me. When Legionnaire's disease took 29 lives in 1976, it made instant front-page news, and the government made immediate pronouncements about its medical significance. For the first 30 days of the Legionnaire's epidemic, the *New York Times* included stories on every day but one and put the story on the front page 11 times. With AIDS, news coverage was scanty for years in mainstream papers. By the end of 1982, two years into the epidemic, the *New York Times* had printed only six articles about the epidemic, none of them on the front page. By the time President Reagan first mentioned AIDS in a public address in 1987, more than 20,000 people had already died of the disease (Shilts, 1987, p. 596). That it was mostly gay men and IV drug users who were the first victims of the illness surely accounted for this lack of media coverage. Yet, over 10,00 hemophiliacs were also infected with HIV, because of reckless behavior of government agencies and corporations in not adequately testing and monitoring the blood supply. Such negligence has often been settled legally, but that will not cure the "Committee of 10,000" hemophiliacs with AIDS.

Because of the government's irrationality, many people involved in the AIDS epidemic became political activists. In the 1980s, political activities definitely helped many AIDS patients whom I saw in psychotherapy to feel hopeful and supported by the community. And to a certain degree, in the 1980s, this hope seemed justified. That was the era when the cure was thought to be just around the corner. Every few months, there was a new great hope, a new magic medicine. There was Suramin, which turned out to be ineffective and extremely toxic. Thinking that it was the great cure that was available only to the rich and well-connected, people flew to Paris to get HPA-23. They were wrong; it didn't work. AL-721, a derivative of egg yolks from Israel, was another great hope, and it did not have a high level of toxicity. People began to drink homemade egg-yolk concoctions, which did virtually no harm but ultimately not much good, either. There were also the Chinese cucumber, Ribaviran, thermal treatment of the blood, and many others so-called cures. With each, there was a flurry of great hope and then, when the results did not hold up, first denial, then disappointment.

There was even the belief that psychological ministrations would turn the disease around. People like Louise Hay, a prominent AIDS "healer," told large groups of patients that AIDS could be healed by positive thinking; and, while this affirmation gave many people hope, it was especially cruel when they became sicker. Then, not only did they have to deal with a worsening medical condition, but they also felt a personal and moral failure.

By the early 1990s, there was less anger and less hope. The popular slogan, "Be here for the cure" started to take on a cruel sound; AIDS patients in psychotherapy spoke much less confidently that a cure would be found in their lifetime. There was still rage, but it became more diffuse and was less clearly directed at any available "enemy." This despair became almost institutionalized at the 1994 International AIDS Conference when scientists agreed to hold the conference only every two years instead of annually. This decision was tantamount to a public acknowledgment of loss of hope by science and government, and the effect of this public despair on individual psychology was very debilitating.

Nevertheless, there was a great deal of medical progress, especially in treating and preventing individual opportunistic infections. And we have learned much better how to tell where someone is in the progress of the disease, thanks to T-cell counts and other markers of the capacity of the immune system and of the viral load (Mellors et al., 1996). These markers have allowed more sophisticated medical attacks directly against the HIV virus. In 1996, the best strategy for treating AIDS became to switch between combinations of various kinds of antiviral medications, including the protease inhibitors. There was still no cure, but people with AIDS could live much longer, and there began to be renewed hope.

PSYCHOTHERAPY WITH AIDS PATIENTS

With the significant medical advances, most people who are HIV-positive can count on living for years, often 10 or even more, and that is enough time for a patient with longstanding interpersonal difficulties to make very good use of psychotherapy. The question is, how should one conduct psychotherapy with people with AIDS? What modifications are necessary in our work, and what does work with AIDS patients teach us about doing better psychotherapy with all patients?

At the William Alanson White's HIV Clinical Service, we have been adapting the principles of interpersonal psychoanalysis to working with AIDS issues. The interpersonal approach to psychopathology is guided by the fundamental question of William Alanson White: "What is the patient trying to do?" (Sullivan, 1924, p.8). We need to formulate this question with the patient and then determine whether we can and should help him or her to do it, and, if so, how (Blechner, 1995). Psychotherapy of a person with AIDS usually has three basic aims: 1) to help him or her take advantage of life-enhancing medical care; 2) to resolve or come to terms with whatever psychological issues are troubling; and 3) to make the best use of the time that remains.

The therapist of a person with AIDS needs to have two kinds of knowledge: medical and psychological (Blechner, 1997). The therapist needs a good basic knowledge of the facts of AIDS, how the illness progresses, what the signposts of significant changes are, and how psychological factors can influence the patient's relationship with his internist. The therapist also needs an understanding of psychological defenses, including the fact that some defenses, like denial, can serve patients well in going on with their lives. And, just as important, the therapist needs to have self-knowledge.

In the early days of psychoanalysis, an analyst's own emotional reaction, the countertransference, was thought to be an impediment to effective treatment. Today, we know that the countertransference is one of an analyst's most useful tools. By examining your own emotional reactions, no matter how irrational or disturbing, you can learn important things about the psychodynamics of your patient and those of his family and caregivers. When Bertram Schaffner and I started to teach psychotherapists who work with AIDS patients, we discovered that the problems they face most frequently is not knowing how to use their countertransference productively and not having a setting where they can safely and openly discuss their emotional reactions. Most therapists do not have trouble when their countertransference emotions are kindly, good feelings. But, when working with severely ill and dying patients, a therapist can have uncanny, dreadful, or painful emotions and shameful thoughts that seem totally unacceptable, and yet there they are. You may think that your thoughts and feelings are so bad that you must suppress them—but that is the worst thing to do. In the long run, it is much better to admit them into consciousness, let them percolate in your mind, and see how you can analyze them yourself. Sometimes it is good to have a trusted set of colleagues, a peer supervision group or something of that nature, where you can talk about your countertransference emotions, so you can find out that what you thought was a terrible reaction is nevertheless fairly common and may be ultimately useful to the treatment.

Typical Clinical Situation

Let us consider a patient who has just discovered that he is HIV-positive. His T-cell count is high, his physical health seems fine, but he is having a very serious psychological reaction to the diagnosis, which may range from anxiety to panic. He may wonder, is this a death sentence? Should I end my life now, before I have to face any suffering?

It is important that the clinician be able to counsel the patient on the realities of AIDS: that there is great uncertainty as to the course of the illness for any individual; that it is possible for those with HIV infection but no opportunistic infections to live symptom free for 10 years or more; that some people seem never to progress from HIV infection to AIDS as currently defined, although most people do (Buchbinder et al., 1993); that people can live with AIDS itself for 10 years or more; that, once the T-cell count does reach 200, it is possible to head off many opportunistic infections with prophylactic medications; and that the best strategy for living is to do those things that one wants to do as best one can for as long as one can, while making informed choices on all those issues that one can influence. It is also important to educate AIDS patients about how to be active participants in their medical care. The medical treatment of AIDS does not fit the model that many modern Westerners expect—that the doctor diagnoses the ailment and prescribes a treatment, which, if followed faithfully, leads to cure. Instead, there are gaps of knowledge and great uncertainty about much of AIDS diagnosis, treatment, and outcome, and patients benefit from active involvement in treatment decisions. But that strategy has to be adapted to each patient's personality style—some people prefer to let their doctors take charge, while others prefer more collaboration.

Once a patient has stabilized and resolved the initial panic reaction to the HIV-positive diagnosis, he may engage in the whole range of psychotherapeutic efforts. I have seen quite a few patients undergo unusually rapid and profound characterological changes and accomplish in a few years life goals that they had been putting off for decades. It had already been observed that reaching middle age and getting closer to feelings of mortality enables some very resistant patients to make good use of psychotherapy (Kernberg, 1980; King, 1980; Myers, 1987). Now we are observing that people of all ages, when confronted with mortality, can do the same thing. I have worked with blocked writers who published several books, and people who had spent most of their lives single formed committed and loving relationships. Some people managed to make peace with estranged family members and confront parental homophobia and other prejudices. Some people who had lived marginal lives of poverty, drugs, and aimlessness found themselves clearing their system of drugs and becoming able to restructure their lives with great drive and intensity of purpose. And some AIDS patients from deprived backgrounds who made their way into some of the better treatment programs found that they were being given close and caring professional attention, the likes of which they had never received in their lifetimes.

Some patients may come to a psychotherapist for the first time when they are already in the late stages of AIDS. Often they are referred by a physician who has identified a serious depression that does not respond to medication alone. Patients who come for therapy in this situation often have great difficulty confronting the changes in their experience of life, and they may be having a different kind of panic—the panic of uncertain but close mortality. Such patients are not likely to be interested in fundamental character change; and they are more likely to be seeking support. I should say that good supportive psychotherapy is at least as difficult to do as good exploratory psychotherapy. It requires that you always stay close to the emotional situation of the patient in the moment. A patient who is in deep despair about a medical setback does not need confrontation; he needs empathy, with perhaps a gentle reminder of a previous time, when his medical condition got worse and then was turned around. Many patients fear not death itself but, rather, intractable pain and the loss of functioning and mobility. Especially difficult is blindness caused by cytomegalovirus infection, persistent pain in the extremities from neuropathy, drastic loss of weight and bowel control, and AIDS dementia. A therapist may find herself needed for some unusual functions with the demented patient, including collaborating with the patient in fantasizing about a hopeful future that the therapist knows is not possible.

It is very common for patients to form the fantasy, during psychotherapy, that the psychotherapist will somehow be able to cure the AIDS. Most therapists have also had such fantasies. Studies have shown that the psychological treatment increases the average survival time of people with different kinds of cancer (e.g., Spiegel et al., 1989; Fawzy et al., 1993), and I suspect that it is also true of AIDS. But, although survival time may increase, I have never seen psychological treatment cure anyone of AIDS.

A patient with advanced AIDS told me that as a teenager he had been severely ill for four years and seemed near death. The doctors were confused, but finally a specialist determined that he had a very rare illness that was curable. He was then properly treated and recovered. So he had great trust in Western medicine but believed that the patient had to stay one step ahead of the physician. This adolescent experience shaped his approach to having AIDS as an adult. He read medical textbooks constantly and often impressed his physicians with his knowledge. I saw him question a planned intervention more than once and ultimately prove that he was right. When he said to me, "The doctors thought I was supposed to die two years ago, and yet here I am. I think I will be the first one to beat this thing," I thought, "I know it has never happened, and probably it will not. But maybe . . ." Unfortunately, when it started to look as though his death was inevitable, I became very depressed. These fantasies of rescue have a great function in maintaining enthusiasm in both the patient and the therapist, but if you believe them too strongly, you may burn out.

One of the most serious problems of patients in the late stages of AIDS may be extreme loneliness. Some may have been abandoned by family or friends, but loneliness can occur even when there is an apparently large personal network. The loneliness may come when the patient's caregivers start to panic about their own mortality and keep a certain distance from his experience. Also, women with AIDS often feel required to maintain their role in supporting their family's function and so try to hide their physical and psychological distress from family members, which makes them feel even more lonely.

For some patients, the hardest and loneliest times are periods of relative health *after* a serious hospitalization. A patient of mine was hospitalized with AIDS for over two months with five difficult-to-treat infections. He had an extraordinary set of friends and relatives who visited him and cared for him round the clock. I myself visited him in the hospital once a week, and more often during a period when he was psychotic. We had sessions in his hospital room, and in one session I thought he would die in front of my eyes. But he didn't. As happens not infrequently, people in the late stages of AIDS are given up for lost only to rebound. The postrebound period can be very difficult. The patient was eventually discharged from the hospital, regained the weight he had lost, and looked quite healthy. Suddenly, the tremendous support network that had surrounded him in the hospital thinned out, and he felt lonely, rejected, and depressed. He spoke nostalgically of his time in the hospital, of the peak emotional experiences he had had. His early life had been one of the most deprived I have ever heard of. He and his five siblings had been abandoned by both parents for a year and lived by begging, stealing, and sleeping in unoccupied dwellings. It was useful in his psychotherapy that we clarified the patterns of abandonment that he had grown used to in his childhood and that he tended to accept passively, so that he could change now and actively talk to his friends and relatives about his isolation.

It is not unusual for psychotherapists to abandon their roles with AIDS patients and to get directly involved in their patients' lives. One of the assistants of Kübler-Ross (1987) has described her total personal involvement and commitment to a dying patient. It reminds one of Sechehaye's (1951) extraordinary devotion to her schizophrenic patient, Renée, a devotion that led to great therapeutic gains but could not become a general method of working, because of the enormous demands put on the therapist's time and energy; such limitless devotion would quickly lead to burnout. Although AIDS patients often need extraordinary caregiving, there is a good case to be made for the psychotherapist to maintain a therapeutically neutral position while other caregivers meet the other needs of the patient. This situation allows the patient to bring her most painful and destructive fantasies and emotions to the therapist, such as wanting to kill the person who gave her AIDS or to kill people who don't have HIV and who are stigmatizing and treating people with AIDS badly. The sessions can then function as a kind of crucible for these unmentionable feelings, and allow the patient to carry on productively outside the sessions. If the patient actually needs the psychotherapist for caregiving outside the sessions, this crucial therapeutic function of the clinician is compromised. The psychotherapist must be sure that the AIDS patient has set up such an independent support network.

A therapist needs to help the AIDS patient to make peace with the life he or she has lived. What has he done of value? How has he lived? Why did he make the choices that he did? At times, there is a need to resolve longstanding conflicts, to settle old scores, to right certain wrongs. The patient may want to make reparation to someone he has wronged, to thank someone who has been important, to admonish or cut off someone who has treated him badly. This does not mean that with such patients an exploration of the early history is irrelevant. On the contrary, sometimes an exploration of the past, with a few pointed interpretations, may clarify for a patient who has never before been in psychotherapy how he came to live life as he did. This can sometimes be done effectively in just a few sessions, even in one or two consultations.

For example, a man in the late stages of AIDS came to me because he was having very severe nightmares. As we explored the content of his dreams, it was clear that there were unresolved conflicts with his family, mainly about his always having to be the strong person supporting the other members of the family, a position that was especially painful now that he had AIDS. He got the courage to bring this up with his family and had some very difficult and revealing discussions with them. And then the nightmares stopped.

AIDS has taught us to deal psychoanalytically with a greatly expanded range of problems. Some of these issues are quite new, and some, while ever-present, are difficult topics that many of us avoid as much as possible. Death and mortality are probably the most difficult for us. Most of us avoid thinking about our own death, and many of us superstitiously avoid doing anything related to death, like writing a will. Yet for someone who has AIDS it is very important at least to make preparations like a will and a health-care proxy. I have seen some therapists in supervision who have had to confront their own countertransference squeamishness about death and mortality before they could address them with their patients.

Kübler-Ross (1969) has provided a model of five sequential stages in facing a terminal illness: denial, anger, bargaining, depression, and acceptance. While patients may have all of these experiences, the stages may occur in a different order and not necessarily as separate entities. Theoretical models of death and dying may be of some use in conceptualizing the experience, although they are no substitute for continual self-examination of one's own experience of health, dying, and the priorities of living and of potential blocks to empathy. It is useful for psychotherapists to read psychologically aware first-person accounts of people with AIDS (e.g., Rowland, 1988; Callen, 1991; Monette, 1994).

Some psychotherapists deal with their fear of death by a counterphobic strategy. With a kind of fake bravado, they try compulsively to get their patients to talk about death, even at a time that the patient has other concerns. This countertransference reaction is usually not very helpful to patients. In a similar vein, I once worked with an HIV-positive man whose previous therapist had interpreted every dream in terms of HIV, which at times required a real stretch of the imagination. This is another dangerous countertransference distortion—we have to remember that a person with HIV is still a person, with all kinds of psychological issues besides HIV.

One of the ongoing themes that comes up with AIDS patients and those who are close to them is bereavement. There is great sadness in losing someone to AIDS. The deterioration is horrible to watch, more so if you love the person who is dying. Often, after the illness has progressed for a long time, one wishes consciously or unconsciously for the person's death, and this wish can evoke great guilt. These and related phenomena are all familiar to people who have cared for and lost loved ones to other slow, painful, and disfiguring diseases, like cancer (Eissler, 1955; Kübler-Ross, 1969; Adler et al., 1975). Patients may come to a psychotherapist because of difficulties grieving the loss of a loved one. The source of difficulty can vary enormously and may include unresolved guilt about their caretaking during the illness, unconscious ambivalence about the deceased, and a complex pattern of projection, introjection, and identification with aspects of the deceased (Szalita, 1974). A psychotherapist must be alert to the nature of the relationship between the patient and the loved one before the illness.

Massive Bereavement

A new and special problem with AIDS that has become more common in recent years is what I call massive-bereavement (Blechner, 1993). Because

AIDS has until now been especially concentrated among certain groups, members of those groups have had to face the loss of many or all of their loved ones and acquaintances. Some keep lists, and their losses can number more than 100. The longer the epidemic goes on, the more common is this syndrome, and the more severe. I have heard many gay men claim that they have lost all of their friends to the disease. Such experiences have until now been rare in our society; there are only certain exceptions, such as people who have lost their entire families in wartime or through the Holocaust. I think of such people as "repeated survivors." Over and over, they have succumbed to loss. Psychotherapy with such AIDS survivors is especially difficult because the trauma is not over; repeated survivors cannot set aside the past and make a new beginning as long as the AIDS epidemic still looms large; many fear that they will start new relationships and that those, too, may succumb to AIDS (Goldman, 1989).

I worked with a gay man in his 30s who had had three lovers who had died of AIDS, and the man he was currently dating had just revealed that he was HIV-positive. This man, who was still HIV-negative, felt extreme grief and had made concrete plans for suicide. I raised the question whether he, personally, could have another relationship with someone who is HIV-positive; clearly his own life was at risk, more from suicide than from HIV, and he had to respect his limitations.

I saw another man in treatment who had had a brief period of hallucinations and delusions, that lasted for a few days. He was in his mid-70s and gay, and had been single all his life. He lived alone and had lost most of his friends to AIDS. His closest friend, Bill, who was his only remaining steady human contact, now had late-stage AIDS. One day he came home and hallucinated that his small apartment was filled with mimes in whiteface. When he tried to talk to them, they wouldn't respond. Then he saw his close friend, Bill, lying in his bed with the covers over his head. As I listened to his history, it seemed probable that the psychotic experiences had been triggered by a new medication that he had started; they did in fact stop when the medication was discontinued. But the content of the hallucinations was important; all the different hallucinations involved large crowds of people arriving unannounced. His hallucinations were like wish-fulfillment dreams or like the end of the movie "Longtime Companion," in which the thousands of people who have died of AIDS return. The hallucinations highlighted his current loneliness and his dread of the even greater loneliness to come when Bill would die. Psychotherapy helped him address this anxiety-laden future.

I also sometimes see people with the problem of survivor guilt, which is exacerbated by other people's being judgmental. For example, a man whose lover had died of AIDS began a new relationship two months after the funeral. He had heard several of his friends speak very contemptuously of people who started new relationships too soon after their lovers had died, and so he was engaged in a complicated deception of keeping his new lover secret from nearly all his friends and family. Since the patient was Jewish, I told him that traditional Jewish law requires a mourning period of one year for a parent, but only for 30 days for a spouse.[1] The rationale is that one should get on with one's life and not live singly, in suffering, for too long a time. In this way, we could start with a perspective that what he had done was not sinful in certain cultures, and we could consider the psychodynamics of those who would condemn him. Thus the issue of his guilt was detoxified so that eventually we could look into some of the unformulated emotional reactions he had to his lover's death, including suppressed rage, that made him more vulnerable to other people's assessment that he was guilty. And then we could also look at the characterological issues that were involved in his deceptive way of living.

Suicidal Ideation

Another area of change for psychoanalytic thinking has to do with suicidal ideation. Most mental health practitioners have been trained about the dangers of suicidal ideation and its correlation with suicidal attempts and actual suicides. For patients with AIDS, however, I have found that suicidal ideation can often be *helpful*. With an illness in which unpredictability and loss of control are so pronounced, suicidal fantasies give the patient the freedom to fantasize having final control of his bodily state and his destiny. Paradoxically, the elaboration and exploration of such fantasies within psychotherapy can, in my experience, lessen the likelihood that a patient will actually commit suicide.

For example, I worked with a patient whose health was worsening. He spent hours moping or crying in his apartment, and he began to talk to me about suicidal thoughts. We immersed ourselves in talk of death. I asked him how he was thinking of committing suicide. He told me he was thinking of tying a rope around his neck and tying the other end onto something in his apartment. Then he would jump out the window and hang dead outside his building. The fantasy had several important aspects. Other people would be forced to see his misery. He would be relieved of much of the loneliness he felt, even though he would be dead. He would also be making a public statement about his misery and rage about having AIDS and about what he felt was society's relative indifference to AIDS

---

[1] A rabbi has since told me that my information about the Jewish mourning laws was inaccurate. The actual mourning period may be longer or shorter, depending on whether there are children (Lamm, 1969).

patients. He then told me other fantasies that were even more shocking and destructive, involving public violence. The elaboration and analysis of these fantasies were very helpful to this patient; they brightened his affect, as he felt freer to turn his rage outward rather than inward, and they also led him to see the emotional burdens of his isolation, some of which was self-imposed and which he could change.

Some patients who fear suffering and incapacity may stockpile barbiturates or other medications to allow them to commit suicide at some time in the future. In my view, it may be contraindicated for a therapist to try to stop such preparations for suicide. We find that, paradoxically, those who take concrete steps to prepare for suicide often do not kill themselves when their physical condition deteriorates. But knowing that they could end things is often very helpful in allowing them to tolerate the pains of the illness. As Shakespeare wrote in *King Lear* [IV;i;29-30], "The worst is not so long as we can say, 'This is the worst.' "

Here, as always, analysis of the countertransference is important. The therapist who has trouble with a patient's suicidal thoughts should ask himself or herself, "What are my own experiences with suicidal thoughts and actions, in others and myself? Have I never had a suicidal thought? What would life be like without the possibility of suicide? Is my reaction against the patient's suicidal thinking possibly fueled by an unconscious *wish* that he commit suicide?" If you can answer these questions honestly, you will be able to work more evenhandedly with your patient's turmoil.

The risk of suicide is increased, however, when a patient, grappling with the difficult medical and psychological issues of AIDS, must face the additional threat from managed care that coverage of her medical needs by insurance is threatened or denied. Besides the very real medical dangers that this threat may pose, it can also be experienced as compounding society's prejudice against those with AIDS and a wish for the patient to die.

Unsafe Sex Without Informing the Partner About HIV Status

One of the most troubling situations for the psychotherapist is when a patient who is HIV-positive confides that he is having unsafe sex and lying to his sex partner that he is HIV-negative. The partner's life is thus threatened, and the therapist usually has very strong feelings. One study (Kegeles, Catania, and Coates, 1988) found that 12% of individuals having HIV testing would not tell their primary partners if they turned out to be HIV-positive.

There is no easy solution to such a situation. The medicolegal guidelines offer a good deal of latitude and, in any case, are not an alternative to good clinical judgment (Daniolos and Holmes, 1995; Schaffner, 1997).

At best, one must steer a course between confronting the patient with the meaning of his action and not alienating him from the therapy. Some therapists feel that such deceptive sexual behavior is tantamount to attempted murder and feel that they must take a strong stand with the patient, at times even saying that he must cease such action or terminate the therapy. The risk is that the patient will then feel so judged and threatened that he will stop treatment and continue his behavior anyway. An alternative approach is to try to work with the underlying motives of such a patient. Not infrequently he has tremendous rage that he has been infected and a wish to infect others who have been more lucky. At times the rage extends to society's tactless and often cruel treatment of HIV-positive people. Often, the situation is often not so clearcut. I have worked with one patient who lied to his sex partners about his HIV-status but justified his lie to himself on the grounds that 1) no one would have sexual relations with him otherwise and 2) in his opinion, he was not engaging in any sexual practices that would put his partners at risk for infection. He felt rage at a society that makes the HIV-infected feel like pariahs. Usually such situations require a good deal of work by the psychotherapist on his countertransference, which, if he is HIV-negative, may involve a fantasied identification with the patient's sex-partner. It is useful to consider not only the destructive aspects of the patient's behavior, but also the possibly unexpressed needs that it is covering over. Many AIDS patients feel physically shunned and yearn most of all for physical contact, which, if it does not involve the exchange of body fluids, is perfectly safe; yet their family and friends may irrationally avoid giving them even a hug.

HIV-RELATED ISSUES IN HIV-NEGATIVE PATIENTS

Another area of psychoanalytic thinking that has been greatly expanded has to do with the pathological consequences of denying, dissociating, and repressing fears of AIDS. The fear of AIDS is having pervasive effects on the mental health of many psychotherapy patients who may be only dimly aware of such fear or who are too afraid to talk about it with the psychotherapist, let alone with their families and friends. The effect of this unconscious or unacknowledged fear of AIDS may take many clinical forms, including depression, an inability to plan one's life, anxiety attacks, schizoid withdrawal, counterphobic sexual exploits, or psychosomatic symptoms. For example, Lucy, a wealthy, young, beautiful, married woman, was referred to me by a physician because of serious physical symptoms that could not be explained medically. As we developed a trusting psychotherapeutic relationship, Lucy "confessed" that there had been one night when she was extremely angry at her husband, went to a bar, got drunk, and woke up the next morning in a hotel room with a man whom she did not know. She had no memory of the night's events but was terrified from then on that she had contracted AIDS. She had never had the HIV-antibody test (by now, several years had passed), and her anxiety only increased.

She asked me how likely it was that she had contracted HIV. I could tell her that it is estimated that the chance of contracting HIV from one act of unprotected heterosexual vaginal intercourse with an infected person is 1 in 500 for a woman, 1 in 700 for a man; from one act of receptive, unprotected anal intercourse with an infected partner, the risk of transmission is 1 in 50 to 100 (Auerbach, Wypijewska, and Brodie, 1994). Often, when patients have engaged in risky behavior and are afraid of contracting AIDS, they ask for such statistics, and it is helpful for the clinician to provide them. But generally, even if the likelihood of transmission is relatively small, the patient's anxiety will not be calmed, and one has to analyze the psychological weight of such statistics.

In the next few sessions, Lucy and I explored her fantasies about AIDS, which were of extreme suffering and were related to religious fantasies of sin and retribution. I eventually told her that I thought her medical symptoms might never resolve without her clarifying the HIV issue. I also told her where and how she could obtain the test privately and confidentially. She had the test, and the result was seronegative. That finding, plus a good deal more psychoanalytic exploration, resolved many of her physical symptoms.

Lucy, like many people, had put her life on hold, while she ruminated about her fears of AIDS and procrastinated about getting the test. In retrospect, she realized that her unconscious presumption was that she did have AIDS and would die soon, so no major life decisions needed to be made. Usually, people become aware of the extent to which they have "put life on hold" only after they receive a seronegative test result.

I have seen this phenomenon so often in my practice that I think it might be worth calling it a syndrome—the syndrome of "depression secondary to HIV anxiety." The initial presentation of such patients can be extremely varied, but often in some way they seem to be paralyzed. They are going through the motions of life without any clear sense of directing their life course. While there can be many other determinants of such a clinical picture, in the era of AIDS, a major, and often unconscious, determinant is the fear of having been infected. Such people may not get past their difficulties until they can resolve their terror of being tested. It is important for the clinician to recognize that this syndrome is very pervasive not only among the so-called risk groups. It can and does appear in anyone. I have often heard that someone like Lucy, a wealthy married woman, asks her wealthy doctor about AIDS fears and is told, 'Oh, *you* don't need to worry about that." The doctor is involved in a kind of projected denial. He seems to be thinking, "AIDS is not threatening you. Not us. Not me." But anyone who asks about AIDS is worried about it, and, if the doctor avoids talking about it or denying the fear, all sorts of psychiatric complications may result.

People like Lucy often want to know how long the incubation period is between HIV infection and the appearance of HIV-antibodies on the test. Seroconversion usually occurs within three months, at most six months. Today we generally advise patients to have the HIV test three months after the last risk behavior, and then again three months later. Further research may refine or change this procedure. It is also a good idea for patients to obtain the test results immediately before a psychotherapy session. For very anxious patients, the drawing of blood is also best arranged to precede a psychotherapy session.

Dissociated fears of AIDS affect not only patients, but also their psychotherapists. About eight years ago, I saw a therapist in supervision who was being uncharacteristically avoidant of the HIV anxieties that were appearing in her patient's dreams. The therapist came to realize that she had unacknowledged fears of HIV herself, and that these fears were blocking her exploration of HIV issues with her patient. The resolution of this deadlock was that my supervisee had the HIV test herself. Once she had worked through her own dissociated terror about HIV, she was freed to work effectively with her patient's fears.

Since then, I have seen many psychotherapists in supervision whose work has been constrained, in different ways, by their own fears of AIDS that have usually not even been acknowledged, let alone worked through. From these experiences, I have come to a principle that applies to every psychotherapist working with AIDS issues, which today is every psychotherapist. *You must have the HIV-test yourself.* It is the only way you will gain empathy, not only with your patients' experiences but also with your own unacknowledged fears and illusions. From the moment you make the appointment to have the blood drawn, you will find your mind flooded with special anxieties that are very specific to you. For example, perhaps you feel protected from HIV by the walls of a long-standing monogamous marriage. You may find, during the wait between the time the blood is drawn and when you receive the result, that no one is fully confident in their mate's fidelity. You will also realize the stigma and embarrassment, and countless other unpleasant feelings, involved in just going for the test.

After the Cure

As I was preparing this chapter, I realized that I was having a recurrent fantasy—what if a cure for AIDS is discovered before this chapter is published? How will all of these observations and discoveries change? Will any of them matter? I think this fantasy has many functions, but it is primarily a wish. The wish and the hope that this nightmare called AIDS will end keeps me from burning out. And when it does end, we will all have learned some important lessons. We will have learned that modern medicine is not omnipotent and that nature will always have a few tricks up her sleeve. We will have learned that psychoanalytic principles of psychotherapy can be adapted to the most dire situations in living. And we will have learned that, however long or short is our time on earth, our personal integrity, love, and human attachment are what make life worth living for all of us.

REFERENCES

Adler, G., Beiser, M., Cole, R., Johnston, L. & Krant, M. (1975), Approaches to intervention with dying patients and their families: A case discussion. In: *Bereavement,* ed. B. Schoenberg, I. Gerber, A. Wiener, A. Kutscher, D. Peretz & A. Carr. New York: Columbia University Press.

Auerbach, J., Wypijewska, C. & Brodie, H., ed. (1994), *AIDS and Behavior.* Washington, DC: National Academy Press.

Blechner, M. J. (1986), Transmission of AIDS from female to male. Letter to the *New York Times,* July 31.

—— (1993) Psychoanalysis and HIV disease. *Contemp. Psychoanal.,* 29:61-80.

—— (1995), Schizophrenia. In: *Handbook of Interpersonal Psychoanalysis,* ed. M. Lionells, J. Fiscalini, C. H. Mann & D. B. Stern. Hillsdale, NJ: The Analytic Press, pp. 375–396.

—— (1997), *Hope and Mortality: Psychodynamic Approaches to AIDS and HIV.* Hillsdale, NJ: The Analytic Press, pp. 3–62.

Buchbinder, S., Mann, D., Louie, L., Villinger, F., Katz, M. & Holmberg, S. (1993), Healthy long-term positives (HLPs): Genetic cofactors for delayed HIV disease progression. *Abst. 9th Internat. Conf. on AIDS* (Abstract No. WS-B03-2), Berlin.

Callen, M. (1991), *Surviving AIDS.* New York: HarperCollins.

Daniolos, P. & Holmes, V. (1995), HIV public policy and psychiatry: An examination of ethical issues and professional guidelines. *Psychosomat.,* 36:12–21.

von Domarus, E. (1944), The specific laws of logic in schizophrenia. In: *Language and Thought in Schizophrenia,* ed. Kasanin, J. S. New York: Norton.

Eissler, K. (1955), *The Psychiatrist and the Dying Patient.* New York: International Universities Press.

Fawzy, F., Fawzy, N., Hyun, C., Elashoff, R., Guthrie, D., Fahey, J. & Morton, D. (1993), Malignant melanoma: Effects of an early structured psychiatric intervention, coping, and affective state on recurrence and survival 6 years later. *Arch. Gen. Psychiat.,* 50:681–689.

Freud, S. (1900), The interpretation of dreams. *Standard Edition,* 4 & 5. London: Hogarth Press, 1953.

——— (1901), The psychopathology of everyday life. *Standard Edition*, 6. London: Hogarth Press, 1960.

Goldman, S. (1989), Bearing the unbearable: The psychological impact of AIDS. In: *Gender in Transition*, ed. J. Offerman-Zuckerberg. New York: Plenum, pp. 263–274.

Hausman, K. (1993), Needle-exchange programs effective but controversial. *Psychiat. News*, Sep. 3, p. 11.

Herek, G. & Capitanio, J. (1993), Public reaction to AIDS in the United States: A second decade of stigma. *Amer. J. Pub. Health*, 83:574–577.

HIV Center for Clinical and Behavioral Studies Report (1991). New York: New York State Psychiatric Institute, Vol. 1, May.

Karel, R. (1993), Needle-exchange program yielding great success. *Psychiat. News*, Jan. 1, pp. 10–11.

Kegeles, S., Catania, J. & Coates, T. (1988), Intentions to communicate positive HIV-antibody status to sex partners. *J. Amer. Med. Assn.*, 259:216–217.

Kernberg, O. (1980), *Internal World and External Reality*. New York: Aronson.

King, P. (1980), The life cycle as indicated by the nature of the transference in the psychoanalysis of the middle-aged and the elderly. *Internat. J. Psycho-Anal.*, 61:153–160.

Kingsley, L. A., Rinaldo, C., Lyter, D., Valdiserri, R., Belle, S. & Ho. M. (1990), Sexual transmission efficiency of hepatitis B virus and human immunodeficiency virus among homosexual men. *J. Amer. Med. Assn.*, 264:230–234.

Kübler-Ross, E. (1969), *On Death and Dying*. New York: Macmillan.

——— (1987), *AIDS: The Ultimate Challenge*. New York: Macmillan.

Lamm, M. (1969), *The Jewish Way in Death and Mourning*. Middle Village, NY: Jonathan David.

Mellors, J., Rinaldo, C., Gupta, P., White, R., Todd, J. & Kingsley, L. (1996), Prognosis in HIV-1 infection predicted by the quantity of virus in plasma. *Science*, 272:1167–1170.

Monette, P. (1994), *Last Watch of the Night*. New York: Harcourt Brace.

Myers, W. (1987), Age, rage, and the fear of AIDS. *J. Geriat. Psychiat.*, 20:125–140.

Osborn, J. (1992), Interview with June Osborn. *The Advocate*, Sep. 8, pp. 40–43.

Pantaleo, G., Menzo, S., Vaccarezza, M., Graniosi, C., Cohen, O., Demarest, B., Montefiori, D., Orenstein, J., Gox, C., Schrager, L., Margolick, J., Buchbinder, S., Giorgi, J. & Fauci, A. (1995), Studies in subjects with long-term nonprogressive human immunodeficiency virus infection. *New Eng. J. Med.*, 332:209–216.

Rowland, C. (1988), A view from the moon: A message from one person with AIDS. In: *The Sourcebook on Lesbian/Gay Health Care*, ed. M. Shernoff & W. Scott. Washington, DC: National Lesbian/Gay Health Foundation, pp. 183–186.

Schaffner, B. (1997), Modifying psychotherapeutic methods when treating the HIV+ patient. In: *Psychodynamic Approaches to AIDS and HIV*, ed., M. J. Blechner. Hillsdale, NJ: The Analytic Press, pp. 63–79.

Sechehaye, M. (1951), *Symbolic Realization*. New York: International Universities Press.

Shenon, P. (1996), AIDS epidemic, late to arrive, now explodes in populous Asia. *New York Times,* Jan. 21, pp. 1, 8.

Shilts, R. (1987), *And the Band Played On.* New York: St. Martin's Press.

Spiegel, D., Bloom, J., Kraemer, H. & Gottheil, E. (1989), Effect of psychosocial treatment on survival of patients with metastatic breast cancer. *Lancet,* 2:888–891.

Sullivan, H. S. (1924), Schizophrenia: Its conservative and malignant features. In: *Schizophrenia as a Human Process.* New York: Norton, 1962, pp. 7–22.

——— (1953), *The Interpersonal Theory of Psychiatry.* New York: Norton.

Szalita, A. (1974), Grief and bereavement. In: *American Handbook of Psychiatry,* Vol. 1, ed. S. Arieti. New York: Basic Books, pp. 673–702.

Washington, R. A. (1995), The challenge for behavior science assisting AIDS service organizations to do HIV prevention work. *Psychol. & AIDS Exch.,* fall, pp. 3–4.

FIFTEEN

The Effectiveness Of Long-Term Intensive Inpatient Treatment Of Seriously Disturbed, Treatment-Resistant Young Adults

SIDNEY J. BLATT
RICHARD Q. FORD

Those who work with seriously disturbed patients appreciate the importance of long-term, intensive inpatient treatment for these patients, most of whom have been relatively unresponsive to extensive outpatient treatment or to brief psychiatric hospitalizations. But it has been difficult for many other health care professionals to appreciate fully the investment of time, effort, and money required for long-term care because generally it has been difficult to provide systematic evidence for the constructive effects of this type of treatment. Especially in times of severe cutback in mental health services, it is essential to identify those patients who can benefit from such treatment, to demonstrate the therapeutic gain that can occur with these patients and to demonstrate these gains in ways that will convince those responsible for planning mental health services of the value and effectiveness of this form of treatment for seriously disturbed, treatment-resistant patients.

Our investigation of therapeutic change in the long-term, intensive, inpatient treatment of 90 severely disturbed, treatment-resistant young adult inpatients (Blatt and Ford, 1994) was conducted through a series of systematic analyses of clinical case records and psychological test protocols that had been established as part of routine clinical procedures at the Austen Riggs Center. Thus, the research findings discussed in this chapter reflect not only the effectiveness of the treatment program at the Austen Riggs Center, but also the quality of the clinical observations and case records available in this treatment facility.

This research was guided by two fundamental assumptions that are relatively novel in treatment research:

1) We assumed that patients come to treatment with different problems, preoccupations, needs, character styles, defenses, and adaptive capacities. And we expected that different types of patients might express therapeutic gain in different ways and through different modalities. Attempts to identify universal expressions of therapeutic change, applicable to all patients, fail to appreciate important clinical differences among patients. We sought instead to identify different types of patients and to allow for the possibility that they might change in different ways (e.g., Cronbach, 1967).

2) Our research was also novel in its focus on evaluating the quality of object relations and object representations. We assumed that object representations, the cognitive-affective schemas of self and other that derive from the internalization of significant interpersonal experiences, express important dimensions of the individual—aspects of their cognitive processes, their general developmental level, and relevant aspects of significant interpersonal relationships (Blatt and Lerner, 1983). We assumed that a systematic assessment of object representations would provide important evidence for therapeutic change in long-term intensive treatment (Blatt and Wild, 1976; Blatt, Wild, and Ritzler, 1975).

DIFFERENTIATION AMONG PATIENTS

We decided not to differentiate among patients using the usual distinctions made in the diagnostic and statistical manuals (*DSM*) prepared by the American Psychiatric Association. These manuals provide an essentially atheoretical taxonomy, a categorization of manifest symptoms established by consensus among a diverse panel of experts. Thus, these manuals are primarily lexicons, a series of political agreements about the use of various diagnostic terms or concepts. As a consequence of this consensus, clinicians and investigators can now be generally consistent in their use of various diagnostic terms, but there is relatively little support for the validity (or meaningfulness) of many of the diagnostic distinctions in *DSM* (Blatt and Levy, 1998).

Seriously disturbed patients, for example, often meet criteria for four, five, six, or more separate personality disorders. The frequency of overlapping and multiple diagnoses in this taxonomic system (sometimes euphemistically called "comorbidity") indicates that these distinctions are ineffective for differentiating among patients. Rather than using the symptom-based atheoretical system of the *DSM*, we sought instead to differentiate among patients by using more theoretically based distinctions derived from psychodynamic and interpersonal formulations—differentiations based on differences in primary instinctual or motivational focus (libidinal versus aggressive), in primary types of defensive organization (avoidant versus counteractive), and in predominant character style (i.e., emphasis on object relations versus an emphasis on self, and on affect versus cognition).

Prior to the initiation of the research presented here, we (Blatt, 1974, 1991, 1995; Blatt and Shichman, 1983) had conceptualized personality development as evolving through the interaction of two fundamental developmental lines: (a) an anaclitic or relatedness line involving the development of the capacity to establish increasingly mature and mutually satisfying interpersonal relationships, and (b) an introjective or self-definitional line involving the development of a consolidated, realistic, essentially positive, differentiated, and integrated self-identity (Blatt and Blass, 1990, 1996). In normal personality development, these two developmental processes evolve in an interactive, reciprocally balanced, mutually facilitating fashion from birth through senescence. An increasingly differentiated, integrated, and mature sense of self is contingent on establishing satisfying interpersonal relationships, and, conversely, the continued development of satisfying interpersonal relationships is contingent on the development of a more mature self-concept and identity. These formulations are consistent with a wide range of personality theories ranging from more clinically oriented psychoanalytic conceptualizations (e.g., Freud, 1930; Erikson, 1950; Balint, 1959; Shor and Sanville, 1978; Blatt and Blass, 1990, 1996) to more empirically oriented investigations of personality development (Angyal, 1951; Bakan, 1966; McAdams, 1980, 1985; McClelland, 1980, 1986; Wiggins, 1991).

Various forms of psychopathology can be conceptualized as expressions of a distorted overemphasis and exaggeration of one of these developmental lines and the defensive avoidance of the other. This distinction enables us to define two fundamentally different configurations of psychopathology, each containing several types of disordered behavior ranging from relatively severe to relatively mild. On the basis of these developmental and clinical considerations, one configuration of disorders can be identified as "anaclitic"—disorders in which patients are primarily preoccupied with issues of interpersonal relatedness, from infantile dependent attachments to more mature relationships. These patients use primarily avoidant defenses (e.g., withdrawal, denial, repression) to cope with psychological conflict and stress. Anaclitic disorders involve extensive pre-occupations with interpersonal relations—with issues of trust, caring, de-pendability, intimacy, and sexuality. These disorders, extending developmentally from more to less disturbed, include nonparanoid schizo-phrenia, borderline personality disorder, infantile (or dependent) character disorder, anaclitic depression, and hysterical disorders (Blatt and Shichman, 1983; Blatt, 1991, 1995). In contrast, a second configuration of disorders can be identified as "introjective"—disorders in which the patients are concerned primarily with establishing and maintaining a viable sense of self, from a basic sense of separateness, through concerns about autonomy and control, to more complex internalized issues of self-worth. These patients employ primarily counteractive defenses (e.g., projection, ratio-nalization, intellectualization, doing and undoing, reaction formation, and overcompensation). Introjective patients are more ideational and exten-sively preoccupied with establishing, protecting, and maintaining a viable self-concept, with little investment in the quality of their interpersonal relations. Issues of anger and aggression, directed toward the self or oth-ers (or both) are usually central to their difficulties. Introjective disorders, from more to less severely disturbed, include paranoid schizophrenia, the schizotypic or overideational borderline, paranoia, obsessive-compulsive personality disorders, introjective (guilt-ridden) depression, and phallic narcissism.

In summary, anaclitic psychopathologies are disorders preoccupied primarily with issues of interpersonal relatedness such as trust, caring, inti-macy and sexuality; people with these disorders use primarily avoidant defenses (e.g., denial and repression). In contrast, introjective psycho-pathologies are disorders concerned primarily with establishing and main-taining a viable sense of self, ranging from a basic sense of separateness, to concerns about autonomy and control, to issues of self-worth; people with these disorders use primarily counteractive defenses (e.g., projection, do-ing and undoing, intellectualization, reaction formation, and overcom-pensation) (Blatt and Shichman, 1983; Blatt, 1991, 1995). In our research, the differentiation of these two types of psychopathology was made reli-ably by clinical judges reviewing typical clinical case records prepared early in the treatment process. We anticipated that these two groups of patients would express therapeutic change in different ways.

ASSESSMENT OF OBJECT REPRESENTATION

The second basic assumption made in our research was the importance of assessing the quality of interpersonal relationships and object representa-tions in the study of therapeutic change. Object representation, the cognitive-affective schemas of self and other, is a theoretical construct central in psychoanalytic theory and research, in developmental and social psychology, and in cognitive science. Investigations in these areas indicate that children transform early interactions with primary caregivers into cognitive-affective schemas of self and other and that these cognitive-affective schemas regulate and direct subsequent behavior in a wide range of circumstances, especially in interpersonal relationships (e.g., Blatt, Auerbach, and Levy, 1997).

This development of interest in interpersonal relations and object representations within psychoanalysis involved a major shift in theoretical emphasis from a one-person psychology that assumed a basically closed biological system involving transformations of drives in interaction with tension thresholds (e.g., defenses) to a more open-system, relational model focused on interpersonal interactions and their internalization as cognitive-affective schemas (Blatt and Lerner, 1983). From this new psychoanalytic perspective, cognitive-affective schemas or mental representations of self and other are viewed as bearing the imprint of significant interpersonal interactions and as expressing the developmental level and other important aspects of the individual's psychic life (e.g., drives, defenses, affects, and fantasy). These cognitive-affective schemas develop over the life cycle and have conscious and unconscious cognitive, affective, and experiential components. They can be veridical representations of consensual reality, or idiosyncratic and unique constructions, or contain primitive and pathological distortions that suggest psychopathology. They become the templates or prototypes that structure how one thinks and feels about others and about oneself. They derive from and determine the experience of the self in the interpersonal world (Beres and Joseph, 1970; Blatt and Lerner, 1983).

Beginning with the early infant–caregiver relationship, these schemas unfold in response to experienced perturbations in interpersonal interactions. When developmental demands are age appropriate and not too severe, existing cognitive structures accommodate experienced perturbations and result in the construction of more mature cognitive-affective schemas that usually develop in a natural, well-defined sequence (e.g., Piaget, 1945). Increasingly differentiated and articulated schemas of self and other more effectively organize, shape, and guide subsequent interpersonal behavior. Life demands that are severe or developmentally inappropriate, however, can overwhelm the child's capacities for accommodation and distort the development of adaptive interpersonal schemas (Blatt, 1991, 1995).

Theory and research from several different perspectives have addressed the role of early caregiving relationships in the development of representations of self and others in normal and in disrupted development. The subtleties of the relational attunement between caregiver and infant in patterns of engagement and disengagement observed during the first three or four months of life (e.g., Stern, 1985; Beebe, 1986) and the establishment of patterns of attachment and separation observed in the first half of the second year (e.g., Ainsworth, 1982; Bowlby, 1988a) demonstrate the contribution of early interpersonal bonds to the development of representations of self and other. These early interpersonal experiences lead to the development of cognitive-affective schemas that organize a person's emerging conceptions of significant caring figures and of the self in intimate relationships (Stern, 1985; Bretherton, 1987; Zeanah and Anders, 1987; Levy, Blatt, and Shaver, 1998). When these cognitive-affective structures derive from relatively satisfactory caring experiences, they facilitate an increasingly mature interpersonal relatedness and a differentiated and cohesive identity (Blatt, Auerbach, and Levy, 1997).

These cognitive-affective schemas of self and other have been discussed as mental representations in psychoanalytic theory or as representations of interactions that have become generalized (Stern, 1985), or as internal working models of caring experiences by attachment theorists (e.g., Ainsworth, 1969, 1982; Bowlby, 1988b). These observations in psychoanalysis, developmental psychology, and attachment theory are consistent with the recent focus in cognitive science, information processing, and social cognition on the importance of understanding the development of these enduring schemas of self and others as prototypes for social interaction and behavior.

Attachment theory and research provide perhaps the clearest examples of the relationship between the quality of early interpersonal interactions and the construction of cognitive-affective schemas. On the basis of the quality of attachment between mother and child, and on their capacities to tolerate separation and to reestablish relatedness upon reunion, Ainsworth and colleagues identified three types of infant-mother dyads: 1) a *securely attached* dyad, in which the caretaker provides a secure base that enables the infant to explore the world beyond the relationship with mother and to seek contact and reestablish interaction with her after separation; 2) an *insecurely avoidant* attachment, in which the infant can explore the environment without the caretaker but who then actively ignores and avoids involvement with the caretaker upon her return after separation, and 3) an *insecurely anxious-resistant (or preoccupied)* attachment, in which the infant focuses his or her attention on the caretaker, is reluctant to separate, and is clinging and dependent on reunion.

Securely attached infants as preschoolers are cooperative, popular with peers, and highly resilient and resourceful (Sroufe, 1983), and at age six they are relaxed and friendly and converse with their parents in a free-flowing and easy manner (Main & Cassidy, 1988). Insecure avoidant infants as preschoolers appear emotionally insulated, hostile, and antisocial

(Sroufe, 1983), and later tend to distance themselves from their parents and to ignore their parents' initiatives in conversation (Main and Cassidy, 1988). Anxious-resistant or preoccupied insecure infants are tense and impulsive as toddlers and passive and helpless in preschool (Sroufe, 1983) and later show a mixture of insecurity and hostile behavior in interaction with their parents (Main and Cassidy, 1988). These three attachment patterns are relatively stable over time (Ainsworth, 1982; Bretherton, 1985) even into early adolescence (age 10) (Elicker and Sroufe, 1992).

These attachment patterns also have cross-generational continuity, as indicated by the fact that mothers report caring experiences with their own mothers that are similar to the caring experiences they have established with their infants. Pregnant women, for example, report early childhood caring experiences that are congruent with the subsequent care they provide their own infants (Fraiberg, 1969; Main, Kaplan, and Cassidy, 1985; Fonagy et al., 1991; Slade and Aber, 1991; Steele, and Steele 1991; Virtue, 1992). These patterns of secure and insecure attachment observed in children and adults are also congruent with differences in cognitive processes, for example, with the degree of cohesion and consistency of narrative reports that adults construct about their early life experiences (Main et al., 1985). Securely attached adults have greater coherence and consistency in their narrative reports than do insecurely attached adults.

These behavioral and cognitive consistencies of attachment patterns across the life cycle suggest that, in the first 18 months of life, the child begins to establish mental representations or internal working models of attachment relationships—"a set of conscious and unconscious rules for the organization of information relevant to attachment and for obtaining or limiting access to that information, that is, to information regarding attachment-related experiences, feelings and ideations" (Main et al., 1985, p. 67). Main and colleagues view the internal working model established by the end of the first year of life as a "template of previously unrecognized strength" (p. 94) that is "related not only to individual patterns in nonverbal behavior, but also to patterns of language and structures of mind" (p. 67). Similarly, Bowlby (1988b) noted:

> The working models a child builds of his mother and her ways of communicating and behaving towards him, and a comparable model of his father, together with the complementary models of himself in interactions with each, are being built by a child during the first few years of his life and, it is postulated, soon become established as influential cognitive structures [p. 130].

These mental representations, formed early in life, vary dramatically in their level of flexibility, adaptiveness, and maturity, and they have a pervasive influence on the nature and quality of significant attachments throughout the entire life cycle.

A basic postulate of both attachment theory and psychoanalytic object relations theory is that the quality of the relationship with primary caregivers has an essential role in the development of these cognitive-affective schemas. Consistent, positive affective experiences between child and attachment figures result in relatively integrated and well-differentiated internal working models of attachment relationships in which stable attributes of the attachment relationship—attributes of self and others—become elaborated and consolidated. New experiences over succeeding developmental periods are integrated into these earlier mental representations, resulting in advances over prior stages, such as the development of object and self-constancy and of symbolic activity more generally. Significant fluctuations, inconsistencies, disruptions, and negative experiences in caretaking interactions, however, can lead to less differentiated, integrated, and consolidated representational schemas organized with a more limited focus as individuals attempt to establish a sense of security in distorted and maladaptive ways.

These formulations about the role of early interpersonal experiences in the construction of cognitive-affective schemas in normal and pathological development may have important implications for the study of the therapeutic process. If various forms of psychopathology involve distortions of object and self-representation, and if satisfactory childhood attachments in normal development result in the formation of increasingly mature interpersonal schemas, then significant constructive interactions between patient and therapist should facilitate relinquishing more distorted representations of self and other and lead to important revisions of representations and to the development of a more integrated and mature sense of self and of others. Thus, the therapeutic relationship should create a process through which pathological interpersonal schemas are recognized, reworked, relinquished, and transformed into more adaptive cognitive-affective representations of self and other (Blatt, Wild, and Ritzler, 1975). Research evidence indicates that toward the end of treatment, representations become more differentiated and integrated, with indications of a more differentiated sense of self and a greater capacity for reciprocal interpersonal relatedness (Blatt et al., 1991; Blatt et al., 1996; Blatt, Auerbach, and Aryan, 1998).

On the basis of these theoretical formulations, we systematically evaluated the quality of object representations by assessing Rorschach responses that contain human or humanoid features. We assumed that Rorschach responses of human figures would convey essential information about the quality of a person's representational world and his or her interpersonal relationships. In earlier research (Blatt et al., 1976), we had established a method, based on developmental concepts from Heinz Werner and Jean Piaget, for systematically assessing the quality of the human figure on the Rorschach. We evaluated the degree of differentiation, articulation, and integration of Rorschach responses that contained human characteristics. Specifically, we assessed 1) the degree to which the response was a fully human figure rather than a partial human detail or a quasi human figure; 2) the degree to which the figure was articulated in its perceptual characteristics (i.e., its size, physical details, clothing, hair style, and posture) and functional characteristics (i.e., age, sex, role, and specific identity); 3) whether the figure was seen in action and if the action attributed to the figure was unmotivated, reactive, or proactive and intentional; 4) whether the action attributed to the figure was fused with the figure, incongruent with the definition of the figure, or congruent with the figure; 5) whether the nature of the action was malevolent or benevolent; and 6) whether the interaction of that figure with another figure was such that one figure was passive or reactive or whether both figures were actively engaged in mutually initiated and shared activity.

In addition to evaluating these developmental dimensions in the representation of the human figure, we also evaluated whether the human figure was accurately perceived—whether the form of the figure conformed to the outline of the inkblot. Thus, we evaluated two fundamental dimensions of human responses: 1) the degree of accuracy or reality testing of the response as expressed in the degree to which the definition of the figure conformed to the form of the inkblot and 2) the developmental level of the perceived human figure, that is, the degree to which these human forms were represented as well articulated, full human figures, engaged in intentional, congruent, benevolent activity, and in mutually active and reciprocal interactions with others.

In prior longitudinal research (Blatt et al., 1976), over the course of normal development in a sample of well-functioning individuals from ages 10-11 to age 30, we found that human responses to the Rorschach became increasingly more full human forms that were extensively articulated with both perceptual and functional features and were increasingly represented as involved in activity that was intentional, congruent, and benevolent. We also evaluated the representation of human forms on the Rorschach within a sample of seriously disturbed inpatients and found that the severity of the patients' psychopathology was significantly related to the degree to which their human responses were quasi-human forms that were minimally articulated and were represented as involved in activity that was unmotivated, incongruent, and malevolent.

Surprisingly, however, we found a subgroup of patients within our seriously disturbed inpatient sample whose responses represented human forms at higher developmental levels than did those of normals (more differentiated, articulated, and integrated), but only when the human forms were inaccurately perceived. This subgroup of patients gave representations of full human figures that were highly articulated and engaged in intentional, congruent, and benevolent activity, but only when there was little justification for the response in the form of the inkblot (see Ritzler et al., 1980 for a replication of these findings). These inaccurately perceived but highly elaborated and integrated human figures on the Rorschach were usually found in preformed, mythic, idealized, benevolent figures such as a princess resting by a stream, a knight on a white horse, or Abraham Lincoln. Although these responses were developmentally advanced—that is, they were highly differentiated, articulated, and integrated, they had little justification in reality—they did not conform to the outline of the inkblot. They were inaccurately perceived and seemed to be serving a restitutive function. They seemed to be an island of safety split off from a very painful reality, a place in which seriously disturbed patients could still maintain some image and hope of positive interpersonal interactions (Blatt, Schimek, and Brenneis, 1980). Thus we interpreted the tendency to give inaccurately perceived human responses at both high and low developmental levels as indicating the tendency to become involved in inappropriate, unrealistic, possibly autistic, types of relationships (Blatt, Tuber, and Auerbach, 1990).

On the basis of earlier findings, we expected the seriously disturbed inpatients in our study of long-term, intensive treatment to express therapeutic gain primarily by a decreased investment in the representation of inaccurately perceived human forms. As expected, we found that clinical improvement was expressed in a decreased investment in the representation of these inaccurately perceived human forms. Although a decreased investment in inaccurately perceived human forms occurred throughout our entire sample of 90 patients, it was more apparent in anaclitic patients, that is, in those patients whose pathology focused primarily on their concerns about disrupted interpersonal relationships. This decreased investment in inaccurately perceived human form on the Rorschach was paralleled by marked behavioral improvement in interpersonal relationships.

In addition to assessing change in the quality of object representation on the Rorschach, we also evaluated therapeutic change on the Thematic Apperception Test (TAT), Human Figure Drawings (obtained on only a subset of the sample), the Wechsler Intelligence Test, and ratings made of independently established clinical case records (Blatt and Ford, 1994). After an average of 15 months of treatment, these seriously disturbed, treatment-resistant young adults, especially the introjective patients, manifested significantly less frequent and less severe clinical symptoms; better interpersonal relations; increased intelligence; a reduction in thought disorder and of fantasies about unrealistic, possibly autistic, interpersonal relations on the Rorschach; decreased defensiveness on the TAT; and more differentiated and organized representations of the human figure. These significant differences were maintained even after we controlled statistically for initial severity of the patients' psychopathology and their premorbid level of adjustment, the use of medication in treatment process, and the level of experience of their therapist.

Extensive follow-up data were also available on a substantial number of the patients in our sample, long after they left the treatment program. Plakun (1989; Plakun, Burkhardt, and Muller, 1985) conducted a mail survey of patients who had been in long-term, intensive treatment at Riggs, and about half of our sample was included in Plakun's survey. Thirteen years after treatment, on average, the patients reported on their current status. The results indicate that the behavioral and psychological gains we noted in our sample after 15 months of inpatient treatment are consistent with Plakun's reports of substantial long-term improvement. A majority (>75%) of these formerly seriously disturbed patients were living in a private residence apart from their families, were gainfully employed, had at least one close friend, and reported having satisfactory relations with the opposite sex. And a majority of the nonpsychotic patients (but only 37% of the formerly psychotic patients) were or had been married. This is an impressive level of adaptation in previously seriously disturbed, treatment-resistant patients some 13 years, on average, after discharge from a long-term, inpatient treatment program.

In summary, the findings of our study indicate substantial therapeutic change in the sample of 90 seriously disturbed, treatment-resistant patients as a consequence of long-term, intensive, psychodynamically oriented inpatient treatment. In addition, on the basis of a differentiation of two broad configurations of psychopathology and from the systematic assessment of object representations, we were also able to make more differentiated statements about the nature of therapeutic change. The two groups of patients that we had differentiated revealed therapeutic change in different ways. Therapeutic change was expressed in anaclitic and introjective patients primarily in the modalities of their major concerns and preoccupations. The assessment of the quality of object representation was particularly important for assessing therapeutic change in the more interpersonally oriented anaclitic patients.

In addition to demonstrating therapeutic gain in these seriously disturbed inpatients, we were able to evaluate whether aspects of the psychological assessment of object representations gathered at the onset of treatment could predict the extent of therapeutic change across the 15 months of intensive inpatient treatment. One of the more important questions for psychotherapy research, as well as for managed care, is the prediction of which seriously disturbed patients are likely to gain from the treatment experience. Still applicable today are Frank's (1979) observations that we know relatively little about the determinants of therapeutic outcome: "Research . . . to date suggest[s] that the major determinants of therapeutic success appear to lie in aspects of patients' personality and style of life . . ." (p. 312). Lambert and Asay (1984), like Frank, stress that the psychological qualities a patient brings to the treatment situation are probably the most important factors determining the therapeutic outcome. Two of the primary psychological qualities influencing treatment outcome are the severity of the patient's pathology and the patient's capacity to become involved in a therapeutic relationship (Gomes-Schwartz, 1978).

Most studies indicate that more integrated and less disturbed patients are more likely to have a positive therapeutic outcome. In an early review of this literature, Luborsky and colleagues (1971) concluded that "initially sicker patients do not improve as much with psychotherapy as the initially healthier" (p. 146). Lambert and Asay (1984), however, noted that a significant body of knowledge also supports the opposite view, that more seriously disturbed patients show the greatest amount of therapeutic gain (p. 335). Yet another set of studies indicate that there is no relationship between degree of maladjustment and therapeutic gain. Lambert and Asay concluded that, though the bulk of research indicates that better therapeutic outcome is obtained with less disturbed patients, there are frequent contradictory findings: "Although better adjusted patients bring more personal resources to the therapeutic situation, they do not necessarily show more therapeutic gain" (p. 340).

In our study of the long-term, intensive treatment of seriously disturbed inpatients, we used Rorschach protocols to assess systematically the severity of psychopathology as well as the patient's potential for establishing meaningful interpersonal relationships. We (Cook, Blatt, and Ford, 1995) tested empirically if these psychological test variables, obtained at the beginning of treatment, provide effective predictors of therapeutic gain in seriously disturbed young adults after a substantial period of long-term, intensive inpatient treatment. We used path analysis as the statistical procedure for evaluating the relationship of these test variables to outcome effects.

The application of the path analytic method to the ratings derived from clinical case records and the assessment of the quality of object representation from Rorschach protocols yielded impressive predictions of therapeutic change. Severely disturbed patients who appear to benefit most over the course of 15 months of comprehensive inpatient treatment, including intensive, four times weekly individual psychotherapy, are those who at admission are able to express disrupted thinking and portray interactions as malevolent and destructive, but who at the same time are able to maintain the structure of human representations at a high developmental level. These results indicate that the prognosis for seriously disturbed young adults to gain from long-term, intensive inpatient treatment is indicated by an initial capacity or willingness to communicate disordered thinking and disruptive experiences as well as a capacity for establishing appropriate and constructive interpersonal relationships. More disordered thinking and the representation of more malevolent, unilateral interactions, as well as more differentiated and integrated representations of the human figure on the Rorschach early in treatment, were related to less intense and frequent clinical symptoms and more intact and appropriate interpersonal relationships after approximately 15 months of intensive inpatient treatment.

In summary, the data from our investigation suggest that seriously disturbed, treatment-resistant patients are quite responsive to long-term, intensive, psychodynamically oriented inpatient treatment. In addition, our findings indicate that there are consistent patterns in the response of seriously disturbed patients to long-term, intensive treatment. In the current climate of significant curtailment of mental health benefits and increased attempts to treat seriously disturbed patients either briefly or primarily with pharmacological interventions, the results of this study could potentially contribute to the decision-making process in identifying those seriously disturbed, treatment-resistant patients who might benefit more fully from more intensive and sustained therapeutic interventions.

For some it may seem that we have spent a lot of time and effort demonstrating the obvious—that long-term, intensive, psychodynamically informed inpatient treatment is effective for seriously disturbed, treatment-resistant patients—particularly at a time when the current emphasis of the entire mental health system is on short-term care. But it is important to recognize that our study is one of the first systematic demonstrations of the efficacy of long-term, intensive inpatient treatment for seriously disturbed young adults, patients who had been relatively unresponsive to a variety of brief interventions, including extensive outpatient psychotherapy and brief psychiatric hospitalizations that also included the use of psychoactive medication. These findings should convince others about the importance of this type of treatment for these seriously disturbed patients, who are usually considered treatment resistant.

The distinction between anaclitic and introjective patients, which was so productive in the study of therapeutic change in the long-term, intensive, inpatient treatment of seriously disturbed treatment resistant patients, was also applied to the data of the Menninger Psychotherapy Research Project (MPRP). For the first time, after many prior analyses of the data gathered as part of the Menninger Psychotherapy Research Project, significant and systematic differences were identifed in outcome between psychoanalysis and supportive-expressive psychotherapy (Blatt, 1992).

Anaclitic patients had significantly greater clinical gain in supportative-expressive psychotherapy, while introjective patients had substantially greater gain in psychoanalysis. Most recently, the anaclitic/introjective distinction was applied to the widely acclaimed, as well as much criticized, NIMH sponsored Treatment of Depression Collaborative Research Program (TDCRP). This well designed and carefully conducted extensive multisite research project compared the therapeutic efficacy of four types of brief (16 weeks) outpatient treatment for depression (cognitive-behavioral therapy, interpersonal therapy, and imipramine and placebo, both with clinical management). Despite numerous prior analyses of these data, minimal differences had been found at termination of treatment among these different brief outpatient treatments for depression (e.g., Elkin, 1994). The introduction of the concepts of anaclitic and introjective personality and these two configurations of psychopathology into the analysis of this extensive data set, however, revealed that outcome in the brief outpatient treatment of serious depression is significantly influenced by pretreatment personality characteristics of the patient. Introjective patients, those patients who are highly self-critical and perfectionistic as measured by the perfectionism factor of the Dysfunctional Attitudes Scale (Weissman and Beck, 1978), did relatively poorly in all four forms of brief outpatient treatment for depression (Blatt et al., 1995). In contrast, the analysis of therapeutic gain in the long-term treatment of inpatients in the data from The Austen Riggs Center (Blatt and Ford, 1994) and of outpatients seen in the MPRP (Blatt, 1992) indicate that introjective, self-critical, perfectionistic patients do relatively well in long-term, intensive, psychodynamically oriented therapy. Taken together, the findings from these three studies suggest that we can identify patients who are likely to be resistant to short-term interventions, but who are likely to benefit extensively from long-term, intensive treatment in both inpatient and outpatient settings.

These findings confirm a very important point made over 40 years ago by the distinguished statistician and research methodologist Lee Cronbach (1967), who stated that we must begin to think of treatment in a more differentiated way, allowing for the possibility that different types of patients may be responsive to different types of treatment and that they might demonstrate clinical change in different ways. It is to be hoped that the findings from these analyses of seriously disturbed, treatment-resistant patients in long-term, intensive inpatient treatment will have a substantial impact on the people who manage the delivery of mental health services and will encourage them to think in more differentiated ways about a wide range of clinical services and to appreciate the relative contributions of both short- and long-term care and when and how these different types of treatment might be utilized most appropriately with different types of patients.

REFERENCES

Ainsworth, M. D. S. (1969), Object relations, dependency, and attachment: A theoretical review of the mother-infant relationship. *Child Develop.*, 40:969–1025.

—— (1982), Attachment: Retrospect and prospect. In: *The Place of Attachment in Human Behavior*, ed. C. M. Parkes & J. Stevenson-Hinde. New York: Basic Books, pp. 3–30.

Angyal, A. (1951), *Neurosis and Treatment*, ed. E. Hanfmann & R. M. Jones. New York: Wiley.

Bakan, D. (1966), *The duality of human existence.* Chicago: Rand McNally.

Balint, M. (1959), *Thrills and Repression.* London: Hogarth Press.

Beebe, B. (1986), Mother-infant influence and precursors of self and object representations. In: *Empirical Studies of Psychoanalytic Theories, Vol. 2*, ed. J. Masling. Hillsdale, NJ: The Analytic Press, pp. 27–48.

Beres, D. & Joseph, E. (1970), The concept of mental representation in psychoanalysis. *Internat. Journal of Psycho-Anal.*, 51:1–9.

Blatt, S. J. (1974), Levels of object representation in anaclitic and introjective depression. *The Psychoanalytic Study of the Child*, 24:107–157. New York: International Universities Press.

—— (1991), A cognitive morphology of psychopathology. *J. Nerv. & Mental Dis.*, 179:449–458.

—— (1992), The differential effect of psychotherapy and psychoanalysis on anaclitic and introjective patients: The Menninger Psychotherapy Research Project revisited. *J. Amer. Psychoanal.*, 40:691–724.

—— (1995), Representational structures in psychopathology. In: *Rochester Symposium on Developmental Psychopathology, Vol. 6*, ed. D. Cicchetti & S. Toth. Rochester, NY: University of Rochester Press, pp. 1–33.

—— Auerbach, J. S. & Aryan, M. (1998), Representational structures and the therapeutic process. In: *Empirical Studies of the Therapeutic Hour*, ed. R. Bornstein & J. Masling. Washington, DC: American Psychological Association, pp. 63–107.

—— —— & Levy, K. N. (1997), Mental representations in personality development, psychopathology, and the therapeutic process. *Rev. Gen. Psychol.*, 1:351–374.

—— Blass, R. B. (1990), Attachment and separateness: A dialectic model of the products and processes of psychological development. *The Psychoanalytic Study of the Child*, 45:107–127. New Haven, CT: Yale University Press.

—— & —— (1996), Relatedness and self definition: A dialectic model of personality development. In: *Development and Vulnerabilities in Close Relationships*, ed. G. G. Noam & K. W. Fischer. Hillsdale, NJ: Lawrence Erlbaum Associates, pp. 309–338.

—— Brenneis, C. B., Schimek, J. G. & Glick, M. (1976), The normal development and psychopathological impairment of the concept of the object on Rorschach. *J. Abn. Psychol.*, 85: 364–373.

—— Ford, R. (1994), *Therapeutic Change.* New York: Plenum.

—————— Lerner, H. D. (1983), Investigations in the psychoanalytic theory of object relations and object representation. In: *Empirical Studies of Psychoanalytic Theories, Vol.1,* ed. J. Masling. Hillsdale, NJ: Erlbaum Associates, pp. 189–249.

—————— Levy, K. N. (1998), A psychodynamic approach to the diagnosis of psychopathology. In *Making Diagnosis Meaningful,* ed. J. W. Barron. Washington, DC: American Psychological Association Press.

—————— Quinlan, D. M., Pilkonis, P. A. & Shea, T. (1995), Impact of perfectionism and need for approval on the brief treatment of depression. *J. Consult. Clin. Psychol.,* 63:125–132.

—————— Schimek, J. & Brenneis, C.B. (1980), The nature of the psychotic experience and its implications for the therapeutic process. In: *The Psychotherapy of Schizophrenia,* ed. J. Strauss, M. Bowers, T. W. Downey, S. Fleck, S. Jackson & I. Levine. New York: Plenum, pp. 101–114.

—————— Shichman, S. (1983), Two primary configurations of psychopathology. *Psychoanal. Contemp. Thought,* 6:187–254.

—————— Stayner, D., Auerbach, J. & Behrends, R. S. (1996), Change in object and self representations in long-term, intensive, inpatient treatment of seriously disturbed adolescents and young adults. *Psychiat.,* 59:82–107.

—————— Tuber, S. B., & Auerbach, J. S. (1990). Representation of interpersonal interactions on the Rorschach and level of psychopathology. *J. Personal. Assess.,* 54:711–728.

—————— Wiseman, H., Prince-Gibson, E. & Gatt, H. (1991), Object representation and change in clinical functioning. *Psychother.,* 28:273–283.

—————— Wild, C. M. (1976), *Schizophrenia: A Developmental Analysis.* New York: Acedemic.

—————— —————— & Ritzler, B.A. (1975), Disturbances in object representation in schizophrenia. *Psychoanal. Contemp. Sci.,* 4:235–288.

Bowlby, J. (1988a), Developmental psychology comes of age. *Amer. J. Psychiat.,* 145:1–10.

—————— (1988b), *A Secure Base.* London: Routledge.

Bretherton, I. (1985), Attachment theory: Retrospect and prospect. In: *Growing Points in Attachment, Monographs of the Society for Research in Child Development,* ed. I. Bretherton & E. Waters, 50:3–35.

—————— (1987). New perspectives on attachment relations: Security, communication, and internal working models. In: *Handbook of Infant Development,* ed. J. Osofosky. NY: Wiley, pp. 1061–1100.

Cronbach, L. J. (1967), Instructional methods and individual differences. In: *Learning and Individual Differences,* ed. R. Gagne. Columbus, OH: Merrill, pp. 23–39.

Cook, B., Blatt, S. J. & Ford, R. Q. (1995), The prediction of therapeutic response to long-term extensive treatment of seriously disturbed young adults. *Psychother. Res.,* 5:176–188.

Elicker, J. & Sroufe, L.A. (1992), Predicting peer competence and peer relationships in childhood from early parent-child relationships. In: *Family-Peer Relationships: Modes of Linkage,* ed. R. Parks & A. Ladd. Hillsdale, NJ: Lawrence Erlbaum Associates.

Elkin, I. (1994), The NIMH Treatment of Depression Collaborative Research Program: Where we began and where we are now. In: *Handbook of Psychotherapy and Behavior Change*, ed. A. E. Bergin & S. L. Garfield. New York: Wiley, pp. 114–135.

Erikson, E. H. (1950), *Childhood and Society*, New York: Norton.

Fonagy, P., Steele, M., Moran, G., Steele, H. & Higgit, A. (1991), Measuring the ghost in the nursery: A summary of the main findings of the Anna Freud Center-University College London Parent–Child Study. *Bull. Anna Freud Centre*, 14:115–131.

——— & Steele, M. (1991), Maternal representations of attachment during pregnancy predict the organization of infant–mother attachment at one year of age. *Child Devel.*, 62:891–905.

Fraiberg, S. (1969), Libidinal object constancy and mental representation. *The Psychoanalytic Study of the Child*, 24:9–47. New York: International Universities Press.

Frank, J. D. (1979), The present status of outcome studies. *J. Consult. Clin. Psychology*, 47:310–316.

Freud, S. (1930), Civilization and its discontents. *Standard Edition*, 21: 64–145. London: Hogarth Press, 1957.

Gomes-Schwartz, B. (1978), Effective ingredients in psychotherapy: Prediction of outcome from process variables. *J. Consult. Clin. Psychol.*, 46:1023–1035.

Lambert, M. J. & Asay, T. P. (1984), Patient characteristics and their relationship to psychotherapy outcome. In: *Issues of Psychotherapy Research*, ed. M. Hersen, L. Michelson & A. S. Bellack. New York: Plenum, pp. 313–359.

Levy, K. N., Blatt, S. J. & Shaver, P. (1998), Attachment styles and parental representations. *J. Personality & Soc. Psychol.*, 74:407–419.

Luborsky, L., Chandler, M., Auerbach, A. H., Cohen, J. & Bachrach, H. M. (1971), Factors influencing the outcome of psychotherapy: A review of quantitative research. *Psychol. Bull.*, 75:145–185.

Main, M., & Cassidy, J. (1988), Categories of response to reunion with the parent at age 6: Predictable from infant attachment classifications and stable over a 1 month period. *Devel. Psychol.*, 24:415–426.

——— Kaplan, N. & Cassidy, J. (1985), Security in infancy, childhood and adulthood: A move to the level of representation. In: *Growing Points of Attachment Theory and Research. Monographs of the Society for Research in Child Development*, ed. I. Bretherton & E. Waters, 50:60–104.

McAdams, D. P. (1980), A thematic coding system for the intimacy motive. *J. Res. Personal.*, 14:413–432.

——— (1985), *Power, Intimacy, and the Life Story*. Homewood, IL: Dorsey.

McClelland, D. C. (1980), Motive dispositions: The merits of operant and respondent measures. In: *Review of Personality and Social Psychology*, ed. L. Wheeler. Beverly Hills, CA: Sage.

——— (1986), Some reflections on the two psychologies of love. *J. Personal.*, 54:335–353.

Piaget, J. (1945), *Play, Dreams and Imitation in Childhood*. New York: Norton, 1962.

Plakun, E. M. (1989), Narcissistic personality disorder: A validity study and comparison to borderline personality disorder. *Psychiatric Clin. North Amer.*, 12:602–620.

Ritzler, B., Zambianco, D., Harder, D. & Kaskey, M. (1980), Psychotic patterns of the concept of the object on the Rorschach test. *J. Abn. Psychol.*, 89:46–55.

Shor, J. & Sanville, J. (1978), *Illusions in Loving.* Los Angeles: Double Helix.

Slade, A., & Aber, L. J. (1991), Attachment, drives and development: Conflicts and convergences in theory. In: *Interface of Psychoanalysis and Psychology,* ed. J. Barron, M. Eagle, & D. Wolitsky. American Psychoanalysis and Psychological Association Press, pp. 154–185.

Sroufe, L. A. (1983), Infant-caregiver attachment and patterns of attachment in pre-school: The roots of maladaptive competence. In: *Minnesota Symposium on Child Psychology,* Vol. 16, ed. M. Perlmutter. Hillsdale, NJ: Lawrence Erlbaum Associates, pp. 41–83.

Stern, D. N. (1985), *The Interpersonal World of the Infant.* New York: Basic Books.

Virtue, C. (1992), The effects of maternal object representations and psychological differentiation on early mother-infant feeding-interactions. *Dissertation Abstracts International,* 52:3917.

Weissman, A. N. & Beck, A. T. (1978), Development and Validation of the Dysfunctional Attitude Scale: A preliminary investigation. Presented at meetings of the American Psychological Association, Toronto, Canada.

Wiggins, J. S. (1991), Agency and communion as conceptual coordinates for the understanding and measurement of interpersonal behavior. In: *Thinking Clearly About Psychology, Vol. 2,* ed. W. W. Grove & D. Cicchetti. Minneapolis: University of Minnesota Press, pp. 89–113.

Zeanah, C. H. & Anders, T. F. (1987), Subjectivity in parent-infant relationships: A discussion of internal working models. *Inf. Mental Health J.,* 8:237–250.

———— Burkhardt, P. E. & Muller, J. P. (1985), 14-year follow-up of borderline and schizotypal personality disorders. *Comprehen. Psychiat.,* 26:448–455.

SIXTEEN

Managed Care Discovers The Talking Cure

ERIC M. PLAKUN

A chapter about the role of psychoanalysis in hospital settings in the 1990s sounds at first like a very short chapter indeed. Psychoanalysis in hospitals? In the managed care 1990s? This must be a joke! To be sure, few if any hospitalized patients ever received classical psychoanalysis. Generally patients disturbed enough to require hospital treatment are not candidates for the deprivation and deemphasis of the real relationship that is part of psychoanalysis. In that sense, psychoanalysis in hospital settings is a misnomer. Psychoanalytic psychotherapy, however—also called psychodynamic psychotherapy or expressive psychotherapy—was offered as part of the treatment program of numerous hospitals in the past. It has largely disappeared.

One might be tempted to offer a fitting eulogy and accusatory condemnation of the forces that killed the noble endeavor of psychoanalytic psychotherapy in hospital settings, but that is not the focus of this chapter. Instead, the chapter reviews, contextualizes, and interprets the process that led to the current state of affairs in behavioral health care in the United States; then offers a surprisingly optimistic report on how and why one psychoanalytically oriented treatment facility, the Austen Riggs Center, is not only surviving, but thriving in the managed care era. In fact, for a subset of treatment-resistant patients, managed care seems to be discovering that the talking cure is a medically necessary and cost-effective treatment.

The author wishes to thank Drs. Edward Shapiro, Craig Piers, Christopher Fowler, Robert Tittmann, and Mr. Ave Schwartz for their helpful editorial comments on earlier drafts of this chapter.

The chapter concludes with predictions about the future role of psychoanalytically oriented clinicians in inpatient treatment.

PSYCHOANALYSIS AND CONTEXT

Freud (1917a; Jones, 1955) proposed three discoveries in human history that so offended human narcissism that those responsible could not be forgiven for their deeds. The discoveries are those of Copernicus, who brought the world the unhappy news that the earth was not the center of the universe; Darwin, who demonstrated that mankind had evolved from more primitive life forms and was not simply created in God's image; and Freud himself, who demonstrated that man's impressive intelligence and rationality are powerfully affected by an irrational dynamic unconscious. Freud was reacting to the hostile response that greeted the introduction of his theories. His ideas have had a profound impact on the 20th-century in numerous domains ranging from the clinical to the arts. Even his most vitriolic detractors reveal the power of his ideas in the heat of their passion and the intensity of their hostility.

As unwelcome as Freud's theories were, they arose when they did, instead of a century or millennium earlier or later, because they fit the *Zeitgeist* of his time. Psychoanalysis, then, arose within a larger context in the outer world. The early history of psychoanalysis was powerfully shaped by an adversarial climate that included elements of antisemitism and outrage at Freud's focus on infantile sexuality in manifestly straitlaced Viennese society. Despite the external adversarial context, psychoanalysis thrived by attending to the study of the previously inadequately understood notions of the mind and the therapeutic dyad. Most of the major theoretical contributions in the field during the 20th century have focused on intrapsychic processes or on the dyad of analyst and analysand. Out of this focus has come the understanding of concepts like transference, countertransference, and enactment, which are so essential to psychoanalytic and psychodynamic therapeutic work.

Despite the focus on inner experience, the place of psychoanalysis itself and of any analyst and analysand pair has always existed within the broader context of the outer world, sometimes referred to as "the third" to the psychoanalytic dyad (Ogden, 1994; Muller, 1996). Within the walls of the consulting room, the notion of the third is often overlooked and taken for granted. For the most part, this does not pose a problem, until the context becomes, for example, a political climate that cannot tolerate psychoanalytic inquiry. The history of 20th-century totalitarian regimes' intolerance of psychoanalysis illustrates the extreme of the impact of the societal third on the psychoanalytic consulting room.

It is not only the societal third that affects the psychoanalytic dyad. Shapiro (1996) has argued that, despite being overlooked and taken for granted, the third is always present in the form of the psychoanalyst's dedication to the task of psychoanalysis and in his or her management of the psychoanalytic frame around such issues as time boundaries, fees, and vacations. The lack of attention to the frame was not often a problem in the treatment of neurosis, except, as Shapiro notes, when an analyst so forgot the connection to the frame of the field's standards, and to the need for commitment to the analytic task, that he or she would lose the therapeutic role and become fused with the patient; with sexual behavior with patients or other comparable boundary violations as a result.

The notion of context has recently become more important because societal trends are once again creating an adversarial climate for psychoanalysis. As an example of this, one need only recall that, at one point in the 1994 debate on national health insurance, it looked as if the conduct of fee-for-service psychotherapy might become illegal. Changes in reimbursement patterns have led to frequent intrusion into the consulting room, with demands for justification of "medical necessity." In the current adversarial context, an isolated psychoanalytic dyad can no longer fail to pay attention to the impact of context and the place of the third. Without greater attention to the integrating and anchoring concept of the third in psychoanalytic work, the dyad is in danger of becoming lost, irrelevant and forgotten by the larger world.

INTERPRETATION AND MANAGEMENT

Shapiro (1996) makes a strong case for conceptualizing treatment interventions into two types, those which focus on management and those which focus on interpretation of meaning. In psychoanalysis, interpretive interventions are a central concept, while management interventions dealing with the frame and the alliance, that is, those which tend to the third, are often taken for granted.

For most of the 20th century, when psychoanalysis was in ascendency, much of the focus in mental health was on interpretation of meaning. The field has now shifted away from interpretation and toward a management focus that targets symptoms and behaviors but ignores meaning. It is this shift toward management and away from interpretation of meaning that is at the conceptual heart of the move away from psychanalytic and psychodynamic treatments and toward the somatic, cognitive, and behavioral interventions that are currently favored. It is not the efficacy of these latter treatments that is the current focus, but rather how to understand them in a broader context.

An example that illustrates the implications of the differences between the management and interpretation foci occurred a few years ago at a meeting of the International Society for the Study of Personality Disorders in Boston. In a symposium on the treatment of self-destructive borderline patients, Charles Swensen, then of New York Hospital-Westchester Division, presented a paper on the use of Dialectical Behavior Therapy, or DBT (Linehan, 1991), in their borderline treatment unit. I presented a paper proposing principles in establishing and maintaining a workable therapeutic alliance in the psychoanalytically oriented psychotherapy of these often suicidal patients (Plakun, 1994). In the discussion that followed, Marsha Linehan spoke from the audience about the similarity between the DBT focus on self-destructive behaviors and the psychoanalytically based principles I had presented without use of psychoanalytic technical jargon. Indeed, her observation seemed accurate. Nevertheless, the difference between the two treatment approaches was also apparent. DBT began and ended with managing the symptoms, whereas the principles I offered had been presented only as a way of managing the therapeutic framework in order to allow the essential interpretive work to proceed.

THE TRANSFORMATION OF BEHAVIORAL HEALTH FROM CLINICAL DISCIPLINE TO INDUSTRY

After World War II, psychoanalytic thinking was the conceptual basis for mental health care in the United States. Most doctoral programs in clinical psychology had an analytic foundation. It was hard to become a psychiatry department chairman or a successful practitioner without becoming a credentialed psychoanalyst. Most psychiatric hospitals had a psychoanalytic orientation, and a number of prestigious hospitals began to offer an opportunity for quality treatment for patients who had failed as outpatients. Institutions like Chestnut Lodge, the Institute of Living, New York Hospital-Westchester Division, the Menninger Foundation, the Austen Riggs Center, McLean Hospital, and half a dozen others came to symbolize the best treatment available, attracting the best and the brightest trainees and staff from around the country and the world. Patients were seen in psychoanalytic psychotherapy several times a week by skilled senior clinicians or closely supervised trainees. Sophisticated milieu treatment programs evolved on the basis of and consistent with psychoanalytic principles. There was time available to offer staff the essential reflective and integrative spaces required for psychoanalytic work in a hospital setting through supervision and case conferences. Treatments were often extended and gradually became more expensive. The expense arose, in part, because of the need to respond to ever-increasing governmental regulations and accreditation requirements.

By the 1970s, a struggle had begun in the field between the interpretive focus of psychoanalysis and the management focus of biological psychiatry. Striking benefit was available to patients through the use of ever-improving psychopharmacologic agents. The struggle between psychoanalysis and biological psychiatry is a manifestation of the struggle between interpretation and management. Biological psychiatry's clear advantages in providing the greatest good to the greatest number, its ready applicability to the emerging community mental health center movement, and its comfort with and easy adaptability to phenomenologic empirical research (as compared with the puzzling aversion to statistical methodology that emerged and persisted in some quarters of psychoanalysis) led to the virtual elimination of the interpretive psychoanalytic point of view from mainstream psychiatry, in favor of a management approach focused on controlling symptoms.

Concurrent with and as part of this transformation, there was a profound change in psychiatric diagnosis. Robert Spitzer and others began to focus on the possibility of developing a reliable and valid diagnostic nosology, culminating in the publication of DSM-III in 1980. The reliable, researchable diagnostic criteria of DSM-III made it possible for the first time for clinicians and researchers in different mental health disciplines and with different treatment approaches to share a common diagnostic language. On the other hand, DSM-III and its descendants, DSM-IIIR and DSM-IV, are not quite the atheoretical documents that their authors propose them to be. The focus on symptoms, the avoidance of criteria requiring inference, the elimination of the notion of neurosis, and other features of the DSM do not allow the easy inclusion of a psychoanalytic interpretive point of view in the diagnostic schema. Even the structure of the multiaxial system of DSM-III creates a hurdle for psychoanalysis. Although not the intent of the authors of the DSM, location of the major psychiatric syndromes on Axis I and of the personality disorders on Axis II inevitably gives second-class status to the often profoundly disabling personality disorders. Most insurance companies view Axis II disorders as having second-class status when it comes to reimbursement for treatment.

DSM bashing is popular in psychoanalytic circles, but I have no intention of adding my voice to that chorus. In spite of its limitations, the development of the contemporary diagnostic and statistical manuals offers an opportunity for psychoanalysis to find its place in the new clinical context. For example, with appropriate caveats about the danger of labeling and categorization in mind (Vaillant, 1992; Fromm, 1995), it is worth noting that the designation of a borderline personality disorder as a diagnostic entity in DSM-III allowed researchers like McGlashan (1983, 1985), Stone (1987; Stone, Hurt, and Stone, 1987), Paris, Brown, and Nowlis (1987), and Plakun (1989, 1991; Plakun, Burkhardt, and Muller, 1985) to establish this disorder as a valid and distinct clinical entity by using the methodology of empirical psychiatry. The view that borderline personality disorder is simply a variant of affective disorders (Akiskal, 1981) has largely disappeared. Additional research has demonstrated that this disorder is often severe and disabling, that it carries a lifetime suicide risk of 5 to 10% (Paris et al., 1987; Stone et al., 1987), and that comorbidity with this Axis II disorder can greatly complicate treatment response to the management-focused interventions of general psychiatric care (Stone, 1987; Friedman et al., 1992). The fact that DSM-IV has included defense mechanisms in an appendix offers a new and exciting opportunity for psychoanalysis to find its place in the new context.

In the 1980s psychiatric hospital treatment became a growth industry, attracting venture capitalists who developed successful for-profit psychiatric hospital chains. Mary Jane England (1993), a recent president of the American Psychiatric Association, noted that these private for-profit hospitals sometimes engaged in unfortunate marketing campaigns that resulted "in many unjustified and even harmful hospitalizations as well as sharply increased costs." In his comprehensive overview of trends in behavioral health care funding, John Iglehart (1996) reports that from 1986 to 1990 there was a 50% increase in mental health and substance abuse expenditures in the United States. Iglehart reports that Americans spent an estimated $85.1 billion for the direct costs of treatment for behavioral health disorders in 1990, an amount approximating 10% of all personal health expenditures in the United States. In much the same way as the world had to begin to come to terms with the limits of other resources, whether the ozone layer, petroleum reserves, or rain forests, by 1990 the nation was approaching the limit of the possible funding resources for mental health treatment. The world had to change, and it did—with the introduction of "managed care" as a means of managing the tension between the need for care and the limitation of resources to fund it. As Iglehart points out, the introduction of managed care had a profound effect on the provision of mental health services, particularly inpatient mental health services. There was money to be made by reducing the health care expenditures of large corporations. Suddenly venture capitalists began to leave the psychiatric hospital business in favor of the managed care business.

Managed care of behavioral health services applies to a number of methodologies. There is a dizzying and ever-changing array of means of management of service provision, including health maintenance organizations, preferred provider organizations, and "carve-ins" and "carve-outs" of mental health coverage. Health maintenance organizations have been criticized for their provision of managed behavioral health care because their expenditures on these services represent only 3%–5% of their total health expenditures, whereas the national average for these services accounts for about 10% of total costs (Iglehart, 1996). Recently health maintenance organizations have begun to show a willingness to increase expenditures for behavioral health care. For example, Iglehart reports that one large HMO, Kaiser Permanente Medical Care Program, is investing $100 million over a period of five years to upgrade its behavioral health services. These services were neglected within the plan, and Kaiser was losing corporate and individual customers.

Whereas health maintenance organizations often provide their own mental health services (the so-called carve-in of benefit), for many large insurance companies the solution has been to turn to specialized managed behavioral health care companies that "carve-out" behavioral health care as a specialty. There is a rapidly changing shell game in managed behavioral health care that has the feel of speed chess, as large managed care organizations have won then lost major corporate contracts and then gone through a frenzy of merger and acquisition of one another. By 1996, the 10 largest managed care organizations generated an estimated 90% of the total revenue collected for behavioral health care (Iglehart, 1996). What these large managed care organizations tend to have in common is 1) a strictly limited benefit package emphasizing acute care, typically offering 20 outpatient visits and 30 hospital days annually; 2) a great deal of clout because of their large size and the large number of lives for which they control mental health expenditures; 3) close monitoring of the provision of services and focused monitoring of high cost cases; and 4) various forms of placing providers of mental health services at financial risk (Frank, McGuire, and Newhouse, 1995; Iglehart, 1996).

During 1993 and 1994 the national debate on health care reform led to an important shift in perspective on mental health policy. The Clinton administration plan ultimately was not adopted and will likely be viewed as a failure of that administration, but nevertheless the plan had a number of important effects. Out of the proposals and related debate came an acceptance of new approaches beyond inpatient and outpatient treatment alone. The notions of residential care and partial hospitalization achieved credibility. Behavioral health care services were also solidly moved into the mainstream of health care funding. The health care debate also led to a decrease in the barrier between public and private sector funding for treatment. Later in the decade the dramatic shift to Republican control of Congress moved the nation inexorably toward an effort to eliminate the Federal budget deficit by early in the 21st century, with talk of spending reductions of nearly half a trillion dollars in Medicare and Medicaid by 2002 (Iglehart, 1996.)

As a means of managing a limited resource, managed care appears to be a success. Battagliola (1994) reports that IBM saw a decline in mental health expenditures from $97.9 million in 1992 to $59.2 million in 1993, while other major corporations also reported reductions of 30%–50% in their expenditures for mental health services (Iglehart, 1996). The introduction of flexing of benefits to cover alternative treatment options to traditional hospitalization has been associated with a substantial change in the utilization of mental health and substance abuse services by employees of the Xerox Corporation. In the period between 1987 and 1994, Xerox saw a decline in the number of hospital admissions per thousand employees from 9.7 to 6.1; a decline in the number of hospital days per thousand employees from 327 to 61; a decline in average length of stay from 33.7 days to 9.9 days; and an average payment per episode for mental health and substance abuse services that declined from $377 to $214 (Iglehart, 1996).

These cost savings and changes in service delivery are dramatic and enticing to those with an eye on the bottom line, but there has been surprisingly little attention to how these dramatic changes in service provision affect patient care. For example, Lutz (1995) reported on a 1994 survey by the National Association of Psychiatric Health Systems showing that, although the average length of inpatient stay had been cut to 15.2 days in 1994 from 19.8 days in 1992, the number of overall admissions was rising, up 12% in just one year. It is no surprise to clinicians that the relentless pressure to decrease length of stay puts patients at risk for more readmissions. Other data (Falcon, 1994) suggest that decreasing expenditures for mental health services is associated with an increase in expenditures for medical services. Those in need of care will find it elsewhere if access to mental health treatment is denied.

THE EFFECT OF MANAGED CARE
ON PSYCHIATRIC HOSPITALS

The new bottom line is that hospitals and hospital staffs are working harder and moving faster to stand still or even move backward. Dramatic cutbacks have become a regular part of the psychiatric inpatient experience. The results of the cutbacks have been profound. There has been a dramatic de-skilling of those providing care, such that registered nurses are replaced by licensed practical nurses or nurses aides, and direct providers have shifted from doctoral level psychiatrists and psychologists to masters level social workers to nurses to uncredentialed "therapists." Since time is money, there have been marked cutbacks in the time available for staff to reflect on and integrate their treatment plans. There is less supervision, fewer staff conferences, and few or no case conferences. Treatment has come to mean management of symptoms, with little or no room left for the interpretation of meaning in the lives of human beings. A clinical vignette illustrates this point.

A naive but highly competent young woman in her late 20s had been the primary caretaker of her disabled mother since a divorce when the young woman was in her early teens. The young woman held a responsible corporate job but was sexually harassed by her boss in an escalating way. Only after more than a year did the woman protest to his supervisors, quit the job, and consult with an attorney, by which point she had clear symptoms of a posttraumatic stress disorder. She sought outpatient treatment at the local general hospital department of psychiatry, where a male psychiatrist convinced her that, despite her reluctance to take pills, they were the best treatment. He prescribed a series of trials of anxiolytics. The woman tried the pills, did not like their effect, but did not tell the psychiatrist she had stopped taking them. Frustrated by the apparent failure of anxiolytics to be of help, the psychiatrist referred the patient to a woman psychologist who concurred with the diagnosis of PTSD and recommended biofeedback. Except briefly in the first session, this therapist was not interested in the woman's experience of harassment, but was concerned primarily in teaching, performing, and monitoring various techniques and procedures. The patient felt helpless, ignored, and pessimistic about treatment, but she continued attending sessions with both providers, while concealing her lack of compliance with the treatment recommendations.

Months later the woman was seen by a dynamically skilled psychiatrist as part of an independent forensic assessment. In their two-hour meeting, this psychiatrist observed and interpreted to the patient the enactment in which she and her treaters were engaged. He helped the young woman see that, with both providers as unwitting and unaware participants, she was engaging in unconscious nonverbal interactions that repeated the experience of harassment and her inability to speak up and put a stop to it. Beyond that, her silent, passive, and masochistic surrender to the harasser had important connections to the woman's guilt-ridden attachment to her critical, disabled mother, for whom she had served as a dedicated caretaker for years at considerable personal sacrifice.

The psychiatrist's primary focus was the forensic assessment, not treatment, but in their brief relationship the woman was able to see the repetition in which she was involved, and she began to take charge of her life. She soon told both her psychiatrist and her psychologist that she was unwilling to continue treatment as they had been structuring it. She insisted on referral to someone who would listen to her experience and help her find meaning in it. She was referred to a dynamically oriented clinician and did well.

Of course, clinicians can become skilled only at those techniques for which they receive training. Academic departments of psychiatry have been particularly hard hit by changes in the field because those purchasing behavioral health services are often disinclined to spend their dollars on training or research. In fact, some formerly respected residency programs have become casualties of this shift. An example is the residency program at Timberlawn Hospital in Dallas. The number and quality of medical school graduates seeking residencies in psychiatry have declined substantially. Contemporary training programs often provide a curriculum organized around mastering the field through a command of the diagnostic nomenclature. Little teaching or supervision related to the principles of dynamic psychiatry is available. Most psychiatry residencies offer no real training in how to understand symptoms in the context of a life through development of a psychodynamic formulation. As Perry, Cooper, and Michels (1987) have argued convincingly, the usefulness of a psychodynamic formulation is not limited to those conducting psychodynamic psychotherapy but offers an opportunity for integration of interpretation and management into a sophisticated multidisciplinary treatment plan. This kind of formulation allows for a deeper understanding of how, for example, a patient's poor medication compliance may be a predictable manifestation of mistrust of authority related to a childhood abuse history and is best dealt with by interpretation rather than a court order.

It has become commonplace in my work as an oral examiner for the American Board of Psychiatry and Neurology to see postresidency candidates sitting for board certification who interview patients using a style that ignores the nuances of the interaction, fails to follow affect, and approaches the entire process as if it were a semistructured gathering of answers to questions about various DSM-IV diagnostic criteria. Most candidates seem at a loss when asked if they can provide a psychodynamic formulation of the patient they have just interviewed.

In an address about the future of psychiatry, Robert Michels, M.D. (1994), suggested that it would fall to the psychiatrists of the future to become the experts in difficult or treatment-resistant cases. Many of these difficult cases are treatment challenges because of personality disorder comorbidity with Axis I syndromes. They often stimulate intense staff countertransference reactions. However, the current direction of psychiatric education, with its focus on the biological and the empirical, and on management at the expense of training in the use of interpretive interventions or in the development and use of a psychodynamic formulation, ill equips future psychiatrists for the role of taking on these difficult patients for treatment.

Of the dozen or so psychoanalytically oriented hospitals referred to earlier, most have survived, but their treatment and training programs, and their identities, have often been utterly transformed. One of them claims to have become "the nation's mental health center," rather than a place of psychoanalytic expertise. Another, since its widely published psychoanalyst medical director retired, has been transformed from a leading treatment and training facility for psychoanalytically oriented treatment of difficult patients into a behaviorally focused treatment program. A third, battered by a successful malpractice case organized around the failure to prescribe medication as a departure from the standard of care, has been sold to a community mental health center and all but surrendered its former mission. In a telephone call last year from another of these facilities referring a patient for residential treatment, my question about what kind of treatment had been provided during the week the patient had already been hospitalized was met with the response, "We don't do treatment anymore, just triage. We were hoping you could provide some." A fifth facility has taken on managed care with an "if you can't lick them, join them" approach and is working vigorously to become an organization that "covers lives" through contracts with industry and providers. For the most part, these psychoanalytically oriented treatment centers all made the decision to link their future to providing services primarily within their regional catchment area. Unfortunately, such a decision inexorably links them to the provision of psychiatric primary care and therefore to management rather than interpretation and to a symptom focus rather than a psychoanalytic focus.

An exception is the Austen Riggs Center. The Center was battered like other facilities by the transition to managed care and the virtual shutting off of referrals for treatment in the early 1990s and underwent a painful and dramatic reduction in force as part of a 30% budget cutback. After the frightening realization of the ways the world had changed associated with this experience, however, the Center reconfirmed its psychoanalytically linked mission and has seen the tide begin to turn in its favor.

Riggs is an unusual facility with a long and deeply held tradition of treating patients as responsible adults. The setting is completely open and voluntary, with a sophisticated and highly evolved therapeutic milieu program in which patients take charge of the community program, and with a staff deeply committed to this tradition of openness and to the provision of four-times-weekly intensive psychoanalytic psychotherapy to all patients by a doctor on the staff. There is no use of seclusion or restraint and no system of privileges for patients. All patients have all privileges at all times, just as would any citizen under the Constitution. This description might make Riggs sound like the probable first casualty of the managed care revolution, but this was not the case. It became clear that Riggs, located on the main street of Norman Rockwell's small town of Stockbridge,

Massachusetts, had no reason to exist if it were simply to provide services to sparsely populated Stockbridge (population 5,000 year round) or even to Berkshire County, with a total population of not much more than 100,000 far-flung rural and small-town residents already served by three other inpatient psychiatric units. Riggs instead reviewed its mission and renewed its commitment to an identity as a national center of excellence for work with treatment resistant patients.

For many of these patients, prominent Axis II pathology puts them at risk to become part of the small percentage of patients whose treatment takes an inordinate proportion of the managed care organizations' resources. For these patients, whose personality disorders complicate Axis I mood, anxiety, eating, substance use, and psychotic spectrum disorders, definitive treatment of their repetitive self-destructive and maladaptive behaviors requires an interpretive, psychodynamic focus, and not a symptom management focus alone (Plakun, 1996; Shapiro, 1996). Riggs approached the large managed care organizations to discuss our specialized treatment program for this group of patients, but discovered they were too busy treating the largest group of less ill patients to notice these outliers. We waited for managed care to discover high costs associated with the treatment of these patients. We have heard from one large managed care organization that 10% of their patients use 70% of the resources for treatment. The most enlightened of the managed care organizations have begun to notice these outliers and to seek more effective treatment for them, instead of squandering resources on more of the same treatment that has led to a chronic cycle of repeated crisis and rehospitalization. This has led to a number of referrals for extended treatment at Riggs funded by managed care. However, we have also had the experience of negotiating a contract or an understanding about the treatment of such outliers with the leaders of a managed care organization, only to find those leaders soon replaced as a second and larger managed care organization purchases the first. It is an ongoing struggle, but Riggs remains busy. In part this is because families have gradually come to lower expectations of what their insurance will cover, and many middle-class families have elected to fund a different and more intensive treatment out of their own resources. In these situations, treatment often begins with funding from the limited insurance benefits available in a contract, then is extended by a combination of family resources, and moves to less expensive step-down programs and fee reductions based on financial need

The Riggs plan is working because Riggs has identified and become committed to a unique clinical mission that includes an emphasis on interpretation in addition to management, while paying careful attention to the individual patient within his or her context. The treatment program extends the offerings of general psychiatric programs by adding intensive, four-times-weekly individual psychodynamic psychotherapy by a doctor on the staff and participation in a sophisticated and highly evolved milieu program. One way that Riggs holds to the interpretive model is through the work of the interdisciplinary treatment teams, which use a psychodynamic formulation for a rich integration of the individual psychotherapy, psychopharmacology, nursing, substance abuse, and family interventions of the treatment plan.

Riggs has given up the notion of being a long-term "hospital," an identity that served it for several decades from the 1960s until the beginning of the 1990s, but it still offers long-term treatment. On an average day, Riggs seldom treats more than 10% of its 50 patients as inpatients. Instead, Riggs has developed a continuum of care, with six distinct programs. In addition to the inpatient program, there are three residential programs, a day treatment program, and an aftercare program. As patients move through the programs, continuity of care is maximized by having the patient continue treatment with the same therapist and the same treatment team throughout all programs. Thus, from the outside, there are six discrete programs with distinct criteria, differentiated goals and foci, and costs, but from the inside a patient's experience is of participation in an unusually seamless continuum of care.

Riggs integrates interpretation, management, and attention to context in an unusual way. A clinical financial interface group, now called the Resource Management Committee, was organized in 1991 with the specific mission of finding the clinical issues embedded and enacted in financial issues. The committee was established because of the recognition that shifts in reimbursement strategies often left the patients out of the tension over resource limitation and relocated it to the dialogue between clinician and funder of care. As Shapiro (1996) and I (Plakun, 1996) have argued, treatment of patients with personality disorders has as one goal the achievement of an improved ability to adapt to the limits of reality. Experiencing the tension over the limitation of resources offers patients with Axis II psychopathology an important opportunity to make sense of and to struggle adaptively with limits. Regardless of length of stay, examination and dynamic interpretation of this tension provides an opportunity for growth and change. The therapist has an obligation to "incorporate the reality of limitations into his framework and interpret within that space" (Shapiro, 1996). He or she does well to avoid the pitfall of projecting evil onto the managed care organization or, for that matter, the family payor, just because there is a resource limitation. As Shapiro notes, "when therapist and patient develop a shared recognition that resources are limited, the patient often directs his rage at the therapist as representative of that reality. Working through this rage leads to grief, mourning and a genuinely intimate engagement around treatment and its limitations" (p. 20).

A clinical example is a patient whose mother continually rescued him, both emotionally and financially, from taking charge of his life. Since childhood she had repeatedly bailed him out when he extended himself beyond his emotional or financial resources. He had become dependent on these rescues but was also enraged at her for them. In the hospital when his insurance coverage was ending, the patient's behavior worsened. He requested a fee reduction from the hospital to stay longer and demanded that his mother pay for his continuing treatment. The financial officer of the Resource Management Committee was inclined to grant his request, but in the ensuing discussion of clinical and financial issues, the clinical staff recognized and interpreted the patient's repetition of his family dynamic. The hospital was now in the position of joining the patient's mother in rescuing the patient. The rescue sought was to include a fee reduction by the hospital as well as the mother's expenditure of her retirement savings on his treatment, and included elements of retaliation and revenge against her. As a result of the work of the Resource Management Committee, an interpretation was made to the patient, who was able to step down to a less expensive program, obtain a job to support himself and continue treatment, with a small fee reduction from the hospital and a contribution from his mother. The patient began to see his pattern of blaming his mother for her overprotectiveness while demanding through regression that she continue to meet his needs. This was the beginning of his taking charge of his life and of this conflict, and it marked the start of the dramatic turnaround that followed.

THE FUTURE OF PSYCHOANALYSIS AND HOSPITALS

What does all this mean for the future of psychoanalysis and hospital treatment? Both resource limitation and treatment-resistant patients are here to stay. Given the reality that resource limitation is here to stay, it is likely that the management-based, symptom-focused treatment approach of psychiatric hospitals will continue. Where psychotherapies are provided, they will most likely be short term, cognitive, or behavioral, rather than psychoanalytically based. The skill of those providing the therapy will sometimes be less than optimal. No room will be created for psychoanalytic clinicians in this framework unless we demonstrate the value of our skills. It is within our grasp to demonstrate that the interpretive focus included in a psychodynamic formulation offers a better way to conduct treatment, even when the treatment is management focused. Psychoanalytic clinicians on a hospital or consulting staff will be in a position to consult with patients and their providers to construct a psychodynamic formulation that integrates, organizes, and coordinates an otherwise chaotic set of problems and treatment interventions. These clinicians will need psychoanalytic skills to unearth the ways that actualization of the transference or enactment around the patient's characterologic liabilities may be leading to a repetition of the underlying dynamic problem without an opportunity to understand its meaning. This role may well fall to psychoanalytically trained psychologists, since psychiatrists receive little training in this area.

The trend in hospital treatment toward patient empowerment also offers an opportunity to psychoanalytic clinicians. Since resource management issues will arise frequently, psychoanalytic clinicians who can apply their skills to these issues should be able to demonstrate the value of this kind of interpretive approach to the task of helping patients take charge of their resources and their treatment in the service of taking charge of their lives. Recognizing the role of resource management issues and bringing them to treatment team discussions, hospital administrators, and patients may provide an opportunity for psychoanalytically based interpretive work to make its way back into the management focus of even short-term psychiatric hospitals in the future.

Although many patients will get better with the management-based treatment approach, it will become increasingly clear that a significant minority of patients will require the expenditure of a disproportionately large share of resources for their treatment, requiring repeated rehospitalization, without significant benefit. Although some will suggest that these patients are chronic and untreatable, it will gradually become clear that a substantial subset of these treatment-resistant patients have significant characterologic contributions to their difficulties. It will be essential for facilities that provide first-line psychiatric inpatient care to develop and maintain the capacity to detect these patients and provide them with or refer them to appropriate treatment.

Finally, as appears to be the case with the Austen Riggs Center, there will be a continuing role for one or more psychoanalytic, hospital-based treatment centers as national referral centers for a proportion of treatment-resistant patients. As managed care companies and HMOs recognize that a small percentage of their patients require a large expenditure of resources, they have begun to seek out Riggs. We believe this trend is likely to continue, especially if a commitment is made to conducting empirically based research to study and demonstrate the results of treatment. Facilities like Riggs will also come to serve as training centers for clinicians who wish to develop the ability and expertise to become consultants or therapists for patients whose treatments repeatedly fail.

Although the relationship between psychoanalysis, hospitals, and the managed care environment of the 1990s has been a difficult one, filled with mutual projection and misunderstanding, managed care has begun to discover that the talking cure may be the best way of tending both to some of their patients and to their bottom line. Despite the fact that an earlier era of psychoanalytic preeminence in hospital treatment is over, there are encouraging hints that psychoanalysis may find a way back into psychiatric hospitals in a more differentiated, specialized, and focused way than in the past.

REFERENCES

Akiskal, H. S. (1981), Subaffective disorders: Dysthymic, cyclothymic and bipo-
    lar II disorders in the "borderline" realm. *Psychiat. Clin. North Amer.*, 4:25–
    60.
Battagliola, M. (1994), Breaking with tradition. *Business and Health*, June 6:53–
    56.
England, M. J. (1993), Health reform and organized systems of care. In: *New
    Directions for Mental Health Services*, ed. M. J. England & V. V. Goff. San
    Francisco: Jossey-Bass, pp, 5–12.
Falcon, S. (1994), Finances and insurance. Presentation at the annual meeting of
    the American Psychiatric Association, Philadelphia.
Frank, R. G., McGuire, T. G. & Newhouse, J. P. (1995), Risk contracts in man-
    aged mental health care. *Health Affairs* 14:50–64.
Freud, S. (1917a), A difficulty in the path of psycho-analysis. *Standard Edition*,
    17:135–144. London, Hogarth Press, 1955.
——— (1917b), Introductory lectures on psycho-analysis. *Standard Edition*,
    16:273–285. London, Hogarth Press, 1963.
Friedman, S., Jones, J. C., Chernen, L. & Barlow, D. H. (1992), Suicidal ideation
    and suicide attempts among patients with panic disorder: A survey of two
    outpatient clinics. *Amer. J. Psychiat.* 149:680–685.
Fromm, M. G. (1995), What does borderline mean? *Psychoanal. Psychol.* 12:233–
    245.
Iglehart, J. K. (1996), Health policy report: Managed care and mental health.
    New Eng. J. Med., 334:131–135.
Jones, E. (1955), *The Life and Work of Sigmund Freud*, Vol. 2. New York, Basic
    Books.
Linehan, M. M., Armstrong, H. E., Suarez, A., Allmon D. & Heard, H. L. (1991),
    Cognitive-behavioral treatment of chronically parasuicidal borderline pa-
    tients. *Arch. Gen. Psychiat.*, 48:1060–1064.
Lutz, S. (1995), Inpatient stay lengths drop sharply. *Mod. Healthcare*, August 21,
    1995:24.
McGlashan, T. H. (1983), The borderline syndrome, I: Testing three diagnostic
    systems; II: Is it a variant of schizophrenia or affective disorder? *Arch. Gen.
    Psychiat.* 40:1311–1323.
——— (1985), The prediction of outcome in borderline personality disorder: Part
    V of the Chestnut Lodge follow-up study. In: *The Borderline: Current*

Empirical Research, ed. T. H. McGlashan, Washington, D.C., American Psychiatric Press, pp. 63–98.

Muller, J. P. (1966), *Beyond the Psychoanalytic Dyad*. New York: Routledge.

Michels, R. (1994), The future of psychiatry. Lecture at the annual meeting of the American Psychiatric Association, Philadelphia.

Ogden, T. H. (1994), The analytic third: Working with intersubjective clinical facts. *Internat. J. Psycho-Anal.* 75:3–20.

Paris, J., Brown, R., Nowlis, D. (1987), Long-term follow-up of borderline patients in a general hospital. *Comp. Psychiat.*, 28:530–535.

Perry, S., Cooper, A. M. & Michels, R. (1987), The psychodynamic formulation: Its purpose, structure, and clinical application. *Amer. J. Psychiat.*, 144:543–550.

Plakun, E. M. (1989), Narcissistic personality disorder: A validity study and comparison to borderline personality disorder. *Psychiat. Clin. North Amer.*, 12:603–620.

—— (1991), Prediction of outcome in borderline personality disorders. *J. Personality Disord.*, 5:93–101.

—— (1994), Principles in the psychotherapy of self-destructive borderline patients. *J. Psychother. Prac. Res.*, 3:138–147.

—— (1996), Economic grand rounds: Treatment of personality disorders in an era of resource limitation. *Psychiat. Serv.*, 47:128–130.

—— Burkhardt, P. E. & Muller, J. P. (1985), 14-year follow-up of borderline and schizotypal personality disorders. *Comprehen. Psychiat.*, 26:448–455.

Shapiro, E. R. (1996), The boundaries are shifting: Renegotiating the therapeutic frame. In: *The Inner World in the Outer World*, ed. E. R. Shapiro. New Haven, CT: Yale University Press, pp. 7–25.

Stone, M. H. (1987), The course of borderline personality disorder. In: *American Psychiatric Press Review of Psychiatry*, Vol. 8, ed. A. Tasman, R. E. Hales & A. J. Frances. Washington, DC, American Psychiatric Press, pp. 103–122.

—— Hurt, S. W. & Stone, D. K. (1987), The PI-500: Long-term follow-up of borderline inpatients meeting DSM-III criteria, I: Global outcome. *J. Personality Dis.* 1:291–298.

Vaillant, G. E. (1992), The beginning of wisdom is never calling a patient a borderline. *J. Psychother. Pract. Res.*, 1:117–134.

SEVENTEEN

Psychoanalytic Perspectives On Clinical Work In the Inner City

NEIL ALTMAN

In this chapter, my effort is to bring together two worlds, that of psycho-analysis and that of the inner city public clinic, which have traditionally been very separate indeed. In these days of cost containment, managed care, and abandonment of the public sector, psychoanalysis and inner city public clinics may easily seem to share only an anachronistic status. I hope to reinforce, or inspire, opposition to the trends in today's society that seek to marginalize both psychoanalysis and our inner cities. I seek to demonstrate that a psychoanalytic perspective is absolutely essential for clinical work in inner city public clinics. I consider how a psychoanalytic point of view contributes to an understanding of the dynamics of the thera-peutic work that takes place in such clinics, with a particular focus on race, social class, and culture. I also look at how a psychoanalytic-systemic per-spective can illuminate the dynamics of the clinic itself as a bureaucratic and interpersonal system and how systemic dynamics interact with the therapeutic work that takes place in the clinic.

First, let us consider briefly how psychoanalysis and public clinic work came to inhabit different, nonoverlapping worlds for the most part. Given the labor intensiveness of the process, there has always been a tendency for psychoanalysis to be expensive (in a free market, in monetary terms) and thus selectively available to people with money and time to devote to it. Impoverished residents of inner city communities are, of course, last on the list of such people. This tendency was reinforced in the United States as psychoanalysis became a lucrative medical specialty taking place almost entirely in private practice.

In Europe before World War II, psychoanalysis was enlisted in socially engaged causes. Left-wing social theorists (from the Frankfurt School, such as Marcuse, 1964, 1966) drew heavily on psychoanalysis to locate a part of the psyche (the id) that existed in opposition to existing social structures. Psychoanalysis was thought to hold the potential for personal liberation from the oppressive effects of social programming. Having emigrated to the United States to escape the Nazis, some of the more politically radical analysts, such as Otto Fenichel, were intimidated during the McCarthy era into silence (see Jacoby, 1983, for a complete account of these events). Thus, one potential source of social commitment on the part of psychoanalysts fell by the wayside.

Another development that contributed to the isolation of psychoanalysis from large segments of society had to do with exclusionary "criteria of analyzability" as developed under the influence of psychoanalytic ego psychology. (These were systematized by Bachrach and Leaff, 1978.) These criteria reflect Calvinist values, such as tolerance for frustration and a tendency to inhibit action in favor of thought and verbalization. Given the culture-boundedness of the underlying value system, it is not surprising that Third World people and others with non-Northern European cultural backgrounds easily came to be seen as not possessing the attributes of a suitable analytic patient.

The aforementioned criteria of analyzability are linked to a psychoanalytic technique that became increasingly rigid in the United States. This technique was organized around analytic anomymity, abstinence, and neutrality. Frustration tolerance became a criterion of analyzability in the context of analytic abstinence, while verbal skill became important in the context of a technical approach that restricted the analyst's behavior to making verbal interpretations. Such a rigid, classical analytic technique is both inappropriate and not viable in an inner city public clinic. Analytic abstinence is not likely to be appropriate when one is dealing with impoverished people who may turn to a therapist for material help or advocacy in obtaining social services. In a community clinic context, anonymity may be impossible to maintain. As it evolved, then, classical technique in its more puristic versions seemed suitable only for private offices serving well-to-do, culturally mainstream patients (and staffed by well-to-do culturally mainstream analysts).

In the current cost-conscious, results-oriented, climate, the forces of managed care have made great inroads in both private and public practice. Public clinics, nearly universally, impose severe limits on the number of times a patient can be seen, making it difficult to conceive of most forms of psychoanalytic treatment. Long-term treatment can be contemplated mostly by those who can pay out-of-pocket, and these are nearly always private patients.

This litany of problems may seem to move inevitably toward the conclusion that "never the twain shall meet" when it comes to psychoanalysis and the public sector. But there is another side to the story. Contemporary developments in psychoanalysis, affecting all schools, from Freudian to self-psychological, have opened up new possibilities for what might constitute a viable psychoanalytic technique and what attributes a viable psychoanalytic patient may possess. Contemporary psychoanalysis sees the analyst as a participant-observer rather than a detached observer. The analyst is seen as inevitably influencing the patient and the patient's transference, even if only by his silence. Abstinence and anonymity are thus seen as impossible to attain and misconstrued as ideals. Technical questions revolve around how the analyst is to interact with the patient to facilitate an analytic inquiry and promote an interactional context in which the patient can change and grow. In this model, the provision of concrete assistance in the public clinic, as well as the analyst's exposure as a person in the clinic setting, does not, prima facie, disqualify the clinic as a setting for psychoanalytic work.

Many contemporary analysts question the distinction between action and verbalization; they regard a verbal comment as having an metacommunicational, or action, level. Seeing the analytic situation as an interaction changes the terms of the discussion of what promotes change and growth in the patient. In the classical model, the patient was thought to use the content of the analyst's intepretations to make the unconscious conscious. In the contemporary model, the patient is thought to use the interaction to try out new ways of behaving, thinking, and feeling with a significant other person. The analyst's work is not only to provide information, but also to foster an interpersonal environment in which inquiry and experimentation can occur.

What makes for an analyzable patient then? Clearly, verbal intelligence is no longer the prime factor. A relational perspective, with its focus on the dyad rather than on the patient as an individual, would lead us to wonder about the viability of the dyad rather than the viability of the patient. Can this particular patient and this particular analyst work out a way of interacting that provides the patient with opportunities to explore and change? Consider, from this point of view, the patient from a traditional Third World culture, or who is from an impoverished socioeconomic group, or who has had few formal educational opportunities. The question is no longer whether the person has the verbal skill, or the freedom from material need, to engage in an analytic process. Rather, the question is whether the two people will be able to negotiate an agreement about how they can work together to promote flexibility and change. Given the analyst's responsibility for the creation of a viable psychoanalytic context, the focus is heavily on the analyst to take account of the patient's meaning-making system, as influenced by the patient's culture and unique personal history, and to find a way of working with this person that makes sense to the patient. It must also make sense to the analyst, given his or her own values, his or her own commitments as an analyst, preferred ways of working, and so on. If patient and analyst can find a way of working that makes sense to both of them, there is a strong foundation for a viable psychoanalytic situation.

RACE, CLASS, AND CULTURE AS PARTS OF THE TRANSFERENCE–COUNTERTRANSFERENCE MATRIX

From a relational point of view, a cultural difference becomes a difference in perspective, a difference in meaning-making system, comparable to any other difference in perspective within the dyad. The analyst's job at many moments is largely to decenter enough to appreciate that the meaning of an event, an action of the analyst's, for example, means something to the patient that the analyst never would have anticipated. The analytic task, for the analyst, is to step outside of his own meaning-making system enough to see the interaction from the point of view of the patient, while retaining his own perspective and analytic orientation. This ability to straddle two perspectives simultaneously is essential both to the analytic work in general and to cross-cultural understanding and communication in particular. Put another way, cross-cultural communication is a special case of cross-person communication and thus is, in principle, no different from what occurs in ordinary analytic work.

With respect to race and social class, as well as culture, there are preconceptions, personally and societally generated, that structure and influence the transference–countertransference field. Elsewhere (Altman, 1995) I have outlined a neo-Kleinian projective-introjective model within which to conceptualize the workings of these social factors in the analytic situation. Consider race as paradigmatic. Race is socially constructed as a dichotomy (black and white), based on variations in physical features (e.g., skin color, facial features) which, in fact, occur on a continuum. The dichotomous structure of race is a consequence of the use to which we put race; that is, in the service of self-definition, we construct a group of people "like me" and another group of people whom we define as "other" or "unlike me." The "not me" group then becomes a convenient focus for the disowning and projection of psychic characteristics that people perceive as problematic for one reason or another. An example would be the way in which white people in the United States tend to project aggression and criminality onto African-American people. These projective and introjective processes tend to create self-fulfilling prophecies and vicious circles as people identify with the characteristics that are attributed to them and as social conditions are created and maintained (e.g., poverty and unemployment) that tend to induce the expected characteristics.

In the clinical psychoanalytic situation, patient and analyst similarly construct "self" and "other" in various ways. The analyst may be defined as "knowledgeable," "powerful," "healthy," and so on within the dyad, while the patient may be defined as "sick," "victimized," and the like. Likewise, a difference in race, social class, or culture can become a focus for such self–other definition. The ways in which patients from Third World cultural backgrounds become defined as ego deficient, as discussed earlier, would be a case in point. The exploration of the transference–countertransference field, then, must include inquiry into the ways in which social characteristics are used within the dyad to structure perceptions of self and other.

While it is true that such distinctions as "healthy" analyst versus "sick" or ego-deficient patient are maintained by self-fulfilling prophecies, it is also true that such distinctions have a way of unravelling within the interaction. For example, the patient's holding on to a "sick" role may be seen as a way of supporting the analyst, who may be perceived as potentially vulnerable. Whether one is looking at the occupants of the subordinate category in gender, racial, or class terms, one can often find ways in which a covert bolstering of the occupant of the "superior" category occurs. In a marital relationship, a woman, feeling that the man would be too threatened by evidence of her autonomy, for example, may hold on to a dependent position. It is the responsibility of the analyst working with "minority" group patients to be aware of the ways in which there may be such covert maintenance of a hierarchy within the dyad that both serves defensive purposes and reflects oppressive hierarchies in society at large.

CLINICAL ILLUSTRATION

I was assigned a patient at the Bronx clinic where I worked, an eight-year-old girl, whom I shall call Taisha, whose symptom was school refusal. This child, having been abandoned in infancy by her crack-abusing mother, lived with her maternal grandmother, Ms. A. Her mother would show up once or twice a year to see Taisha but never expressed an interest in raising her. Taisha's father had never been part of the picture; the grandmother did not even know who he was. Ms. A had worked for many years as a domestic employee; now she was retired. Grandmother and granddaughter lived together in a high-rise, middle-income housing project on the edge of a severely poverty-stricken and decaying neighborhood. A couple of blocks away lived the grandmother's younger sister, a very intelligent but severely disturbed, paranoid woman. The great-aunt was convinced that there were listening devices in her wall, for example. These were long-standing, stable delusions. She had had a hospitalization or two over the years but did not seem unstable at the time. Taisha would be sent to stay with Ms. A's sister sometimes for a day or two or over a weekend. Taisha seemed content to visit her great-aunt; the whole arrangement seemed quite stable and satisfactory.

Exploring the onset of the school refusal, I discovered that it began around the time that Ms. A's son, Taisha's uncle, Mr. B, showed up drunk at the apartment one midnight, threatening to hurt Ms. A as he ranted and raved. Mr. B was a severe and chronic alcoholic who disappeared for months at a time. But, when least expected, he would show up drunk in the middle of the night, stay for a few days, then disappear again. Ms. A thought Taisha had slept through the most recent incident, but it was shortly thereafter that Taisha began refusing to go to school. Taisha denied remembering this most recent visit of her uncle. I decided that I would try to help the grandmother prepare herself to "set limits" with her son; I advised her to confront him and inform him that he was welcome to visit, but only when he was sober. The grandmother said she didn't know where to find him, she would have to wait until the next time he showed up, when he would surely be drunk. I saw Taisha once a week for individual therapy. I saw the grandmother once a week to counsel her on getting Taisha back into school and to discuss how she would handle her son the next time he showed up drunk. I also began meeting occasionally with the maternal aunt. The aunt proved able to take Taisha to school, and the immediate crisis passed.

I had a feeling of nearly unbearable sadness about Taisha and her family. I thought, from time to time, that I was getting a sample of the legacy of slavery and subsequent oppression and discrimination in the form of the drug addiction, alcoholism, and mental illness in this African-American family. Ms. A was a very passive, gentle, church-going woman. Her meek and proper demeanor struck me as yet another legacy of slavery and oppression, although it stood in stark contrast to the chaotic lives of her children. Ms. A once told me about the rich people for whom she had done domestic service on Fifth Avenue and on Central Park West in New York City. She had left her children during the week with other family members, and I remember being struck by how she had accommodated to an inequitable social order by suppressing her aggression, not speaking up, not protesting. I thought how much her children might have paid the price for what she had to do to make a living. Her passivity seemed most manifest in her relationship with her son, and it seemed to me that Taisha, as well as Ms. A, was paying a heavy price.

My hypothesis was that Taisha's school refusal reflected her anxiety that her uncle would hurt her grandmother; I thought that Taisha was staying home to make sure she was all right. Over time, I became aware of the problems associated with identifying Mr. B as the source of the problems in this family. Making the uncle the problem simplified matters, to be sure. Doing so made it possible to have a relatively simple and coherent treatment plan. In the face of the overwhelming breakdowns that had occurred in this family's functioning over the years, it was possible to say, "Set limits with (if not get rid of) the uncle, and things will get better." If one regards Mr. B (not to mention Taisha's mother) as the "identified patient," as the family therapists say, then excluding him would be a futile exercise in isolating the problem. And, indeed, Ms. A raised complications. At first, in her compliant way, she agreed with the plan. But as soon as Mr. B showed up at her door, she (again, compliantly) let him in, drunk as he was. When, on hearing of the incident, I showed disappointment in my face, Ms. A, crying, said to me, "But he's my son. It's not so easy." I felt sympathetic, helpless, impatient. I ended up urging her to go with him to a detox program, to research A.A. programs, to insist that he follow a treatment plan if he wanted to be able to come to her home. She said that he had been over all those routes before, many times, but she would try again. Then she said she was afraid he would kill her if she refused to let him in to the apartment. He had been violent toward her when he was drunk. He was always terribly remorseful when he was sober, but that did not stop him from being violent the next time around.

When Ms. A said, "He's my son. It's not so easy," I began to realize how much I was excluding Mr. B. I was regarding him as hopeless, shrinking from trying to engage him myself, advocating that Ms. A deal with him while I failed to offer even to meet him. This put Ms. A in an untenable position. There was a mother–son bond that could not be denied. Ms. A's protest was also perhaps her first assertive act in relation to me. She further called to my attention the level of rage that she knew could be called forth in her son if she tried to send him away. I shifted gears at this point, as I have indicated, and suggested, not that she simply send him away, but that she go with him to a detox program and A.A., making his participation a condition of his being able to come to her apartment. But, as she pointed out, this course of action was easier said than done.

As I thought about the situation later, I realized that I was asking Ms. A to deal with her son in a way that I was not prepared for myself. I realized that the last thing in the world I wanted was to confront Mr. B myself. As the "identified patient," he embodied for me too much individual and social pathology. But then I imagined Ms. A politely going about her business, taking care of the homes of well-to-do people on Fifth Avenue, while her children suffered in the Bronx. Most of the time most of us can ignore the human suffering generated by social inequities of this kind. Meeting Mr. B would have made it all too explicit for me. I would have been face-to-face with some of the rage, despair, and self-destructiveness produced by life in the South Bronx. But I could not continue trying to operate by proxy through Ms. A, and I could not simply wish that Mr. B and the problems he represented would go away. By failing to meet with him, I was also acting out of an implicit belief that it was useless to make a claim on him to take personal responsibility for his own behavior and its consequences. I did not really believe that he would go to a detox program and A.A.; I was really suggesting that Ms. A take a tenable position from which she could get rid of him. One could try to get rid of Mr. B, as Ms. A had tried to rid herself of her own rage and despair by adopting a polite, inoffensive way of being in the world. The result, however, was untenable and unstable, as all efforts at defensive exclusion of psychic pain tend to be in the long run.

From this vantage point, Taisha knew, unconsciously, that her sense of security with her grandmother was illusory. Her uncle's appearance confronted her with the rage and chaos that lurked around her, in her family, in her neighborhood, in her school. The only way to help Taisha in a more fundamental way was to acknowledge what there really was to be afraid of, not simply to get her to go back to school. For me, the first step in this process was to acknowledge that Mr. B was a member of this family and needed to be dealt with. I asked Ms. A, therefore, if she could find a way to get a message to Mr. B that I would like to meet with him. These efforts were unsuccessful, but I think I succeeded in conveying to Ms. A that I had recognized her position in relation to her son and that I had wrestled with my own anxiety and conflict about dealing with him.

Meanwhile, my individual work with Taisha was organized around the idea that Taisha was struggling, on one hand, with fear of her uncle and injury to her grandmother and, on the other, with the fantasized destructive consequences of her own unconscious rage, which presumably was stimulated by the current events as well as much in her past history. Not surprisingly, Taisha's play (with human figures) was full of destructive attacks by "bad guys" on a family. At Taisha's request, I took on the role of the bad guy. Viewing this figure as the representative of Taisha's uncle as well as her own destructive self, I tried to humanize him, to draw Taisha out about how he had come to be such a bad guy, what he felt, what motivated him. Over time, Taisha was able to identify with the bad guy, to take on his role in the play, to see him in more than a one-dimensional way. The process here paralleled my own process of coming to recognize Mr. B as a human being. I believe that the play helped Taisha both to think about her uncle as a person, making him thus less monstrous to her, and to recognize and own her rage and her destructive impulses. (See

Caspary, 1993, for a full discussion of this way of working with fantasy play in order to help children reclaim disowned parts of themselves.)

I worked with this family until they decided to move to a small town in the South where there was some family, after Ms. A heard that her son had died in the street, most likely of liver failure. Taisha stayed in school. She was a reserved, kind, and gentle girl like her grandmother, but somewhat more assertive and less fearful.

DISCUSSION OF THE CASE MATERIAL

Psychoanalytic one-person (intrapsychic), two-person (interpersonal), and three-person (systemic) psychologies are all necessary for an adequate understanding of this case, considered as representative of those encountered in public clinics. The individual work with Taisha, focusing as it did on intrapsychic dynamics, fits well into a traditional one-person psychoanalytic framework, despite the once-a-week frequency. The work that went on with Ms. A, and within my countertransference to Ms. A and to Mr. B, required a two-person or three-person perspective but was nonetheless both essential to the work and essentially psychoanalytic.[1] A one-person approach in isolation from two- and three-person perspectives, focusing solely on Taisha's conflicts over her own aggression, for example, runs the risk of pathologizing Taisha by failing to recognize the reactive elements in her fear. On the other hand, a systemic perspective without the one-person point of view tends to render the patient a victim of circumstance. To focus solely on the external threat would have been to collude in a defensive process of denial of Taisha's and Ms. A's own aggression.

All psychoanalytic theories deal with both one-person and two-person dimensions of the analytic field. Drive theory, which is basically about intrapsychic elements, includes the other person as object of drive energy. Interpersonal theory, which is basically about a two-person interaction, includes the intrapsychic domain in terms of "personifications" (Sullivan, 1953). The difference between such extreme positions has to do with the priority given to intrapsychic and interpersonal factors, which of them is considered primary and which of them is considered secondary or derivative. There are also differences in the role that the second person, the analyst, is considered to play in the analytic field.

From my own relational perspective, the analyst's experience is a crucial part of the analytic field. Like Aron (1996), I prefer not to marginalize

---

[1] By psychoanalytic I refer here to that aspect of my approach that addresses that which is unconscious, that is, those elements of the psychic world that are repressed, dissociated, or disowned.

this experience by calling it countertransference, that is secondary to the patient's transference. I believe that the patient's experience, or transference, is seen through the prism of the analyst's experience, or countertransference. The focus of the work is the patient's behavior and experience, not the analyst's; but epistemologically speaking, the experiences of the two participants are fully interwoven.

One-Person Factors

Among one-person psychologies, there are nonpsychoanalytic ones such as the behavioral model and the medical model. From a behavioral point of view, of course, it would have been possible to achieve a successful and complete result in a much shorter time. Taisha was, in fact, back in school quite quickly after beginning treatment. From a medical-model perspective, there might have been brief interventions that could have been effective. I believe there are times when behavioral and medical interventions are necessary and helpful tools for the psychoanalytic clinician. From a psychoanalytic point of view, however, to work in a purely symptom-focused way would have been to fail to recognize and engage the enormous pain of this family. As I view Taisha as an individual, my hypotheses concerning her conflicts about her own rage fall into the one-person category.

Two-Person Factors

A central part of my participation in this work was my conflict about "taking in" the pain of this family. It would have been only too easy to avoid this pain. For one thing (and here I bring in a systemic factor), the clinic's administrative structure was set up to distract me from an immersion in painful experience by immersing me, instead, in an overwhelming number of cases and an overwhelming amount of paperwork. In fact, much of my time in this clinic was spent in a fairly dehumanized, dissociated state, dealing with charts and symptoms, or simply trying to get through a day in which I was confronted with one impossible situation after another. When one is overloaded with work and human suffering beyond a certain point, one becomes numb, and then the next patient or the next family becomes a persecutory experience. As difficult as this situation is, and as much as clinicians complain about it, I believe it may be less distressing than an acutely emotional response to peoples' lives in the inner city. And so, working in that context, one can rely on the obsessional, dissociated, ambiance of the clinic for some emotional distance.

A psychoanalytic perspective is essential for the recognition of this emotional situation. As an analyst, I was prepared to note my initial dissociative response to the pain of Taisha and her family and to attempt to transcend it by recognizing the pain against which it defended me. My thoughts about the historical legacy of suffering and discrimination represented my initial, still somewhat abstract and distant efforts to connect with the family's suffering. Later, again with the assistance of my analytic training, I was able to recognize the ways in which I was excluding Mr. B and to reflect on what he represented and why I might want to exclude him.

The point is not to use analytic insight simply to overcome "resistance" to recognition of the family's and one's own suffering. Rather, I think the analyst's own resistance and defensiveness in itself connects him or her to the family's conflicts between avoiding and confronting their pain. Thus, while maintaining my awareness of the defensive function of her behavior, I could, for example, attempt to avoid a pejorative attitude toward Ms. A's polite, conventional presentation or her difficulty setting limits with her son.

Three-Person, Systemic Factors

To begin with, there is an influential systemic factor in the clinic's administrative structure that, as I said, overloads the clinician with patients and paperwork. It can be argued on pragmatic grounds that these demands are inevitable. After all, the clinic depends on public funding, and governmental agencies require documentation and are accustomed to measuring productivity in purely quantitative terms. On another level, however, it seems to me that the paper work and the crush of patients are conducive to an obsessive-compulsive and dissociative defense against human contact with people in great psychic pain. Jaques (1955) called such phenomena "social defenses." Menzies (1975) has written a lucid discussion of how such defenses operate in inpatient hospital nursing services. To take just one of many examples, she points out how the assignment of nurses to tasks rather than patients protects the nurses from the pain of emotional contact with suffering people and loss through their death. The nurse ends up taking the temperature of many people, instead of taking care of all the needs of any given patient. Patients are referred to by room number or diagnosis rather than by name. Similarly, when a psychotherapist is overworked, patients become numbers in the roster, a means to the end of meeting one's quota of "numbers" (i.e., number of patients seen in a week), and the object of symptom checklists, goals, treatment plans, treatment plan reviews, and so on. Therapists commonly complain about the crush of work and the way it distracts them from being able to do the clinical work. But it may also serve a defensive purpose to lose oneself in paper work or complaints about paper work. Defensive activity in relation to painful and distressing clinical work thus operates both at the administrative level and at the level of the individual clinician. The boundaries between the two levels of analysis begin to blur as one applies a psychoanalytic perspective to the system as a whole, but I believe there are major clinical advantages to taking this broader perspective. It can be helpful to clinicians trying to be as aware as possible of how they are functioning in the clinic context; it can also be helpful to those who are trying to create or modify administrative systems to facilitate clinical work.

Let us now carry this psychoanalysis of the context further, into the sociocultural field. Having a private practice at the same time as I worked in the public clinic, I was aware of how much stronger the dehumanizing forces were in the latter context. In private practice, fees tend to be higher and administrative overhead lower, so that the therapist in private practice usually has less need to book overwhelming numbers of patients. Paperwork demands may be less (although as managed care has taken over in private practice, private work has become more like clinic work in this respect). The net result is that private patients tend to get more individual attention, more dignified physical surroundings, more respectful treatment, a less preoccupied and harrassed therapist than clinic patients do.

What especially interests me here is how this two-tier treatment of patients replicates the larger social structure. Public funding of mental health treatment for the poor starts out as a well-intentioned effort to make care available regardless of social status and income. But discrimination based on these factors creeps back in as treatment in the public sector is allowed to become increasingly dehumanized. Therapists, however committed they may be to egalitarianism, end up, in one way or another and to one extent or another, treating public clinic patients with relatively less respect, attention, and dignity. One's office in the public clinic may be less comfortable, or one may have to shuttle from office to office. The demands on one's time may make one resent the patient just for being there, or one may feel grateful to the patient for showing up so that one can escape one's supervisor's censure for having "low numbers." A loss of morale is an inevitable consequence as the (perhaps initially idealistic) therapist finds himself or herself having become an agent of a discriminatory social system.

Looking at oneself, as therapist, in a larger social context in this way can sensitize one to critical aspects of the transference–countertransference interaction. The therapist can better understand the ways in which he or she may be distrusted by the clinic patient, of the ways in which the patient may plausibly expect to be treated poorly. Patients may express such distrust overtly or covertly–by missing appointments, by arriving late for sessions, and so on. The therapist's repertoire of ways of understanding such behavior is expanded by a consideration of the therapist as embedded in a social and administrative system. All this is not to say that the therapist will not be able to convey respect and concern for the patient in many ways, despite an unfavorable administrative context, or that the patient will not register these more positive aspects as well. The range of feelings between patient and therapist is as great in clinic work as anywhere else. The negative feelings I have mentioned, however, may be more implicit, subtle factors, requiring an expanded perspective for their full appreciation.

Finally, putting present-day interactions into historical perspective is essential, especially when members of groups that have been oppressed are involved. Just as the behavior of a traumatized person cannot be fully understood without reference to his or her traumatic history, so the behavior of members of historically traumatized groups needs to be understood in that context, among others. Holocaust survivors, their children, and "hidden" children have received some psychoanalytic attention from this point of view. Gump (1997) has pointed out that the descendants of the African American slaves have rarely been looked at in this light. The legacy of slavery for African Americans lives on in an ongoing traumatic history of violence, discrimination, poverty and its sequelae, and so on. Looking at African American people in impoverished inner-city communities without reference to history and current social oppression would give an unbalanced picture of individual and family pathology. Understanding the historical context is not necessarily to relieve individuals of their responsibility for how they choose to live their lives. Looking at people as victims of history would be as unbalanced as looking at them as unrestricted free agents, solely responsible for their successes and failures. This view of the individual as free to make of himself whatever he chooses is embodied in the American "Horatio Alger" myth. A consequence of overlooking the ways in which we are shaped by history and circumstance is that people of lower socioeconomic status tend to blame themselves overly for their social position, as Sennett and Cobb (1972) have pointed out.

As I have mentioned, one-person, two-person, and three-person (systemic) points of view, if considered in isolation from one another, all give a skewed view of any given clinical situation. Historically, psychoanalysis has emphasized the one-person view at the expense of the two-person, or interpersonal view. This bias is being remedied as the focus in psychoanalytic theory shifts toward the analytic interaction. My argument is that the systemic perspective correcting for biases inherent in the two-person view, further enriches our understanding of our patients and of our interactions with them. The historical perspective operates within the analyst's countertransference. In my clinical example, there was a shift in my countertransference heralded by my seeing Taisha and her family in the light of the legacy of slavery. Repositioned in this way, I could feel less judgmental about Mr. B's alcoholism and Ms. A's failure to set limits with him. I could be less impatient when my therapeutic efforts failed to bear immediate fruit. All these developments facilitated my ability to foster a strong alliance with the members of the family and to understand their experience in productive ways.

CONCLUSION

I will conclude with an anecdote. I attended a workshop at a major psychoanalytic conference in which an analyst was presenting work on violence. In discussing his interviews with convicted, incarcerated murderers, he mentioned that what he heard over and over was that the murder had been triggered by a feeling that the victim had "dissed" (street language for "disrespected") the perpetrator. He went on to describe an intervention project that had resulted in dramatically lower rates of violence in prisons. At this point, one of the analysts in the audience said something like this: "One can't argue with success, but I must point out that the understanding of violence being presented is not psychoanalytic."

My immediate emotional response was a violent one: I wanted to attack the person who spoke. A moment's thought made clear to me that I felt "dissed"; I felt that the analyst was pulling rank by claiming to have a version of psychoanalysis superior to that of the speaker, with whom I identified. The presenter responded quite effectively, pointing out that Kohut and self psychology have quite a bit to say, psychoanalytically, about narcissistic rage.

I want to use this anecdote to make several concluding points. First, excessive purism and elitism about what constitutes a psychoanalytic approach runs the risk of marginalizing psychoanalysis into extinction. Second, I would argue that my point of view as an analyst is illuminating about the incident itself. As Levenson (1982) pointed out, people tend to enact the content of that about which they are speaking. This is one way of defining transference–countertransference as an omnipresent phenomenon in the clinical psychoanalytic situation. If this had been a clinical situation, a group psychoanalysis, for example, the way in which the content, that is, disrespect and rage, was being unconsciously enacted would have made for an interesting and productive discussion. A psychoanalytic perspective is valuable in all sorts of contexts, then, including a psychoanalytic workshop. It can illuminate various sorts of dynamics as well, including the internecine strife that characterizes our field. Likewise, being open to applying a psychoanalytic perspective to whatever work needs to be done in a public clinic deepens and enriches that work. As a psychoanalyst, I cannot conceive of such work without that perspective.

REFERENCES

Altman, N. (1995), *The Analyst in the Inner City*. Hillsdale, NJ: The Analytic Press.

Aron, L. (1996), *A Meeting Of Minds*. Hillsdale, NJ: The Analytic Press.

Bachrach, H. M. & Leaff, L. A. (1978), Analyzability: A systematic review of the clinical and quantitative literature. *J. Amer. Psychoanal. Assn.*, 26:881–920.

Caspary, A. (1993), Aspects of the therapeutic action in child analytic treatment. *Psychoanal. Psychol.*, 10:207–220.

Gump, J. (1997), Discussion of paper by N. Altman, "Black and White Thinking: A Psychoanalyst Reconsiders Race." Presented at meeting of Washington Psychologists for the Study of Psychoanalysis, Washington, DC, November.

Jacoby, R. (1983), *The Repression of Psychoanalysis*. New York: Basic Books.

Jaques, E. (1955), Social systems as defence against persecutory and depressive anxiety. In: *New Directions in Psychoanalysis*, ed. M. Klein. London: Tavistock, pp. 478–498.

Levenson, E. (1982), Language and healing. In: *Curative Factors in Dynamic Psychotherapy*, ed. S. Slipp. New York: McGraw-Hill, pp. 91–103.

Marcuse, H. (1964), *One Dimensional Man*. Boston, MA: Beacon Press.

——— (1966), *Eros and Civilization*. Boston, MA: Beacon Press.

Menzies, I. E. P. (1975), A case study in the functioning of social systems as a defense against anxiety. In: *Group Relations Reader I*, ed. A. D. Colman & W. H. Bexton. Jupiter, FL: A. K. Rice Institute, pp. 281–312.

Sennett, R. & Cobb, J. (1972), *The Hidden Injuries of Class*. New York: Vintage Books.

Sullivan, H. S. (1953), *The Interpersonal Theory of Psychiatry*. New York: Norton.

PART V

Epilogue

A Look Toward the Future

THE EDITORS

The current struggle surrounding the provision of mental health services in the United States reflects several crises of values. First and foremost, there is the conflict of values between managed health care systems and psychotherapeutic care. Managed health care systems are fundamentally profit-oriented cost-management strategies. Although they first came on the scene touted as methods for providing more responsible oversight of care and preventing costs from escalating owing to profligate use of expensive medical technology, it has become clear that fundamentally they are always subject to the temptation to enhance profits by limiting care or by selecting lower-paid providers as deliverers of care. So basic is this conflict that we return to it later in the present discussion.

Second, because the problems of health care will ultimately be handled politically, it is important to acknowledge the existence of the long-standing, value-laden conflict of approaches between the two major political parties in the United States. Although both offer legislation to guarantee protection for consumers, each proposes solutions in keeping with its traditional positions and associated values: Democrats generally favor increased governmental regulation of health maintenance organization and insurance companies, Republicans mostly elect to trust the regulatory effects of market forces and to avoid enlarging centralized governmental authority and bureaucracy. The final result is as yet unknown, but it is clear that, although both parties are aware of the sorry state of affairs under the present systems, it is politics that will determine the shape of the future.

There is also the tension of the public's conflicted desire for health insurance. Few would question the desirability of health insurance as an abstract ideal, but as it operates in the real world it creates problems. On one hand, people today have become accustomed to having some help in shouldering the costs of health care, especially when they are basically well and experience it as their right; on the other hand, they chafe under the restrictions imposed by the agencies that provide it. They chafe all the more when they become ill and find that decisions they consider relevant to their care are out of their—and often their doctor's—hands and, more-

over, may be made on what are ultimately financial grounds. So serious
has this tension become that it has been discussed as a crisis around issues
of personal responsibility (Shore, 1998).

As this volume goes to press, it is obvious that nationwide resentment against many of the practices of managed health care has steadily
risen. Newspapers regularly carry reports of the disaffection of health care
providers as well as the public, and there is constant discussion of possible
approaches to mending or overhauling the system. Much has been made
of the grass-roots anger manifested by audiences cheering when a character in a popular movie[1] inveighs against the inadequacies of the managed
health care available to her family. It has become increasingly clear to most
people that managed care does not operate according to the simple principle
that patients ought to receive the type and length of treatment they need
to relieve their suffering and to have an opportunity to lead productive
lives. Instead, managed care is driven by the notion of the "quick fix" and
the need to maximize profits. In the area of mental health care, the treatment most diametrically opposed to those concerns is psychoanalytically
informed care.

But how to make the case in the face of the forces marshaled against
such treatment? It seems to the editors that the case for psychoanalytic
and psychodynamic treatment is best made not by the direct advocacy of
long-term psychoanalytic treatment specifically, but by fighting for the
principle that people have a right to receive the kind and length of treatment they need. In the area of psychological distress, this means that patients who need and can benefit from extended, long-term psychotherapy
should have it.

It also seems to us, in a world where policies flow from politics as well
as from profits, that psychoanalytic interests will be best met by psychoanalytic practitioners and advocates allying themselves with consumer and
other groups who fight for proper health care despite the risk to profits.
Many such groups exist; many of them are coalitions, either of various
groups of mental health professionals or of professionals as well as concerned members of the public. Although they were just a short while ago
considered by many observers to be fighting an impossible rear-guard action, today it appears that they have kept alive a conscientious opposition
to the limitations of managed health care, have educated both the public
and professionals, and serve as rallying points for advocacy efforts.[2]

---

[1] *As Good As It Gets,* with Jack Nicholson and Helen Hunt.

[2] One of the most visible and vocal examples of such groups is the National Coalition of
Mental Health Professionals and Consumers. Another is the National Association for the
Mentally Ill (NAMI). Many others exist, including those based in the various mental helath
professions.

Still, there is a level on which the case for long-term psychotherapy must be made on the grounds of time-honored, professionally appropriate scientific criteria. To do that, we need to address, more fully than they have hitherto been addressed, issues of effectiveness, accountability, and outcome. The contributors to this book have made a convincing case regarding the range of applicability of psychodynamic treatment—that is, the appropriateness of such treatment to a wide range of problems and populations. Their case needs to be supplemented and strengthened by further research on effectiveness, including cost-effectiveness and broad outcome criteria. An example of what needs to be done appeared in a supplemental issue of *Psychoanalytic Inquiry* (Lazar, 1997) on the daunting topic of "Extended Dynamic Psychotherapy: Making the Case in an Era of Managed Care." In a significant step toward demonstrating the great value of long-term psychodynamic treatment for a wide range of patients, its articles and the literature they cover present important information on a variety of essential matters, including the cost-effectiveness of extended outpatient psychotherapy, the importance of long-term psychotherapy for patients with serious medical illnesses, and the outcome of child psychoanalysis.

Consistent with the implications of those articles is an informative and passionate statement on managed care by Harold Eist, former president of the American Psychiatric Association. Eist (1997) states that, whereas managed care companies have failed to deliver on their promises to reduce cost and improve quality, "they have made good on their pledge to achieve profits" (p.177). Eist observes, "We have ethical, moral, and legal obligations to advocate for the best care for our individual patients and for excellent systems of care" (p. 179) and goes on to state that "in fulfilling these obligations, we will be seen as a moral force fighting to preserve the sanctity of life over the sanctity of the dollar" (p. 179). He notes that, "psychoanalysis, which has been more egregiously raped than many areas of our profession, must broadcast that it is a small cost item critical to the care of many deeply suffering people" and must "challenge biases and prejudices and insist that it remain the core discipline of all psychotherapies including cognitive, behavioral and brief psychotherapies" (p.180).

We would all do well to heed Eist's call to inform the public at large; to work toward appropriate legislation; to challenge publicly the actions of managed care; to engage in public education initiatives; to form and expand strategic alliances; to participate in litigation against certain managed care practices; and to insist on our ethical and professional standards and values. We need to guard against a little-recognized danger: the improper and selective use—what Sleek (1997) refers to as "cherrypicking"—

of treatment outcome research data to justify the inappropriate limits placed on psychotherapy benefits. As editors we note that the research training of psychologists places them in a position of special responsibility in this regard.

Recognition of the abuses of managed care has, of course, not been limited to psychoanalytically oriented critics. What gives psychoanalysis a privileged voice in the fight against managed care, however, is not only that it has been, in Eist's compelling phrase, more egregiously raped than many other areas, but also that, in a fundamental way, psychoanalytic values are opposed to the values of managed care. It is difficult to imagine a discipline more inhospitable and more diametrically opposed to the "quick fix" and the patching-over approach than psychoanalysis. In addition, at its best, psychoanalysis is based on the values of honesty, autonomy, confidentiality, and the supreme importance of the relationship between patient and therapist—all values that are undermined by managed care. As Scholom (1998) puts it, "(T)o have a set of humanistic values placing individuals first is anathema to the imperatives of the corporate market" (p. 10). It is true that, prior to the advent of managed care, psychoanalytic practice itself, particularly in the United States, was embedded in and strongly influenced by a market ideology—except for patients seen in low-cost facilities typically associated with training institutes, only those who could afford to pay would receive long-term treatment. If, however, as the contributions to this volume have attempted to demonstrate, psychoanalytically oriented treatment is applicable to a wide range of problems and populations, then it should be more widely available to people who can benefit from such treatment. Managed care, purporting responsible provision of necessary and appropriate care, has achieved the opposite result.

The crisis of values between psychoanalysis and managed care seems to the editors to mirror a long-standing crisis in the society. As a nation we have always been doers who, believing that anything can be fixed, are certain that the right technique or system will lead to ever-expanding improvement. Yet as a nation we are committed as well to the significance of individual lives and the individual's pursuit of happiness, a commitment that sometimes operates at cross-purposes to the wish for pragmatic solutions. We believe that to avoid deepening this schism, psychotherapists cannot simply insist, as Eist does (1997), that "[p]sychoanalysis . . . remain the core disciplines of all psychotherapies . . ." (p. 180) unless they also provide solid evidence of the cost-effectiveness of long-term treatment. In this matter, we might reluctantly grant that the advent of managed care is a useful spur to the difficult task of studying long-term treatment.

As analytically oriented therapists, we have claimed that long-term treatment is not simply a luxury for the so-called worried well. It is clear from Doidge's contribution that the very notion of the "worried well" is a myth. Further, the effects of medication have proven more modest in many cases than would be realized from the readiness of managed care representatives to urge—indeed, often to insist on—psychiatric consultations for patients who, in their view, are not showing rapid enough improvement. It remains for analytic clinicians to demonstrate that with long-term and intensive treatment we are able to help patients reduce significantly their vulnerability to future psychopathology and impairment in adaptive functioning and improve the quality of their lives. With such evidence in hand we can go beyond the merely face-valid claim that addressing a person's long-standing characterological problems provides a therapy that is cost-effective in the long run.

Such a program of study also addresses the fault lines in several systems of values and has the potential to help heal the rifts in the area of mental health care.

REFERENCES

Eist, H. I. (1997), Managed care: Where did it come from? What does it do? How does it survive? What can be done about it? *Psychoanal. Inq.*, Suppl.: 162–181.

Lazar, S. G. (Issue Editor) (1997), Extended dynamic psychotherapy: Making the case in an era of managed care. *Psychoanal. Inq.*, Suppl.

Scholom, A. (1998), Managed care's assault on our hearts and minds. *Psycholog.-Psychoanal.*, 18:6–10.

Shore, K. (1998), E-mail to Division 42 Independent Practice, American Psychological Association), July 4.

Sleek, S. (1997), The "cherrypicking" of treatment research. *The Monitor (Newspaper of the American Psychological Association)*, 29(12): 1, 21.

Index